Nonpharmacological Management of Atrial Fibrillation

Edited by

Francis D. Murgatroyd, M.A., M.R.C.P.
Senior Registrar
Department of Cardiac Electrophysiology
Glenfield Hospital
Leicester, United Kingdom

A. John Camm, M.D.
Chairman of Medicine and Chief
Department of Cardiological Sciences
St. George's Hospital Medical School
London University
London, United Kingdom

**Futura Publishing
Company, Inc.**
Armonk, NY

Library of Congress Cataloging-in-Publication Data

Nonpharmacological management of atrial fibrillation / edited by
  Francis D. Murgatroyd and A. John Camm.
      p.   cm.
    Includes bibliographical references and index.
    ISBN 0-87993-665-7 (alk. paper)
    1. Atrial fibrillation—Treatment. 2. Catheter ablation.
  3. Cardiac pacing. I. Murgatroyd, Francis D. II. Camm, A. John.
    [DNLM: 1. Atrial Fibrillation—therapy. 2. Catheter Ablation.
    3. Defibrillators, Implantable. WG 330 N8135 1997]
    RC685.A72N66   1997
    616.1′2806—dc21
    DNLM/DLC
    for Library of Congress   97-4340
                                                                  CIP

Copyright 1997
Futura Publishing Company, Inc.

Published by
Futura Publishing Company, Inc.
135 Bedford Road
Armonk, NY 10504-0418

LC #: 97-4340
ISBN #: 0-87993-665-7

Contributors

John Adams, B.S.E.E. InControl, Inc., Redmond, WA, USA

Masood Akhtar, M.D. EP Laboratory, University of Wisconsin Medical School, Milwaukee Clinical Campus, Milwaukee, WI, USA

Jeffrey L. Anderson, M.D. Cardio Renal Advisory Committee, USA Food and Drug Administration and Division of Cardiology, University of Utah School of Medicine, LDS Hospital, Salt Lake City, UT, USA

Robert H. Anderson, M.D. Department of Paediatrics, National Heart and Lung Institute, Imperial College School of Medicine, London, United Kingdom

Gregory M. Ayers, M.D., Ph.D. InControl, Inc., Redmond, WA, USA

Brett M. Baker, M.D. Cardiovascular Division, Washington University School of Medicine, St. Louis, MO, USA

Gust H. Bardy, M.D. Department of Medicine, Division of Cardiology, University of Washington, Seattle, WA, USA

Zalmen Blanck, M.D. EP Laboratory, University of Wisconsin Medical School, Milwaukee Clinical Campus, Milwaukee, WI, USA

Gregory W. Botteron, M.D. Clinical Electrophysiology Laboratory, Washington University School of Medicine, St Louis, MO, USA

Michael E. Cain, M.D. Cardiovascular Division, Washington University School of Medicine, St. Louis, MO, USA

A. John Camm, M.D. Department of Cardiological Sciences, St. George's Hospital Medical School, London, United Kingdom

Ronald W.F. Campbell, M.D. Department of Academic Cardiology, University of Newcastle upon Tyne, Newcastle upon Tyne, United Kingdom

Jonas Carlson, M.Sc. Department of Cardiology, University Hospital, Lund, Sweden

Serge Cazeau, M.D. Département de Stimulation Cardiaque, Centre Chirurgical Val d'Or, Saint-Cloud, France

Jacques Clémenty, M.D. Hôpital Cardiologique du Haut-Lévêque, Bordeaux-Pessac, France

Harry J.G.M. Crijns, M.D. Department of Cardiology, University Hospital, Groningen, The Netherlands

Paul Dorian, M.D. Department of Medicine, St Michael's Hospital and University of Toronto, Toronto, Ontario, Canada

Adam P. Fitzpatrick, M.D., M.R.C.P. Manchester Heart Centre, Manchester Royal Infirmary, Manchester, United Kingdom

Stéphane Garrigue, M.D. Département de Stimulation Cardiaque, Centre Hospitalier Universitaire, Bordeaux, France

Irakli Giorgberidze, M.D. Arrhythmia and Pacing Service, Eastern Heart Institute, Passaic, NJ, USA

A.T. Marcel Gosselink, M.D. Department of Cardiology, University Hospital, Groningen, The Netherlands

Daniel Gras, M.D. Département de Stimulation Cardiaque, Centre Chirurgical Val d'Or, Saint-Cloud, and Centre Hospitalier Régional de Rennes, France

Richard A. Gray, Ph.D. Department of Pharmacology, SUNY Health Science Center at Syracuse, Syracuse, NY, USA

Jerry C. Griffin, M.D. InControl, Inc., Redmond, WA, USA

Richard A. Grimm, D.O. Section of Cardiovascular Imaging, Department of Cardiology, The Cleveland Clinic Foundation, Cleveland, OH, USA

Colette M. Guiraudon, M.D. Department of Pathology, London Health Sciences Center, University of Western Ontario, London, Ontario, Canada

Gerard M. Guiraudon, M.D. Department of Thoracic and Cardiovascular Surgery, Millard Fillmore Hospital, Buffalo, NY, USA

David E. Haines, M.D. Cardiovascular Division, Department of Internal Medicine, University of Virginia School of Medicine, Charlottesville, VA, USA

Michel Haïssaguerre, M.D. Université de Bordeaux, Hôpital Cardiologique du Haut-Lévêque, Bordeaux-Pessac, France

David L. Hayes, M.D. Mayo Clinic, Rochester, MN, USA

Siew Yen Ho, Ph.D. Department of Paediatrics, National Heart and Lung Institute, Imperial College School of Medicine, London, UK

Magnus Holm, M.Sc. Department of Cardiology, University Hospital, Lund, Sweden

Pierre Jaïs, M.D. Hôpital Cardiologique du Haut-Lévêque, Bordeaux-Pessac, France

José Jalife, M.D. Department of Pharmacology, SUNY Health Science Center, Syracuse, NY, USA

Michiel J. Janse, M.D., Ph.D. Department of Clinical and Experimental Cardiology, Academisch Medisch Centrum, University of Amsterdam, Amsterdam, The Netherlands

Mohammad R. Jazayeri, M.D. EP Laboratory, University of Wisconsin Medical School, Milwaukee Clinical Campus, Milwaukee, WI, USA

Mark E. Josephson, M.D. Arrhythmia Service, Beth Israel Deaconess Medical Center, Harvard Medical School, Boston, MA, USA

Raur Kaushik, M.D. Arrhythmia and Pacing Service, Eastern Heart Institute, Passaic, NJ, USA

David Keane, M.R.C.P.I., Ph.D. Cardiac Arrhythmia Service, Massachusetts General Hospital, Boston, MA, USA

Charles R. Kerr, M.D. Division of Cardiology, St Paul's Hospital, Vancouver, British Columbia, Canada

Charles Kirchhof, M.D., Ph.D. Arrhythmia Service, Beth Israel Deaconess Medical Center, Harvard Medical School, Boston, MA, USA

George J. Klein, M.D. Department of Medicine, London Health Sciences Center, University of Western Ontario, London, Ontario, Canada

Ryszard B. Krol, M.D. Arrhythmia and Pacing Service, Eastern Heart Institute, Passaic, NJ, USA

Chu-Pak Lau, M.D. Division of Cardiology, University of Hong Kong at Queen Mary Hospital, Hong Kong

Arnaud Lazarus, M.D. Département de Stimulation Cardiaque, Centre Chirurgical Val d'Or, Saint-Cloud, France

Samuel Lévy, M.D. Service de Cardiologie, Centre Hospitalier Régional et Universitaire, Marseille, France

Philip Mathew, M.S. Arrhythmia and Pacing Service, Eastern Heart Institute, Passaic, NJ, USA

Rahul Mehra, Ph.D. Medtronic, Inc., Minneapolis, MN, USA

Kevin Monahan, M.D. Arrhythmia Service, Beth Israel Deaconess Medical Centre, Harvard Medical School, Boston, MA, USA

Jacques Mugica, M.D. Département de Stimulation Cardiaque, Centre Chirurgical Val d'Or, Saint-Cloud, France

Anand N. Munsif, M.D. Arrhythmia and Pacing Service, Eastern Heart Institute, Passaic, NJ, USA

Francis D. Murgatroyd, MRCP Department of Cardiac Electrophysiology, Glenfield Hospital, Leicester, United Kingdom

Calambur Narasimhan, M.D. EP Laboratory, University of Wisconsin Medical School, Milwaukee Clinical Campus, Milwaukee, WI, USA

David Newman, M.D. Department of Medicine, St Michael's Hospital and University of Toronto, Toronto, Ontario, Canada

Ann-Marie Nilsson, M.Sc. Department of Cardiology, University Hospital, Lund, Sweden

S. Bertil Olsson, M.D., Ph.D. Department of Cardiology, University Hospital, Lund, Sweden

Panagiotis T. Panotopoulos, M.D. EP Laboratory, University of Wisconsin Medical School, Milwaukee Clinical Campus, Milwaukee, WI, USA

Panos Papageorgiou, M.D., Ph.D. Arrhythmia Service, Beth Israel Deaconess Medical Center, Harvard Medical School, Boston, MA, USA

Miney Paquette, M.Sc. Department of Medicine, St Michael's Hospital and University of Toronto, Toronto, Ontario, Canada

Atul Prakash, M.D., MRCP Arrhythmia and Pacing Service, Eastern Heart Institute, Passaic, NJ, USA

Rasmakota Reddy, M.D. Department of Medicine, Division of Cardiology, University of Washington, Seattle, WA, USA

Philippe Ricard, M.D. Service de Cardiologie, Centre Hospitalier Régional et Universitaire, Marseille, France

Philippe Ritter, M.D. Département de Stimulation Cardiaque, Centre Chirurgical Val d'Or, Saint-Cloud, France

Mårten Rosenqvist, M.D., Ph.D. Department of Cardiology, Karolinska Hospital, Stockholm, Sweden

Jeremy Ruskin, M.D. Cardiac Arrhythmia Service, Massachusetts General Hospital, Boston, MA, USA

Alan V. Sahakian, Ph.D. Department of Biomedical Engineering, Northwestern University, Evanston, IL, USA

Sanjeev Saksena, M.D. Arrhythmia and Pacemaker Service, University of Medicine and Dentistry of New Jersey—New Jersey Medical School, Children's Hospital of New Jersey, Newark NJ, and Eastern Heart Institute, Passaic, NJ, USA

Adam T. Schoenwald, M.S. Department of Biomedical Engineering, Northwestern University, Evanston, IL, USA

Dipen C. Shah, M.D. Hôpital Cardiologique du Haut-Lévêque, Bordeaux-Pessac, France

Joseph M. Smith, M.D., Ph.D. Cardiovascular Division, Washington University School of Medicine, St. Louis, MO, USA

John F. Swartz, M.D. Cardiac Arrhythmia Consultants, P.C. and, Department of Medicine, St Francis Hospital, Tulsa, OK, USA

Steven Swiryn, M.D. Department of Medicine, Northwestern University Medical School and Evanston Hospital, Evanston, IL, USA

Robert G. Tieleman, M.D. Department of Cardiology, University Hospital, Groningen, The Netherlands

Maarten P. Van den Berg, M.D. Department of Cardiology, University Hospital, Groningen, The Netherlands

Isabelle C. Van Gelder, M.D. Department of Cardiology, University Hospital, Groningen, The Netherlands

Albert L. Waldo, M.D. Division of Cardiology, University Hospitals of Cleveland, Case Western Reserve University School of Medicine, Cleveland, OH, USA

Hein Wellens, M.D. Department of Cardiology, Academic Hospital, Maastricht, The Netherlands

Harley White, M.S.E.E. InControl, Inc., Redmond, WA, USA

D. George Wyse, M.D., Ph.D. Division of Cardiology, University of Calgary/Foothills Hospital, Calgary, Alberta, Canada

Raymond Yee, M.D. Department of Medicine, London Health Sciences Center, University of Western Ontario, London, Ontario, Canada

Peter Zimetbaum, M.D. Arrhythmia Service, Beth Israel Deaconess Medical Center, Harvard Medical School, Boston, MA, USA

Preface

Atrial fibrillation is far from being the benign alternative to normal sinus rhythm that was tacitly assumed until recently. This cardiac arrhythmia is very common (0.4% of the population, 4% of the hospital population and 40% of patients with congestive heart failure). The risks associated with atrial fibrillation fall into three categories: (1) associated with the underlying disease; (2) consequential to the atrial fibrillation; and (3) due to the (inappropriate) treatment of the condition. Mortality in patients with atrial fibrillation is double that of patients in sinus rhythm and is related to stroke, heart failure, and sudden ventricular arrhythmia.

Some of the symptoms of atrial fibrillation, such as palpitations, breathlessness, and chest pain, result fairly immediately from the loss of atrial transport and the rapid/irregular ventricular response rate. However, atrial fibrillation, like hypertension, is an insidious condition, in which progressive atrial and ventricular cardiomyopathy occurs. Endocardial dysfunction also probably develops slowly when the atria fibrillate due to progressively abnormal atrial electrophysiology. Thus, atrial dilation and absent contractility favors thrombus formation and the possibility of arterial embolism, including cerebrovascular accident. Ventricular myopathy results in a clinical picture which resembles dilated cardiomyopathy and congestive cardiac failure develops because of the underlying atrial fibrillation. The treatment of heart failure and the threat of thromboembolism demands conventional treatment with antifailure and anticoagulant therapy, as well as vigorous attempts to prevent atrial fibrillation or, at the very least, control the ventricular response rate to atrial fibrillation.

Atrial fibrillation is classified according to its temporal pattern and its etiological background. Atrial fibrillation that terminates spontaneously is *"paroxysmal"*; that which can be successfully cardioverted is *"persistent,"* and that which is completely refractory is *"permanent."* Both paroxysmal and persistent atrial fibrillation tend to be recurrent. An isolated, nonsustained attack may not require treatment. Therapies for each of these varieties differ: paroxysmal—prophylaxis against recurrence; persistent—cardioversion and prophylaxis; and permanent—rate control. *"Lone"* atrial fibrillation is not associated with any significant underlying cardiac disease.

Inadequate rate control further promotes ventricular dilation and heart failure. Digoxin is usually insufficient to control the ventricular rate, especially in response to mental stress or physical exertion, and additional therapy with beta blockade, calcium antagonists or nonspecific AV nodal blocking drugs may be needed. Underlying sinus node and AV conduction system diseases may be dangerously aggravated by such treatment. Drugs (quinidine, flecainide and sotalol) are used with some success to prevent the recurrence of atrial fibrillation but all aggravate heart failure, and confer a proarrhythmic risk which, possibly with the exception of quinidine, is not proven but is certainly likely. The proarrhythmic effects are more noticeable in patients with heart disease (cardiomegaly, heart failure, hypertrophy, infarction and/or ischemia) and in women. Amiodarone is probably better at preventing the recurrence of atrial fibrillation but it has a long catalog of potentially serious side effects. Importantly, it has not been shown to carry any significant proarrhythmic or negative inotropic risk. Antiarrhythmic drugs, especially flecainide (iv or po) or ibutilide (iv only) can be used to cardiovert atrial fibrillation. The use of ibutilide is associated with an early proarrhythmic risk. Without careful monitoring anticoagulation may also add risk to the pharmacological treatment of atrial fibrillation.

The pharmacological basis for the management of atrial fibrillation is, therefore, far from satisfactory. This has led to a keen search for new and better antiarrhythmic agents. Many of these ventures have so far failed; bidisomide, sematilide, almokalant, d-sotalol, and many other class III drugs which were known only by manufacturers numbers did not get beyond clinical trials. Some new drugs such as dofetilide and azimilide may make the grade but only time will tell. No doubt the pharmaceutical industry will have other bright ideas, but it will take many years for such therapy to make any significant inroads in the treatment of this common condition. Another therapeutic prospect is, however, on the immediate horizon. It may be possible to treat many aspects of atrial fibrillation with nonpharmacological methods.

Electrical defibrillation was the first and most important non-pharmacological approach to the management of atrial fibrillation. It was introduced in the mid-1960s, when quinidine was almost the only alternative. Electrical cardioversion is a very effective and largely safe procedure, provided that the patient is adequately anticoagulated. In addition to external cardioversion, conversion to sinus rhythm may be achieved using small electrical discharges delivered between electrodes within the right atrium and coronary sinus or pulmonary artery. Temporary, flotation and intraoperative catheter systems have been developed and an implantable atrial defibrillator has been implanted.

Cardiac stimulation with temporary and permanent pacemakers has been successfully used to interrupt single circuit reentrant tachycardias (burst overdrive) and to prevent the recurrence of arrhythmias such as ventricular tachycardia (physiological overdrive). Pacing approaches have also been applied to the management of atrial fibrillation with the notion that they may be used to prevent recurrences of arrhythmia by eliminating bradycardia, suppressing ectopic beats, changing the activation pattern of the atria, stabilizing atrial electrophysiology, etc. Mild overdrive pacing has been successful, especially in those patients with significant underlying or precedent bradycardia and dual-site pacing has met with some success in patients with obvious intra- or interatrial delay.

Surgical ablation was originally used for dividing the accessory pathways responsible for Wolff-Parkinson-White syndrome. The technique was highly successful for this indication but it was rapidly eclipsed by catheter ablation after its introduction in the 1980s. Surgeons then turned their attention to other target arrhythmias, including atrial fibrillation. A number of techniques have been developed, ranging from simple appendectomies and left or biatrial isolation to complex and more specific operations. Such operations were designed to prevent the possibility of atrial fibrillation continuing (Maze and Spiral techniques) or to control the ventricular response rate (Corridor operation). The Maze technique, in particular, has met with success, although it is a major open heart procedure to which most patients with atrial fibrillation would not like to submit.

Catheter ablation is now the technique of choice for the management of Wolff-Parkinson-White syndrome, AV nodal re-entrant tachycardia and atrial flutter. Destructive ablation of the compact AV node and subsequent pacing is a useful technique for patients with a rapid ventricular rate, refractory to other therapy. Partial destruction of the AV node may limit AV nodal conduction sufficiently to control the ventricular rate without the need for subsequent pacing. Recently several groups have begun to apply rows of discrete lesions or linear lesions directly to the atrial myocardium in an attempt to prevent the meandering, interlacing wavelets of conduction that are responsible for atrial fibrillation.

Atrial fibrillation has received scant attention until now, but it is increasingly clear that only an aggressive management strategy will lead to a significant reduction of the cost and mortality associated with the arrhythmia. A wide range of non-pharmacological techniques is now emerging which will provide the first opportunity to tackle this arrhythmia successfully. In this book, the current status of these techniques is comprehensively explored.

A. John Camm
Professor of Clinical Cardiology
St. George's Hospital Medical School
London, United Kingdom

Contents

PART I

Atrial Fibrillation: The Clinical Problem

CHAPTER 1

Why Is Atrial Fibrillation Bad for You?

Consequences of Atrial Fibrillation

Harry J.G.M. Crijns, Isabelle C. Van Gelder,
Robert G. Tieleman, A.T. Marcel Gosselink,
Maarten P. Van den Berg

Introduction

Atrial fibrillation (AF) causes palpitations, chest pain, dyspnea, and fatigue. Some patients experience presyncope or even drop attacks, especially at arrhythmia onset or termination. All patients with longer lasting AF develop left ventricular dysfunction, even those without underlying heart disease, and some of these patients incur a tachycardiomyopathy. Conversely, many patients with AF have preexistent heart failure. Apart from the above, AF is associated with excess thromboembolic complications, especially in the elderly.

Impaired Quality of Life

Quality of life is negatively affected by AF. It is determined by the severity of the arrhythmia but also by the underlying heart disease. Apart from a disturbing irregularity of the heart beat, patients may suffer decreased exercise tolerance. Additionally, symptoms related to thromboembolism and side effects of drugs—including induction of heart failure and proarrhythmia as well as bleeding—may have a profound impact. In paroxysmal AF, many patients suffer from fatigue for several days after the attack, and between attacks most patients live

From *Nonpharmacological Management of Atrial Fibrillation*, edited by F.D. Murgatroyd and A.J. Camm. © 1997, Futura Publishing Co., Inc., Armonk, NY.

in fear of the next one. Frequent visits to the hospital and loss of social contacts due to physical and emotional instability are additional disturbing factors.

There are few data to date concerning objective quality of life measurements in AF. Hamer et al.[1] studied 69 patients with paroxysmal supraventricular tachycardia (26 had AF) and reported that, in the absence of background psychopathology, symptoms were moderately disruptive to quality of life in 47 patients. The latter could not be distinguished from patients without significant disruption on the basis of frequency or duration of symptoms. However, these subjects did report more pain. In terms of coping, subjects who were more disturbed by their symptoms tended to cope by diverting attention and viewing the situation catastrophically. These strategies are considered more primitive and less successful in reducing distress.[1] Recently, at an American College of Cardiology meeting, Jenkins et al.[2] reported on quality of life in 151 patients with symptomatic AF, of whom 45% had chronic arrhythmia. Using several types of questionnaires, AF patients scored significantly below norm scores for patients with congestive heart failure or recent myocardial infarction. Similarly, preliminary data from our institution suggest low quality of life as measured with the RAND-36 questionnaire in a cohort of 60 consecutive patients with chronic AF. Quality of life scores concerning physical and mental role limitations were comparable to those found in crippled rheumatoid arthritis patients.

Kay and co-workers[3] looked at the effect of catheter ablation of the atrioventricular junction combined with rate-responsive pacemaker implantation in 12 patients with drug-refractory paroxysmal AF. Nearly all patients had underlying heart disease, but left ventricular function was relatively preserved (mean ejection fraction 54%). Scores of the physical dimension of the McMaster Health Index Questionnaire and the Psychological General Well-Being Index had increased significantly 6 weeks after ablation, compared to baseline. In a controlled study, Brignole et al.[4] found a significant improvement in quality of life 90 days after atrioventricular junction ablation in 23 patients with chronic drug-refractory AF. This was paralleled by increased exercise performance and improved echocardiographic fractional shortening, in particular in patients with depressed cardiac performance at initial evaluation.

Increased Mortality

Several cohort studies have shown that the relative risk of death in subjects with AF is roughly twice that found in subjects in sinus rhythm.[5–7] The reduced survival presumably relates to underlying cardiovascular disease, but also to excess risk of stroke. However, in the absence of underlying heart disease, mortality may not appear increased. Kopecky et al.[8] followed 97 lone AF patients (paroxysmal in 80%) under the age of 60 at the time of diagnosis and showed a benign prognosis. Still, after a follow-up of 15 years 19 patients died, but mean age at death was 73 years. Gajewski and Singer[5] showed that paroxysmal AF in the setting of a normal heart did not increase mortality, whereas the relative risk was 2 in the presence of cardiovascular disorders. A further increase of mortality risk to at least sevenfold that for subjects in sinus rhythm was found in the subgroup with chronic AF, regardless of whether associated cardiac impairment was identified.

The CASS registry[7] reported survival in relation to rhythm in over 18,000 patients undergoing cardiac catheterization for symptomatic coronary artery disease. The 7-year mortality of patients with AF was twice that of those in sinus rhythm. In addition to higher age, functional class, and male sex, presence of AF at the time of catheterization was an independent predictor of mortality.

Atrial fibrillation is the most common arrhythmia in advanced heart failure, occurring in up to 35% of cases.[9–13] Only two of these studies have suggested that AF is an independent risk factor for sudden death and heart failure death.[11,12] Middlekauff and co-workers reported on 390 patients with severe heart failure of whom 75 had AF (19%). Actuarial death rate was 48% for AF patients compared to 29% in patients in sinus rhythm. AF was correlated with increased mortality and sudden death independently of pulmonary capillary wedge pressure, ejection fraction, and etiology of heart failure. Patients with AF and lower filling pressures had an increased risk of sudden death, whereas AF associated with elevated filling pressures—while on therapy—was not associated with a further impairment of prognosis.[12]

It is probably safe to state that the clinical significance of AF as a marker for prognosis is inversely related to the severity of underlying disease. This is illustrated by the study of Middlekauff et al.[12] who showed that in patients with heart failure and near normal left ventricular end-diastolic pressure, prognosis is negatively influenced by the presence of AF, whereas in patients with more advanced forms of heart failure AF does not further affect prognosis.

It is unknown whether commonly used treatment strategies reduce mortality. Preliminary data from our institution suggest that patients who are referred for cardioversion and who maintain sinus rhythm long-term after the shock have a similar survival compared to those relapsing to AF.[14] Multivariate analysis revealed that mortality was related to coronary artery disease and poor left ventricular function, rather than the presence or absence of AF.

Thromboembolic Complications

AF is the most common cardiac cause of systemic emboli, usually cerebrovascular. The cardiac embolus causing a cerebral infarct often results in occlusion of a major cerebral artery. The ensuing infarct is often large and may be fatal. Risk factors for stroke in AF include rheumatic heart disease,[6] age >65 years, hypertension, stroke or transient ischemic attack, diabetes[15,16], recent heart failure, and echocardiographic atrial or ventricular enlargement.[16] The annual stroke incidence in placebo groups of the recently completed trials ranged from 1% to >5%.[15] Apart from symptomatic strokes, AF has been associated with an excess risk of silent strokes.[17] Using computed tomography, silent brain infarcts have been found in 35% of cases with nonrheumatic AF.

Even in the absence of underlying heart disease, AF may cause a significant increase in stroke compared to arrhythmia-free subjects. According to the Framingham study,[18] the annual risk of stroke in lone AF is 2.5% (i.e., fourfold that found in matched controls). This substudy did not exclude patients with hypertension and diabetes mellitus. By contrast, Kopecky et al. reported a yearly risk of only 0.55%.[8] Mean age at inclusion was only 44 years and they used a more strict diagnosis of lone AF.

The Framingham study has shown that independent from the presence or absence of AF, the risk of stroke increases with age. However, in the presence of AF, the risk shows an approximately fivefold increase unrelated to age.[19] Whereas AF was a significant contributor to stroke at all ages, the impact of the risk factors heart failure, coronary artery disease, and hypertension declined with age. The proportion of AF-related stroke increased significantly with age, from 6.7% for ages 50–59 years, to 36.2% for ages 80–89 years.

Coumarin and aspirin are both effective for the prevention of ischemic stroke in patients with AF. Coumarin is substantially more effective than aspirin but bleeding complications importantly negate its benefit. The Stoke Prevention in Atrial Fibrillation (SPAF) investigators showed that both advancing age and more intense anticoagulation increase the risk of major hemorrhage in patients given warfarin.[20]

Progressive Increase of Atrial Size

Atrial enlargement is a common finding in patients with AF. AF may develop secondary to left atrial enlargement.[21] On the other hand, the left atrium may dilate in response to an increased left atrial pressure in patients with AF.[22] In patients with mitral stenosis, AF accounts for an additional increase in left atrial size.[23] Others have demonstrated a correlation between left atrial dimension and duration of the arrhythmia.[24] Sanfilippo et al. found an increase in atrial size after a mean of 20 months in 15 patients with lone AF, despite normal baseline atrial dimensions.[25] Thus, these studies indicate that atrial enlargement may be both a consequence and a cause of the arrhythmia. The importance of atrial size lies in the fact that atrial enlargement is associated with an increased risk for thromboembolic complications and a high arrhythmia recurrence rate following cardioversion. In addition, drugs used to convert the arrhythmia may be less effective. Restoration and long-term maintenance of sinus rhythm, on the other hand, may reverse the process of atrial enlargement,[26,27] even in patients with mitral heart disease.[28] Hypothetically, reverting atrial enlargement by cardioversion and subsequent maintenance of sinus rhythm may reduce the associated risks.

Hemodynamic and Functional Consequences

Hemodynamic changes associated with AF can be attributed to an excessive ventricular rate and loss of atrial transport function. One experimental study indicated that the very irregularity of the ventricular rhythm may be an additional factor, leading to a 9% reduction in cardiac output,[29] but so far no confirmation has come from human studies. Apart from loss of atrial kick, excessive rate response, and rhythm irregularity, two other—dynamic—factors, potentially leading to decreased functional capacity, should be mentioned. These are especially important in *chronic* AF and include progression of underlying cardiovascular disease and development of tachycardia-related cardiomyopathy. Associated heart disease, in fact, makes up the background hemodynamic derangement which is modulated by the other factors. Time-dependent progression of cardiac disease may provoke decrease of left ventricular function, which may worsen further due to tachycardiomyopathy. Of note, tachycardiomyopathy may be concealed, i.e., heart failure due to tachycardiomyopathy cannot be distinguished from that due

Table 1
Percentage Increase in Cardiac Output Acutely after Cardioversion of Atrial Fibrillation

Study	Patients (n)	CO Change at Rest (%)	CO Change with Exercise (%)
Hansen[33]	14	27*	30*
Graettinger[34]	17	10	7
Kahn[35]	10	22*	27*
Morris[36]	11	16*	18*
Rowlands[37]	12	11*	–
Resnekow[38]	15	2	16*
Kaplan[39]	16	15*	–
Shapiro[40]	11	12	15*
Orlando[41]	15	9*	–

* $p < 0.05$; CO = cardiac output.

to the underlying cardiovascular disease but may be demonstrated after restoration of sinus rhythm.[30]

The hemodynamic consequences of AF have been studied in several ways. Typically, clinical studies evaluated the effects of cardioversion or rate control. Only one study has looked at longer term effects on exercise capacity during persistent AF.[31] Several studies have found an increase of cardiac output immediately after restoration of sinus rhythm, either at rest, during exercise or both (Table 1). Also, atrioventricular pacing models have been used in patients with complete atrio-

Table 2
Functional Capacity before and after Cardioversion of Chronic Atrial Fibrillation in Patients Maintaining Sinus Rhythm

1st Author	Pts (n)	Max. HR (bpm) Baseline	Max. HR (bpm) 1 Month	Peak VO2 (ml/Kg/min) Baseline	Peak VO2 (ml/Kg/min) 1 Month
Lipkin[42]	14	164	132	23	26*
Atwood[43]	11	192	144	21.4	23.3
Lundström[44]	16	174	145	23.0	24.7*
Van Gelder[30]	8	184	147	20.1	25.2*
Gosselink[32]	27	175	140	21.4	23.7

* $p < 0.05$; HR = heart rate; VO2 = oxygen consumption.

Table 3
Changes in Left Ventricular Systolic Function after Rhythm Control

1st Author	Mode of Rhythm Control	n	EF, FS Before (%)	EF, FS After (%)	Change (%)	Follow-up (Months)
Kieny[45]	ECV	12	32	53	66	4.7
Grogan[46]	ECV/RC	10	25	52	108	30
Van Gelder[30]	ECV	8	36	53	47	6
Heinz[47]	HBA	5	21(FS)	31	44	1.5
		5	35(FS)	39	–	
Rodriguez[48]	HBA	12	43	54	22	14
		18	59	59	–	
Twidale[49]	HBA	14	43	49	14	1.5
Edner[50]	HBA	14	32	45	40	7
		15	58	55	–	

Lower line in rows showing 2 lines of figures represents patients with normal left ventricular function before rhythm control.

ECV = electrical cardioversion; EF = echocardiographic or radionuclide left ventricular ejection fraction; FS = echocardiographic fractional shortening; HBA = His bundle ablation; RC = rate control with negative chronotropic drugs.

ventricular block to illustrate the importance of atrial contraction to cardiac output. Direct scintigraphic measurement of atrial contribution to ventricular filling in patients undergoing electrical cardioversion[30] showed that atrial contribution is virtually absent immediately after the shock, normalizing at 1 week (contributing 15% to end-diastolic volume). Other studies looked at maximal oxygen consumption before and after restoration of sinus rhythm (Table 2), or long term after acceptance of AF.[31] In the past few years several investigators have reported progressive increase of left ventricular systolic function after control of the ventricular rate or restoration of sinus rhythm (Table 3).

Concealed and Overt Tachycardiomyopathy

It is our belief that many patients with AF have a *concealed* left ventricular (LV) dysfunction. This is evidenced in particular by a reduced exercise capacity, even in patients without any structural heart disease.[32] In addition, as mentioned above, several studies have shown a significant improvement in ejection fraction or exercise tolerance after adequate rate slowing or conversion to sinus rhythm (Tables 2 and 3). Many of these patients improved to normal.

Van Gelder and co-workers[30] studied the time course of systolic and diastolic hemodynamic changes after conversion of AF to sinus rhythm, with attention also to changes in exercise tolerance. Exercise tolerance, assessed as maximum oxygen consumption, normalized at 1 month. Restoration of (resting) LV ejection fraction followed the same time course. However, both were preceded by restoration of (resting) atrial systolic function at 1 week. This time-dependent dissociation suggests an intrinsic cardiomyopathy. After acute normalization of the ventricular rate and subacute restoration of the atrial kick, there is no obvious reason for persistent left ventricular dysfunction other than an intrinsic cardiomyopathy.

Atrial Fibrillation Is Difficult to Cure

AF is a lifelong condemnation for most patients. Once it has occurred, it will remain, either on a chronic recurrent or a persistent basis. This should be viewed within the framework that even aggressive pharmacological therapy does not prevent relapses of paroxysmal or chronic AF. Similarly, catheter ablation of atrioventricular conduction should be considered a palliative rather than a curative procedure. Although it may improve quality of life and reverse left ventricular dysfunction by effectively controlling heart rate, it does not prevent or abolish AF. Consequently, the risk of thromboembolism remains and atrial transport function is not restored. Likewise, patients with atrial defibrillators continue to have symptoms, unless a transient episode of repeated defibrillation prevents AF from becoming chronic. It remains to be answered whether definitive solutions like the Cox "maze" procedure may cure a patient from AF.

References

1. Hamer ME, Blumenthal JA, McCarthy EA, et al. Quality-of-life assessment in patients with paroxysmal atrial fibrillation or paroxysmal supraventricular tachycardia. Am J Cardiol 1994;74:826–829.
2. Jenkins LS, Ellenbogen K, Kay N, et al. Quality of life in patients with symptomatic atrial fibrillation. Circulation 1995;92(I):490. Abstract.
3. Kay GN, Bubien RS, Epstein AE, Plumb VJ, et al. Effect of catheter ablation of the atrioventricular junction on quality of life and exercise tolerance in paroxysmal atrial fibrillation. Am J Cardiol 1988;62:741–744.

4. Brignole M, Gianfranchi L, Menozzi C, et al. Influence of atrioventricular junction radiofrequency ablation in patients with chronic atrial fibrillation and flutter on quality of life and cardiac performance. Am J Cardiol 1994; 72:242–246.
5. Gajewski J, Singer RB. Mortality in an insured population with atrial fibrillation. JAMA 1981;245:1540–1544.
6. Kannel WB, Abbott RD, Savage DD, McNamara PM. Epidemiologic features of chronic atrial fibrillation. N Engl J Med 1982;306:1018–1022.
7. Cameron A, Schwartz MJ, Kronmal RA, Kosinski AS. Prevalence and significance of atrial fibrillation in coronary artery disease (CASS registry). Am J Cardiol 1988;61:714–717.
8. Kopecky SL, Gersh BJ, McGoon MD, et al. The natural history of lone atrial fibrillation: a population based study over three decades. N Engl J Med 1987;317:669–674.
9. Unverferth DV, Magorien RD, Moeschberger ML, et al. Factors influencing the one-year mortality of dilated cardiomyopathy. Am J Cardiol 1984;54: 147–152.
10. Diaz RA, Obasohan A, Oakley CM. Prediction of outcome in dilated cardiomyopathy. Br Heart J 1987;58:393–399.
11. Hofmann T, Meinertz T, Kasper W, et al. Mode of death in idiopathic dilated cardiomyopathy: a multivariate analysis of prognostic determinants. Am Heart J 1988;116:1455–1463.
12. Middlekauff HR, Stevenson WG, Stevenson LW. Prognostic significance of atrial fibrillation in advanced heart failure: a study of 390 patients. Circulation 1991;84:40–48.
13. Carson P, Fletcher R, Johnson G, Cohn J. Atrial fibrillation/flutter does not decrease survival in congestive heart failure. J Am Coll Cardiol 1991; 17:90A. Abstract.
14. Van Gelder IC, Hillege HL, Gosselink ATM, Crijns HJGM. Mortality in patients with atrial fibrillation is related to underlying heart disease and not to the arrhythmia. Circulation 1994;90:I-541. Abstract.
15. Risk factors for stroke and efficacy of antithrombotic therapy in atrial fibrillation: analysis of pooled data from five randomized controlled trials. Arch Intern Med 1994;154:1449–1457.
16. The Stroke Prevention in Atrial Fibrillation Investigators. Predictors of thromboembolism in atrial fibrillation: I. clinical features of patients at risk. Ann Int Med 1992;116:1–5.
17. Petersen P, Madsen EB, Brun B, et al. Silent cerebral infarction in chronic atrial fibrillation. Stroke 1987;18:1098–1100.
18. Brand FN, Abbott RD, Kannel WB, Wolf PA. Characteristics and prognosis of lone atrial fibrillation: 30-year follow-up in the Framingham study. JAMA 1985;254:3449–3453.
19. Wolf PA, Abbott RD, Kannel WB. Atrial fibrillation: a major contributor to stroke in the elderly. Arch Intern Med 1987;147:1561–1564.
20. The Stroke Prevention in Atrial Fibrillation Investigators. Bleeding during antithrombotic therapy in patients with atrial fibrillation. Arch Intern Med 1996;156:409–416.
21. Abildskov JA, Millar K, Burgess MJ. Atrial fibrillation. Am J Cardiol 1971; 28:263–267.

22. Selzer A, Cohn KE. Natural history of mitral stenosis: a review. Circulation 1972;45:878.
23. Keren G, Etzion T, Sherez J, et al. Atrial fibrillation and atrial enlargement in patients with mitral stenosis. Am Heart J 1987;114:1146–1155.
24. Petersen P, Kastrup J, Brinch K, et al. Relation between left atrial size and duration of atrial fibrillation. Am J Cardiol 1987;60:382–384.
25. Sanfilippo AJ, Abascal VM, Sheenan M, et al. Atrial enlargement as a consequence of atrial fibrillation. Circulation 1990;82:792–797.
26. Manning WJ, Leeman DE, Gotch PJ, Come PC. Pulsed Doppler evaluation of atrial mechanical function after cardioversion of atrial fibrillation. J Am Coll Cardiol 1989;13:617–623.
27. Van Gelder IC, Crijns HJ, Van Gilst WH, et al. Decrease of right and left atrial sizes after direct-current electrical cardioversion in atrial fibrillation. Am J Cardiol 1991;67:93–95.
28. Gosselink ATM, Crijns HJGM, Hamer JPM, Lie KI. Changes in atrial dimensions after cardioversion of atrial fibrillation: role of mitral valve disease. J Am Coll Cardiol 1993;22:1666–1672.
29. Naito M, David D, Michelson EL, et al. The hemodynamic consequences of cardiac arrhythmias: evaluation of the relative roles of abnormal atrioventricular sequencing, irregularity of the ventricular rhythm and atrial fibrillation in a canine model. Am Heart J 1983;106:284–291.
30. Van Gelder IC, Crijns HJGM, Blanksma PK, et al. Time course of hemodynamic changes and improvement of exercise tolerance after cardioversion of chronic atrial fibrillation unassociated with cardiac valve disease. Am J Cardiol 1993;72:560–566.
31. Gosselink ATM, Bijlsma EB, Landsman MLJ, et al. Long-term effect of cardioversion on peak oxygen consumption in chronic atrial fibrillation: a two year follow-up. Eur Heart J 1994;15:1368–1372.
32. Gosselink ATM, Crijns HJGM, Van den Berg MP, et al. Functional capacity before and after cardioversion of atrial fibrillation: a controlled study. Br Heart J 1994;72:161–166.
33. Hansen WR, McClendon RA, Kinsman JM. Auricular fibrillation: hemodynamic studies before and after conversion with quinidine. Am Heart J 1952;44:499.
34. Graettinger JS, Carleton RA, Muenster JJ. Circulatory consequences of changes in cardiac rhythm produced in patients by transthoracic direct-current shock. J Clin Invest 1964;43:2290–2302.
35. Kahn DR, Wilson WS, Weber W, Sloan H. Hemodynamic studies before and after cardioversion. J Thorac Cardiovasc Surg 1964;48:898–905.
36. Morris JJ, Entman M, North WC, et al. The changes in cardiac output with reversion of atrial fibrillation to sinus rhythm. Circulation 1965;31:670–678.
37. Rowlands DJ, Logan WFWE, Howitt G. Atrial function after cardioversion. Am Heart J 1967;74:149–160.
38. Resnekov L. Hemodynamic studies before and after electrical conversion of atrial fibrillation and flutter to sinus rhythm. Br Heart J 1967;29:700–708.
39. Kaplan MA, Gray RE, Iseri LT, Williams RL. Metabolic and hemodynamic responses to exercise during atrial fibrillation and sinus rhythm. Am J Cardiol 1968;22:543–549.
40. Shapiro W, Klein G. Alterations in cardiac function immediately following

electrical conversion of atrial fibrillation to normal sinus rhythm. Circulation 1968;38:1074–1084.

41. Orlando JR, Van Herick R, Aronow WS, Olson HG. Hemodynamics and echocardiograms before and after cardioversion of atrial fibrillation to normal sinus rhythm. Chest 1979;76:521–526.

42. Lipkin DP, Frenneaux M, Stewart R, et al. Delayed improvement in exercise capacity after cardioversion of atrial fibrillation to sinus rhythm. Br Heart J 1988;59:572–577.

43. Atwood JE, Myers J, Sullivan M, et al. The effect of cardioversion on maximal exercise capacity in patients with chronic atrial fibrillation. Am Heart J 1989;118:913–918.

44. Lundström T, Karlsson O. Improved ventilatory response to exercise after cardioversion of chronic atrial fibrillation to sinus rhythm. Chest 1992; 102:1017–1022.

45. Kieny JR, Sacrez A, Facello A, et al. Increase in radionuclide left ventricular ejection fraction of chronic atrial fibrillation in idiopathic dilated cardiomyopathy. Eur Heart J 1992;13:1290–1295.

46. Grogan M, Smith HC, Gersh BJ, Wood DL. Left ventricular dysfunction due to atrial fibrillation in patients initially believed to have idiopathic dilated cardiomyopathy. Am J Cardiol 1992;69:1570–1575.

47. Heinz G, Siostrzonek P, Kreiner G, Gossinger H. Improvement of left ventricular systolic function after successful radiofrequency His bundle ablation for drug refractory, chronic atrial fibrillation and recurrent atrial flutter. Am J Cardiol 1992;69:489–492.

48. Rodriguez LM, Smeets JLRM, Xie B, et al. Improvement of left ventricular function by ablation of atrioventricular nodal conduction in selected patients with lone atrial fibrillation. Am J Cardiol 1993;72:1137–1141.

49. Twidale N, Sutton K, Bartlett L, et al. Effects on cardiac performance of atrioventricular node catheter ablation using radiofrequency current for drug-refractory atrial arrhythmias. PACE 1993;16:1275–1284.

50. Edner M, Caidahl K, Bergfeldt L, et al. Prospective study of left ventricular function after radiofrequency ablation of atrioventricular junction in patients with atrial fibrillation. Br Heart J 1995;74:261–267.

CHAPTER 2

Who Wants to Be Treated for Atrial Fibrillation?

Relationship of Clinical Variables to Symptoms

Charles R. Kerr
For the Canadian Registry of Atrial Fibrillation (CARAF) Investigators

Introduction

Atrial fibrillation (AF) is the most common sustained arrhythmia encountered by physicians. Recently, the increased morbidity and mortality associated with AF has been better appreciated and much attention has been directed towards appropriate management.

When considering potentially aggressive interventions to restore and maintain sinus rhythm, one must examine the potential benefits versus the risks of intervention. Proven rationales for conversion and maintenance of sinus rhythm include the alleviation of symptoms and the control of ventricular rate to prevent ventricular cardiomyopathy.[1-3] Intuitively, restoration and maintenance of sinus rhythm should theoretically decrease the likelihood of thrombosis and embolization but no study to date has addressed this theory, making it an unproven justification. In patients with left ventricular hypertrophic states and in patients with congestive heart failure, the atrial kick may contribute more to cardiac output. However, no methodical study has evaluated the overall benefits of restoration of sinus rhythm compared to rate control alone in these individuals. Therefore, the predominant reason for the restoration and maintenance of sinus rhythm is the improvement in symptoms.

From *Nonpharmacological Management of Atrial Fibrillation*, edited by F.D. Murgatroyd and A.J. Camm. © 1997, Futura Publishing Co., Inc., Armonk, NY.

Some patients may be highly symptomatic from AF, some may have minimal symptoms, and some may be completely unaware of the dysrhythmia, leading completely normal lives. The factors that predict the presence of symptoms in general, and specific symptoms, are largely unknown.

Case Studies

The following two patients demonstrate the diversity of symptoms:

Case 1

G.D. is a 47-year-old man who had AF diagnosed at age 42 years during routine examination. This arrhythmia became "chronic" at age 46 and he has been known to be in continuous AF for 18 months. Even on direct questioning he has absolutely *no* symptoms. He runs 3 to 4 miles 4 to 5 days per week, works out regularly in the gym, and holds a full-time job as a lawyer. His echocardiogram shows a slightly enlarged left atrial size, at 41 mm, but is otherwise normal.

His resting electrocardiogram and strips of his Holter monitors are shown in Figure 1. His resting ECG (Fig. 1A) shows AF with a well-

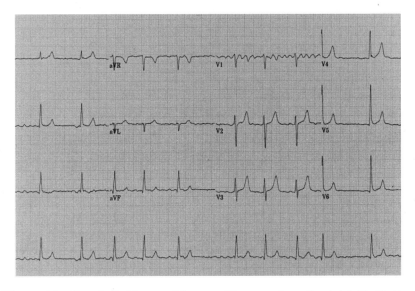

Figure 1A. *Case 1:* A 47-year-old man with asymptomatic atrial fibrillation. At rest his ECG shows a well-controlled ventricular rate.

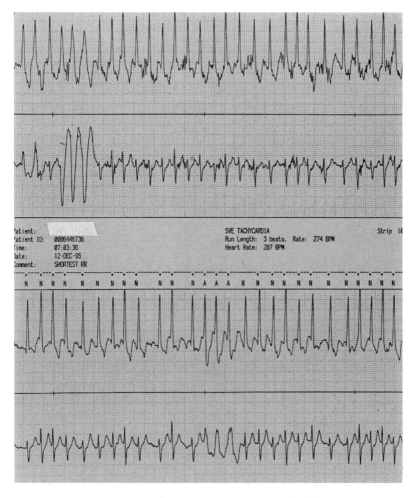

Figure 1B. *(continued)* During exercise, ambulatory monitoring shows a very rapid rate, although no symptoms occurred.

controlled ventricular rate. The Holter monitor (Fig. 1B) shows a severe tachycardia occurring with moderate exercise while working out in the gym. Ventricular rates reached 270 beats per minute. In spite of this rapid rate he remained completely asymptomatic. After discussions with the patient, the decision was made to leave him in AF on no medication.

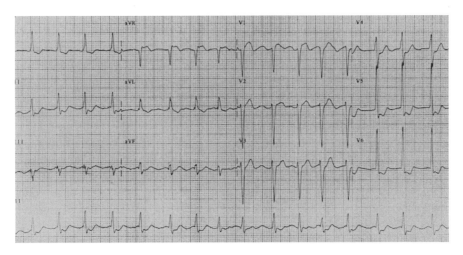

Figure 2. *Case 2:* A 72-year-old woman with severe symptoms during atrial fibrillation. ECG shows a moderate ventricular rate and left ventricular hypertrophy.

Case 2

M.D. is a 72-year-old woman with a 20 year history of paroxysmal AF. She has a past history of significant hypertension, currently controlled on medications. She had been on multiple drugs to prevent AF. She had episodes of AF approximately twice per year. During these episodes, she developed severe anxiety accompanied by pressing central chest pain, and severe awareness of palpitations. She was mildly dyspneic. Her heart rate was observed to vary between 65 and 115 beats per minute. Investigations included an echocardiogram that showed mild left ventricular hypertrophy and a left atrium at 43 mm. Because of recurrent chest pain, a coronary angiogram was performed, showing normal coronary arteries.

Her electrocardiogram (Fig. 2) demonstrates left ventricular hypertrophy and AF with a moderate ventricular response. During this electrocardiogram she was severely symptomatic.

Why do these two individuals vary diametrically with respect to symptoms?

Genesis of Symptoms in Atrial Fibrillation

Various symptoms may arise as the result of hemodynamic disturbances during AF, mainly rapid heart rate, irregular rhythm, and loss

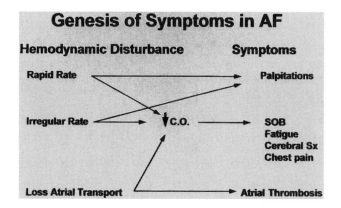

Figure 3. Diagrammatic representation of the relationship of symptoms to hemodynamic change during atrial fibrillation. CO = cardiac output; SOB = shortness of breath; Sx = symptoms.

of atrial contraction (Fig. 3). All of these perturbations lead to decreased cardiac output that, in turn, may lead to breathlessness, fatigue, symptoms of cerebral hypoperfusion, and chest pain. The rapid and irregular heart rate may cause palpitations. The loss of active atrial transport likely contributes to thrombus formation. Thus, the presence of various symptoms relates to the underlying hemodynamic changes. Why some people experience symptoms has remained unclear.

In order to elucidate factors that may contribute to the presence or absence of symptoms, we utilized the data from the Canadian Registry of Atrial Fibrillation.

Canadian Registry of Atrial Fibrillation (CARAF)

The Canadian Registry of Atrial Fibrillation enrolls patients at the time of their first electrocardiographically confirmed diagnosis of AF. Patients were enrolled at seven electrophysiology centers in six cities across Canada. Patients were diagnosed at family physician's or specialist's offices, emergency rooms, cardiology laboratories, and during hospitalizations for other illnesses. At the time of entry, an extensive database was collected including comprehensive medical history and recorded clinical data, laboratory testing including thyroid stimulating hormone (TSH), and echocardiographic data. Patients were then followed by a research nurse at 3 months, 1 year, and annually. Electrocardiograms were recorded annually and echocardiograms were performed every 2 years. This study was observational without directed intervention. However, any interventions were recorded, including drug therapy and cardioversion. Recurrence of AF was documented and major events such as death or stroke were investigated.

Analysis of Results

Data were collected on over 600 patients, approximately 80% with paroxysmal AF and 20% with chronic AF. All were directly interrogated regarding the presence of a variety of symptoms. The frequency of individual symptoms was as follows: palpitations, 50%; chest pain, 29%; fatigue, 28%; dizziness/presyncope/syncope, 27%; anxiety, 17%; dyspnea, 17%; and nausea, 8%. A total of 79% of patients had one or more symptoms. Twenty-one per cent of patients denied all symptoms.

Analysis was then performed to identify baseline variables that led to symptoms in general and to specific symptoms. Five factors were highly predictive of symptoms: young age, higher systolic blood pressure, higher heart rate, female gender, and no history of myocardial infarction. Utilizing these five variables, a theoretical formula was created to predict the likelihood of development of symptoms.

Several specific symptoms were then evaluated. Palpitations were more likely to occur in patients of younger age, of female gender, with normal left ventricular function, and with increased heart rate. Symptoms of cerebral hypoperfusion were more likely to occur in patients with no previous history of myocardial infarction and smaller left atrial dimension. Dyspnea occurred more frequently in patients with higher systolic blood pressures, increased left atrial and left ventricular size, female gender, and younger age. Chest pain was predicted by higher blood pressure, absence of mitral regurgitation, and older age.

Discussion

The variability of symptomatology in AF is well recognized. In a study using ambulatory monitoring to assess recurrence of paroxysmal AF on medication, Page et al. reported that asymptomatic episodes of paroxysmal AF may occur much more frequently than symptomatic episodes.[4] This emphasizes that symptoms may vary with any one patient from time to time. Our study evaluated symptoms only at the time of first diagnosis. One might imagine that symptoms could differ under different states of activity and autonomic control.

Our study has identified five factors that predict symptoms in general: young age, female, higher blood pressure and heart rate, and no history of myocardial infarction. In a study using transtelephonic recordings during follow-up of patients treated for AF, Bhandari et al. found higher rates in symptomatic transmissions than in asymptomatic transmissions.[5] The other factors in our study have not previously been recognized.

Older patients without underlying heart disease or high blood pressure who have AF at a slower heart rate are more likely to be asymptomatic. Nonetheless, these individuals may have a risk of embolic events and identification of recurrence of AF in this patient group is important to monitor the risk of stroke.

Palpitations, the most common symptom, were more frequent in younger patients with normal left ventricular systolic function and increased heart rate. The higher sympathetic tone, combined with good cardiac contractility may increase the awareness of cardiac contractions, particularly in younger patients who are more active.

Symptoms of cerebral hypoperfusion (presyncope, syncope) were more common in the absence of previous myocardial infarction. Myocardial infarction may decrease contractility and damage c-fiber receptors, leading to a loss of neurocardiogenic reflexes that have been suggested to result in decreased blood pressure during AF.[6,7]

Again, dyspnea was more common in younger patients, possibly related to their higher level of activity and increased demand for augmentation of cardiac output. Higher systolic blood pressure, larger left atria, and increased left ventricular diastolic dimension can all increase left atrial pressure and contribute to dyspnea. Furthermore, left ventricular hypertrophy from hypertension may cause diastolic dysfunction, with higher dependency on active atrial transport.

Chest pain was more common in older ages when coronary artery disease is more prevalent, and with higher blood pressure which may increase myocardial oxygen demand.

Other symptoms identified in this study also had variables identified that may lead to these specific symptoms.

Summary

In summary, symptoms during AF vary dramatically from patient to patient and they vary from time to time in the same patient. Careful evaluation of clinical and echocardiographic variables utilizing the Canadian Registry of Atrial Fibrillation has permitted some insight into the genesis of a variety of symptoms in AF.

The ability to identify those patients who may be asymptomatic during recurrences of AF may increase the need to anticoagulate such patients, should they develop recurrent events that go unnoticed.

Although the mechanisms suggested for the development of various symptoms are unproven, the theoretical basis for such symptoms may guide the type of therapy for the different subgroups of patients.

Acknowledgments: I wish to acknowledge the following members of the Canadian Registry of Atrial Fibrillation (authors): Xiaohua Wang, MSc, Susan Mooney, RN, John Boone, MD, FRCPC, Murray Rosenbaum, MD, FRCPC, all associated with the University of British Columbia, Vancouver, B.C.; Stuart Connolly, MD, FRCPC, McMaster University, Hamilton, Ontario; Martin Green, MD, FRCPC, University of Ottawa, Ottawa, Ontario; George Klein, MD, FRCPC, University of Western Ontario, London, Ontario; Robert Sheldon, MD, FRCPC, University of Calgary, Alberta; and Mario Talajic, MD, FRCPC, Montreal Heart Institute, Montreal, Quebec.

References

1. Peters KG, Kienzle MG. Severe cardiomyopathy due to chronic rapidly conducted atrial fibrillation: complete recovery after restoration of sinus rhythm. Am J Med 1988;85:242–244.
2. Grogan M, Smith HC, Gersh BJ, Wood DL. Left ventricular dysfunction due to atrial fibrillation initially believed to have idiopathic dilated cardiomyopathy. Am J Cardiol 1992;69:1570–1573.
3. Kieny JR, Sacrez A, Facello A, et al. Increase in radionuclide left ventricular ejection fraction after cardioversion of chronic atrial fibrillation in iodiopathic dilated cardiomyopathy. Euro Heart J:1992;13:1290–1295.
4. Page RL, Wilkinson WE, Clair WK, et al. Asymptomatic arrhythmias in patients with symptomatic paroxysmal atrial fibrillation and paroxysmal supraventricular tachycardia. Circulation 1994;89(1):224–227.
5. Bhandari AK, Anderson JL, Gilbert EM, et al. and the Flecainide Supraventricular Tachycardia Study Group. Correlation of symptoms with occurrence of paroxysmal supraventricular tachycardia or atrial fibrillation. Am Heart J 1992;123:381–387.
6. Brignole M, Gianfranchi C, Menozzi C, et al. Role of autonomic reflexes in syncope associated with paroxysmal atrial fibrillation. J Am Coll Cardiol 1993;22(4):1123–1129.
7. Leitch J, Klein GJ, Yee R, et al. Neurally-mediated syncope and atrial fibrillation. (Letter). N Engl J Med 1991;324:495–496.

CHAPTER 3

Evaluation of Quality of Life in Atrial Fibrillation

Paul Dorian, Miney Paquette,
David Newman

Leontes: I have tremor cordis on me; my heart dances, but not for joy, not joy.

The Winter's Tale, I, ii

Why Assess Quality of Life?

In the traditional biomedical assessment of physical and cardiovascular illness, clinicians and especially researchers usually concentrate on objective, quantitative attributes of the disease in question; these most often relate to the detailed measurement of organ or system function, for example, left ventricular systolic function, heart rate, or exercise capacity. Patient outcomes are usually quantified with respect to easily defined events, such as myocardial infarction (MI), stroke, or death. However, from both the physician's and patient's perspectives, a very important aspect of a disease is the patient's subjective experience of the malady, which may be expressed as the "illness burden". The distinction between the extent of organ dysfunction and the magnitude of distress it causes in a given patient is especially prominent in chronic illnesses, for example, chronic arrhythmias.

Physicians and caregivers are increasingly recognizing that patients' subjective perceptions of their illness are important considerations in designing management strategies for various diseases, and that many patients consider quality of life to be the most important outcome of treatment.

Because quality of life measurements are subjective and difficult

From *Nonpharmacological Management of Atrial Fibrillation*, edited by F.D. Murgatroyd and A.J. Camm. © 1997, Futura Publishing Co., Inc., Armonk, NY.

to quantify, their importance is often at least implicitly questioned. It is generally assumed that clinical outcomes, such as frequency of recurrence of atrial fibrillation, are inherently valid as a measure of treatment efficacy. However, there is no clear reason to believe that this type of objective outcome is more meaningful as a measure of illness burden than the patient's perception of the condition, although the latter is much more difficult to measure. "To a certain extent, what the psychosocial measure may lack in precision, it may compensate for in relevance."[1]

Quality of life measurements can be used to predict subsequent physical outcomes, or subsequent subjective, psychological outcomes. For example, many psychosocial variables such as depression, social isolation, personality type, coping style, pessimism, and similar attributes are important predictors of subsequent "hard" biological endpoints such as mortality or disease recurrence, and they may also predict long-term patient adaptation to the illness. Social isolation, depression, and psychological well-being have been shown to be important predictors of mortality and rehospitalization following MI, bypass surgery, and during cardiac rehabilitation.[2-4] Personality style, such as the tendency to suppress emotional distress (type "D" personality) is a very important predictor of mortality in patients with coronary artery disease.[5] The predictive ability of quality of life measures affords the opportunity to target patient subgroups with tailored psychosocial or medical interventions. In a meta-analysis of controlled studies of psychosocial interventions following MI, treated patients had a 30% reduction in mortality compared to controls attesting to the importance of behavioral factors in determining physical outcomes.[6]

Quality of life can also be used as an outcome measure, analogous to recurrence of arrhythmia, infarction, or death. However, it is often more responsive to changes in health status than traditional biological indices, and may elucidate meaningful differences between therapeutic interventions which could be obscured by concentrating on mortality outcomes alone. The difficulty in evaluating the meaningfulness of a quality of life change is related to the absence of a "gold standard" against which to compare a particular test result. Useful comparators to place quality of life changes in perspective include: "anchor based interpretations"[7] which compare a change in a quality of life scale to some global measure of distress (e.g., "on a scale of 1–10, how disruptive is the illness?"); comparison with test scores of normal controls or patients with a variety of other illnesses; the strength of a particular quality of life change in predicting an outcome; and the subjective relation of a particular magnitude of quality of life change to life events, as perceived by the patient.

How Is Quality of Life Measured?

As generally conceived, quality of life may be health related and non-health related. Aspects of health-related quality of life are generally thought to include physical functioning, psychological functioning, social and occupational functioning, and somatic sensation (e.g., pain or discomfort). Most quality of life research employs patient self-reports using validated questionnaires, with questions centered around general aspects of health-related quality of life, functional capacity, and disease-specific aspects of health-related quality of life, which focus on symptoms and disabilities specific to the disease in question. Health-related quality of life is inherently multidimensional, and variable over time. Thus, its accurate measurement is complex, and the task of ensuring that the tools we use to measure it are reliable, valid, and reproducible is critical. The instruments should be responsive (able to detect changes within individuals over time), reliable (able to measure in a reproducible and consistent fashion), interpretable (the size of the changes should be meaningful), and valid (should measure that which is intended to be measured). The process of validation is usually an ongoing one with increasing confidence as validation progresses.

A complementary measure of quality of life involves adjusting years of life (years gained from therapy, for example) for the severity of disability. Most patients are prepared to "trade" years of life for an improved quality of life if the symptoms of disease are severe.[8] The concept of "quality-adjusted life years" (QALYs) first evolved from interventions in patients with chronic renal failure who were able to balance quality of life gains and increased mortality risk with a kidney transplant.[9] In addition to providing an integrated measure spanning morbidity (quality) and mortality (quantity), QALYs serve as a measurement unit for cost-utility analyses, a form of economic assessment to evaluate competing therapies. QALYs measure patient preferences for different outcomes and provide researchers with a common unit to make interpretable comparisons across any number of treatments and disease states.

The general consensus among researchers is that two broad types of questionnaires should be included to assess particular domains of health-related quality of life. Generic tests assess a broad range of health domains and are intended for use across a number of different disease states. Assessments of physical functioning, social functioning, psychological functioning, functional capacity, and somatic sensation are usually part of any general health battery. The use of generic scales facilitates comparison across different disease states and the broad approach allows for detection of unexpected results. The most commonly used scale, the MOS SF-36 (Short Form of the Medical Outcomes Study) has been evaluated in numerous trials in over 150 conditions, and normative data is available for comparison.[10] As part of the International Quality of Life Assessment Project, the SF-36 will soon be available in 17 different languages.[11,12]

Disease-specific scales, as the name implies, assess domains specific to the disease in question, including specific symptoms, management strategies, and specific impairments. By design, disease-specific scales are often more responsive to change than generic scales although comparison between different disease groups is sometimes not possible. For example, in a study of patients with ventricular defibrillators, the disease-specific University of Toronto Scale differentiated between patients who had their devices a shorter vs. longer period of time, and also between those with better vs. worse left ventricular (LV) function; the SF-36 did not differentiate between either group of patients.[13]

While outcome scales measure the consequences of a therapeutic intervention, or change in quality of life over time, predictive scales are used to identify subgroups of patients who may be at greater risk for certain outcomes. Predictive scales usually measure stable constructs, including personality factors such as optimism or hostility, as well as coping styles and indices of social support. For example, in patients undergoing radiofrequency ablation for reentrant supraventricular tachycardias, somatization tendencies were correlated with lower quality of life scores at baseline as measured by a generic instrument[14]; patients who tended to suppress emotional distress (type "D" personality type) had higher rates of long-term mortality, independent of other physiological predictors.[5]

Most investigators assessing health-related quality of life use self-administered questionnaires because they allow a cost effective approach to collecting data from a large sample of patients. The need for trained interviewers is eliminated, and self-reporting vs. face-to-face interviews reduces demand characteristics of patients (i.e., the desire to report socially desirable or positive results), as well as biases on the part of the interviewer. It is important to note that although there are countless quality of life questionnaires available for a multitude of purposes, some are more reliable and sensitive than others, and the degree of validation varies widely.

When choosing scales for use in studies, the following issues should be kept in mind. Scales should be appropriate for the population of interest (i.e., type and severity of disease). Scales should be culturally sensitive, and attempts should be made to ensure that scales are appropriate across gender and age groups. In studies where quality of life is assessed across cultures or in different countries, it is imperative to have each scale validated in the language and culture of interest. Except in cases where the educational level of the group is known, reading level of the items should require no higher than a grade eight education. The respondent burden (total number of scales and items needed) should be limited to a reasonable number. When the respondent burden is excessive, reliablility of responses can be jeopardized. Generally, an attempt should be made to use existing, validated scales, rather than constructing new scales which have unconfirmed psychometric properties.

There are several issues which must be addressed prior to beginning a study where primary outcomes are based on perceived health status. The difficulty interpreting subjective measures of health is partly due to the absence of a "gold standard" which could serve to assess the adequacy and appropriateness of the quality of life measures. Consequently, there is a need to relate quality of life measures to objective measures of disease severity, and disease impact. Issues of external validity are at least partially addressed by comparing quality of life ratings with global patient well-being ratings, physician ratings of disease severity (to provide an integrated measure of symptom duration, frequency and severity), and utilization of health care resources (e.g., doctor visits, hospitalizations, drug therapy, days lost from work). In addition, quality of life measures may also be compared to clinical outcomes such as heart failure, stroke, and mortality. For example, in one study, psychological distress (as measured by the Symptom Checklist 90) predicted significantly higher rates of rehospitalization and other "hard" biological outcomes such as death and MI in patients with coronary artery disease.[15]

Why Is Measurement of Quality of Life in Atrial Fibrillation Important?

Atrial fibrillation (AF) exerts its primary adverse effects through impairment of exercise tolerance, its association with symptoms of fatigue, palpitations, and dyspnea, as well as its association with stroke or other thromboembolism. Although AF is associated with an increase in mortality risk, it is unclear if AF itself is an independent risk factor for premature mortality since it is so often associated with other risk factors for coronary artery disease or other risks for cardiac death (e.g., valvular disease, cardiomyopathy, etc.).[16] In randomized clinical trials, anticoagulation with coumadin can reduce stroke risk virtually to that of the baseline risk for patients of similar age without AF; therefore, the chief illness burden to be borne with AF is that which results from the symptomatic effects of the rhythm disturbance as well as the adverse effects of therapy. Despite the lack of clear association between AF and "hard" endpoints such as mortality, AF imposes a major illness and health/economic burden, since it frequently results in hospitalization, physician visits, drug therapy, days lost from work or productive activity, and appears to limit the physical, social, emotional, and occupational activities of many patients. However, the severity of symptoms and degree of life disruption caused by AF are extremely variable. Patients' perception of health-related quality of life usually revolves around factors that are poorly, if at all, related to the more objective measures of cardiovascular function usually employed to assess treatment efficacy or disease burden in AF. For example, there is only limited evidence that ventricular rate control with drugs in AF improves patient well-being,[17] except in selected subsets of patients; treatment designed for maximum exercise tolerance on a treadmill does not necessarily result in improved subjective well-being.[18] Many of the drug treatments applied to patients with AF are expensive, carry a risk of symptomatic side effects, and do not necessarily lead to improved health-related quality of life even if they improve conventional measures of disease severity (e.g., frequency and duration of attacks of AF).[19]

Studies of Quality of Life in Patients with Atrial Fibrillation

There is very limited information on the effect of AF on systematically measured quality of life, using validated measures. In the most highly symptomatic patients, referred for atrioventricular (AV) node ablation and the placement of a permanent pacemaker, there is a substantial improvement in one aspect of quality of life (as assessed with a symptom checklist), as well as in exercise tolerance.[20] In a similar population of patients undergoing AV node ablation, quality of life scores improved markedly after therapy, and disabling symptoms were reported to be less frequent after treatment.[21] Specific activities of daily living such as climbing stairs or carrying groceries, as well as exercise capacity, improved after ablation, and utilization of health care resources (hospital admissions, emergency room visits, physician visits, and antiarrhythmic drug use) decreased significantly.

Not all measures of quality of life are equally useful. Hamer et al.,[22] in a series of patients with supraventricular arrhythmias (supraventricular tachycardia and paroxysmal AF) entering into investigational drug studies, found that measures of psychological distress discriminated poorly between patients whose lives were "disrupted" or "not disrupted" by AF. These investigators measured anxiety, coping with illness strategies, depression, and other emotional attributes of illness adjustment, and found that only a few subscales were able to distinguish between patients who felt that their lives in general were highly, or little disrupted by AF. Notably, there were no differences between these two groups in terms of number of years of symptoms, or number of previous arrhythmic episodes. Furthermore, there were no differences between "low disrupted" and "high disrupted" groups with respect to personality factors including anxiety or locus of control measures. Higher pain and somatization scores in the "high life disruption" group were the only significant differences between these two groups. Other domains of quality of life such as social adjustment, physical well-being, symptoms specific to AF such as palpitations or dyspnea, or general health perceptions were not evaluated, and a control population was not available.

We assessed patients with a variety of paroxysmal supraventricular tachycardias prior to, and 3 months following radiofrequency ablation[14]; the majority had reentrant tachycardias using an accessory pathway or AV nodal reentry. Quality of life at baseline (as measured by a generic scale, the SF-36) was impaired compared to normal or post-MI controls, and improved substantially following successful radiofrequency ablation. Patients reported feeling significantly less pain, had less physical role limitations, better physical functioning, and increased vitality after radiofrequency catheter ablation. In this study, baseline adjustment and the extent of improvement was modulated by psychological characteristics present at baseline, including the extent of somatization. In a preliminary report, Jenkins et al.[23] used the SF-36, the Quality of Life Index for cardiac patients (QLI-C), and the Symptom Frequency and Severity Checklist to assess patients with AF prior to undergoing AV node ablation. All subscale scores of the SF-36 scale were significantly lower for patients with AF than normal controls or cardiac controls (patients with recent MI), and the QLI-C and Symptom Checklist scores were also lower in this group than in other cardiac groups. Although this assessment was limited to a selective group of highly symptomatic patients, it is apparent that the disease burden of AF can be considerable.

It is commonly appreciated that many patients with AF are entirely asymptomatic. In contrast, others have severe and disabling symptoms even though their episodes of AF may be infrequent, of short duration, or without terribly rapid ventricular response. Although the gap between "disease" severity and "illness" severity is occasionally very wide, little is known of the factors which lead to variable patient distress and disability in patients with apparently equivalent disease burden. Treatment strategies aimed at improving patient quality of life will not only have obvious value in improving patient well-being, but are likely to be highly cost effective in that they will likely reduce the number, duration, and cost of hospitalizations and may improve long-term prognosis. A careful examination of the evidence relating ventricular rate control in patients with AF to patient subjective well-being illustrates the difficulties in using a crude biological endpoint to assess clinically relevant patient outcomes. In view of the frequent presence of subjectively distressing palpitations during rapid ventricular responses to AF, and the dramatic increase in heart rate during exercise, a great deal of attention has been paid to drug therapy that controls ventricular response during AF, especially during exercise. It has long been observed that digitalis is relatively ineffective at controlling marked rises in ventricular rate during exercise, even when rate is controlled at rest. This observation has led to a large number of studies which investigated the ability of beta-blockers or calcium channel blocking agents with AV nodal blocking properties (verapamil, diltiazem) in controlling ventricular response. A large number of controlled studies have shown that these latter agents are more effective than placebo or digoxin alone in limiting maximum heart rate during exercise.[17] However, there is no evidence that beta-blockers can increase exercise duration, patient well-being, or maximum oxygen consumption in patients with AF, and some studies suggest that exercise capacity is diminished and subjective effort is increased during peak exercise on beta-blocker therapy.[17,18,24] Following calcium channel blocking drugs, a few studies show improved exercise tolerance[25] but the majority of placebo controlled trials show no improvement in maximum exercise tolerance, subjective effort at maximal exertion, maximum oxygen consumption, or well-being in patients treated with calcium channel blockers as opposed to digitalis alone.[17,18,26,27] These rather disappointing results may be due to the negative inotropic effect of the AV nodal blocking drugs, other symptomatic adverse effects, or a lack of correlation between slower heart rates and better cardiac function. These results do not, of course, indicate that ventricular rate control is inappropriate, but simply that the drugs currently available to achieve this end, at least in many patients, may result in limited or unproven clinical benefit.

It would seem reasonable to assess the effect of therapy for AF not only on objective endpoints such as the frequency and duration of recurrence or heart rate during AF, but also on more subjective (and more difficult to measure) endpoints. These would include, for example, perceived severity of recurrences, and the effects of the illness and its treatment on a composite of physical symptoms, social and emotional function, and general health perception, since it is these latter variables which intrude on the patient's well-being.

How Should the Impact of Atrial Fibrillation Be Assessed?

There are no published studies of the impact of AF on quality of life over time or following treatment. Together with a group of investigators studying implanted atrial defibrillators, we have devised a protocol for measuring quality of life in patients with AF. The questionnaires to be used and related information about the severity of disease are listed below; this approach represents an attempt at systematically assessing quality of life in these patients and may serve as an example of the types of measures that may be useful in assessing quality of life in AF.

Self-Report Instruments

In addition to a standard demographic component which is used to record the patient's age, sex, education, social contacts (marital, family, employment) and socioeconomic status, three predictive scales are used to identify subsets of patients who may be more or less responsive to various interventions. At baseline only, patients receive the following:

• The Life Orientation Test (LOT), a measure of optimism which has been shown to have good internal consistency in past studies, and good discriminant validity with respect to related constructs such as locus of control and psychological adjustment scores.[28]

• The Barsky Somatization Scale, used in a wide variety of cardiac populations, including patients with paroxysmal supraventricular tachycardia.[14]

• The Freiburg Questionnaire of Coping with Illness (FQCI), designed to examine how patients cope with their illness, including their associated emotions and what measures were taken to cope.[29]

The following outcome scales are given to patients at baseline and during follow-up:

• The SF-36, described previously, is a generic health scale measuring several health domains including physical functioning, role functioning, social functioning, mental health, vitality, pain, and general health perceptions. The questionnaire is based on the Rand Corporation's physical and mental health scales used in the Medical Outcomes Study.[10] This shorter, revised version correlates highly with the longer scale, and all scales have been shown to be responsive to a number of medical and psychiatric problems.

• The modified Goldman Specific Activity Scale (SAS) is a functional status scale for patients with cardiovascular disease. The original version of this scale is in a "yes/no" format but the revised version has been Likert-scaled to increase its discriminatory power. Evaluation in a small sample of pacemaker patients suggests good convergent validity and high test-retest reliability.[30]

• The disease-specific University of Toronto Arrhythmia Scale, adapted for use in patients with AF, has been shown to have good discriminant validity in patients with ventricular defibrillators.[13] Preliminary investigations of this instrument suggest good test-retest reliability and good convergent validity with the SF-36. The questions address symptoms specific to patients with arrhythmias, as well as assessing adaptation to the defibrillator.

• The Symptom Checklist quantifies both symptom frequency and severity of symptoms related to arrhythmias. Initial investigations of validity in an AF population suggest good content validity, and it is currently being validated as part of a study in progress ("Ablate and Pace Trial: A Multicenter Registry of A-V Nodal Ablation and Pacing in Atrial Fibrillation",[23] sponsored by Medtronic®, Inc., Minneapolis, MI, USA).

• The Illness Intrusiveness Scale,[31] is a 13-item scale designed for patients with chronic illness. The concept of illness intrusiveness is introduced to represent the disruptions to activities, interests, and general functioning caused by the patient's chronic illness. Often the illness will also compromise psychosocial well-being, and increase emotional distress. This scale has been validated in a number of diverse disease states including end-stage renal disease, multiple sclerosis, rheumatoid arthritis, laryngeal cancer, systemic lupus erythematosus, sleep disorders, mood disorders, and schizophrenia.

A summary score will then be used, based on the assessments listed below, to classify the patient's clinical burden of AF as mild, moderate, or severe. The "clinical disease burden score" will reflect objective and subjective portions of the clinical disease burden and severity obtained from the subject, including: (1) number of emergency room visits, hospitalizations, and cardioversions during the interval since last evaluation; (2) average frequency of AF episodes; (3) average duration of AF episodes; and (4) severity of average episodes of AF (measured on a 10-point visual analog scale).

The physician or study coordinator will record: (1) number of AF related medications (antiarrhythmic and/or anticoagulant) being taken by the subject; (2) number of antiarrhythmic medications that failed during the interval since last evaluation (retrospective 1–2 years at baseline); (3) left ventricular ejection fraction; (4) New York Heart Association classification (NYHA); (5) history of hypertension; (6) left atrial size; (7) etiology of heart disease; and (8) other cardiovascular and medical conditions. These variables combined with patient report variables will provide a matrix of clinical disease severity and a summary score.

Conclusions

Since health-related quality of life is a difficult concept to define, may mean different things to different people, and is difficult to measure accurately, reliably, and reproducibly, it has often been ignored in the standard evaluation of the efficacy of treatments for AF. As we move forward with increasingly complex, adventuresome, and innovative treatments for AF, it is important that the focus be maintained on the overriding purpose of medical care, that is the relief of suffering and the promotion of a productive and satisfying life.

References

1. Shipper HS, Clinch JJ, Olweny, CLM. Quality of life studies: definitions and conceptual issues. In: Spilker B, ed. Quality of Life and Pharmacoeconomics in Clinical Trials. Philadelphia, PA: Lippincott-Raven Publishers; 1996:11–23.
2. Ruberman W, Weinblatt E, Goldberg JD, et al. Psychosocial influences on mortality after myocardial infarction. N Engl J Med 1984;311:552–559.
3. Frasure-Smith N, Lesperance F, Talajic M. Depression and 18–month prognosis after myocardial infarction. Circulation 1995;91:999–1005.
4. Lewin B, Robertson IH, Cay EL, et al. Effects of self-help post-myocardial

infarction rehabilitation on psychological adjustment and use of health services. Lancet 1992;339:1036–1040.

5. Denollet J, Sys SU, Stroobant N, et al. Personality as independent predictor of long-term mortality in patients with coronary heart disease. Lancet 1996;347:417–421.

6. Linden W, Stossel C, Maurice J. Psychosocial interventions for patients with coronary artery disease: a meta-analysis. Arch Intern Med 1996;156: 745–752.

7. Guyatt GH, Jaeschke R, Feeny DH, et al. Measurements in clinical trials: choosing the right approach. In: Spilker B, ed. Quality of Life and Pharmacoeconomics in Clinical Trials. Philadelphia, PA: Lippincott-Raven Publishers; 1996:41–48.

8. Torrance GW. Designing and conducting cost-utility analyses. In: Spilker B, ed. Quality of Life and Pharmacoeconomics in Clinical Trials. Philadelphia, PA: Lippincott-Raven Publishers; 1996:1105–1111.

9. Klarman HE, Francis J, Rosenthal GD. Cost-effectiveness analysis applied to the treatment of chronic renal disease. Med Care 1968;6(1):48–54.

10. Ware JE, Sherbourne CD. The MOS 36-Item Short-Form Health Survey (SF-36) I: conceptual framework and item selection. Medical Care 1992; 30:473–483.

11. Aaronson NK, Acquadro C, Alonso J, et al. International quality of life assessment (IQOLA) project. Qual Life Res 1992;1:349–351.

12. Gandek B. International quality of life assessment (IQOLA) project. The Quality of Life Newsletter 1992;5–10.

13. Ham M, Newman D, Irvine J, et al. Quality of life in implantable defibrillator patients: utility of a disease specific scale. Can J Cardiol 1995;11:84.

14. Davies E, Sheahan R, Bajaj R, et al. A prospective evaluation of catheter ablation for cardiac arrhythmias on quality of life. Can J Cardiol 1995;11: 83.

15. Allison TG, Williams DE, Miller TD, et al. Medical and economic costs of psychologic distress in patients with coronary artery disease. Mayo Clin Proc 1995;70:734–742.

16. Cuddy TE, Connolly SJ. Atrial fibrillation and atrial flutter. Can J Cardiol 1996;12:9A-44A.

17. Brignole M, Menozzi C. Control of rapid heart rate in patients with atrial fibrillation: drugs or ablation? PACE 1996;19:348–356.

18. Lewis RV, Laing E, Moreland TA, et al. A comparison of digoxin, diltiazem and their combination in the treatment of AF. Eur Heart J 1988;9:279–283.

19. Newman D, Gillis A, Gilbert M, et al. Chronic drug therapy to prevent recurrence of atrial fibrillation. Can J Cardiol 1996;12: 24A-28A.

20. Kay GN, Bubien RS, Epstein AE, et al. Effect of catheter ablation of the atrioventricular junction on quality of life and exercise tolerance in paroxysmal atrial fibrillation. Am J Cardiol 1988;62:741–744.

21. Fitzpatrick AP, Kourouyan HD, Siu A, et al. Quality of life and outcomes after radiofrequency His-bundle catheter ablation and permanent pacemaker implantation: impact of treatment in paroxysmal and established atrial fibrillation. Am Heart J 1996;131:499–507.

22. Hamer ME, Blumenthal JA, McCarthy EA, et al. Quality-of-life assessment in patients with paroxysmal atrial fibrillation or paroxysmal supraventricular tachycardia. Am J Cardiol 1994;74:826–829.

23. Jenkins LS, Ellenbogen K, Kay N, et al. Quality of life in patients with symptomatic atrial fibrillation. Circulation 1995;92(8):I-490.
24. DiBianco R, Monganroth J, Freitag J, et al. Effects of nadolol on the spontaneous and exercise-provoked heart rate of patients with chronic atrial fibrillation receiving stable dosages of digoxin. Am Heart J 1984;108: 1121–1127.
25. Lang R, Klein H, DiSegni E, et al. Verapamil improves exercise capacity in chronic atrial fibrillation: double-blind crossover study. Am Heart J 1983;105:820–824.
26. Steinberg J, Katz R, Bren G, et al. Efficacy of oral diltiazem to control ventricular response in chronic atrial fibrillation at rest and during exercise. J Am Coll Cardiol 1987;9:405–411.
27. Lundstrom T, Ryden L. Ventricular rate control and exercise performance in chronic atrial fibrillation: effects of diltiazem and verapamil. J Am Coll Cardiol 1990;16:86–90.
28. Scheier MF, Carver CS. Optimism, coping, and health: assessment and implications of generalized outcome expectancies. Health Psych 1985;4: 219–247.
29. Muthny FA. Illness specificity and coping with illness: an empirical comparison of dialysis and heart infarct patients. Zeitschrift fur Psychosomatische Medizin und Psychoanalyse 1988;34(3):259–273.
30. Newman D, Dorian P, Darling D, et al. The effect of rate responsive functions on quality of life in patients with dual chamber pacemakers. Can J Cardiol 1993;9:69E.
31. Devins G. Illness intrusiveness and the psychosocial impact of lifestyle disruptions in chronic life-threatening disease. Adv Renal Replacement Ther 1994;1(3):251–263.

PART II

Controlling the Ventricular Rate: The Basics

CHAPTER 4

The Anatomy of the Atrioventricular Conduction Axis in Relation to Its Function

Robert H. Anderson, Siew Yen Ho

Introduction

It is salutary to realize that, in 1906, Sunao Tawara[1] provided an original description that, even now, is difficult to improve upon concerning the location and structure of the axis of specialized myocardial tissue responsible for conduction of the cardiac impulse from atria to ventricles. This is even more significant in that morphologists continue to argue among themselves concerning the precise arrangement of cells within the atrioventricular (AV) node.[2,3] With the advent, and widespread acceptance, of interventional techniques for ablation of arrhythmias, including atrial flutter and fibrillation, precise knowledge of this topic has become of paramount importance to clinicians, particularly the location of the so-called slow pathway and its relation to the histologically specialized areas. In this review, we will recapitulate our understanding of the structure of this crucial area. We should emphasize that not only is this very much a restatement of an account given 20 years ago,[4] but it is also a total endorsement of the initial description of Tawara.[1] To provide a framework for our histological findings, we will start our account with a description of the gross anatomy of the right atrium and the AV junctions, since this topic has also been the subject of recent controversies.[5,6]

Salient Gross Morphological Features

To understand the landmarks of the specialized AV junctional area, it is also necessary to understand the structure of the right atrium

From *Nonpharmacological Management of Atrial Fibrillation*, edited by F.D. Murgatroyd and A.J. Camm. © 1997, Futura Publishing Co., Inc., Armonk, NY.

and the components that separate its cavity from the left-sided chambers of the heart. The right atrium is made up of a smooth walled venous component, a broad triangular appendage, a vestibule inserting into the orifice of the tricuspid valve, and the right atrial aspect of the septum (Fig. 1). The septal components are complex. The wall separating the cavities of the right and left atria, in other words the true atrial septum, is relatively small. The larger part of this structure is the floor of the oval fossa (Fig. 2), marking the site of the fetal interatrial communication. This fibromuscular sheet is the remnant of the primary atrial septum which, on its left atrial aspect, overlaps the rims of the fossa. It is often thought that much of the overlapped rim of the fossa is the "septum secundum". In reality, the larger part of the rim is simply the infolded muscular walls between the orifices of the caval and the pulmonary veins (Fig. 2). The inferior rim of the fossa, in contrast, is another component of the true septum, but one which is confluent with two additional septa. One of these is the tissue separating the oval fossa from the coronary sinus, itself confluent with the tissues surrounding the mouth of the sinus which separate it from the left atrium. This is the sinus septum. The other septum is made up of the overlap-

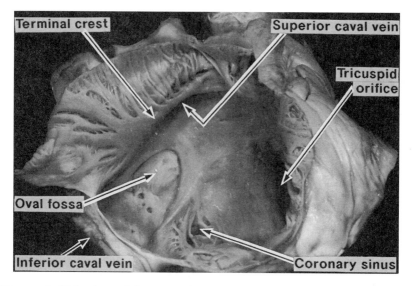

Figure 1. This view of the opened right atrium shows how the anatomical arrangement is dominated by the musculature surrounding the entrances of the great veins, the interatrial communication (oval fossa) and the vestibule of the tricuspid valve.

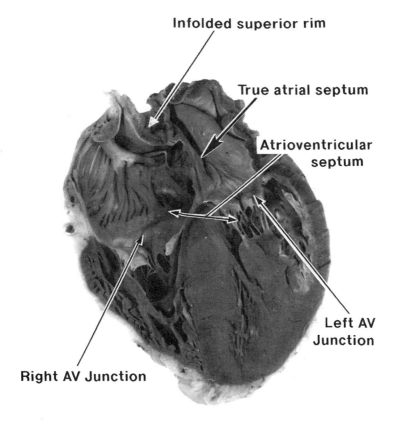

Infolded superior rim

True atrial septum

Atrioventricular septum

Left AV Junction

Right AV Junction

Figure 2. This "four chamber" section close to the crux of the heart shows the relationship of the floor of the oval fossa to its infolded superior rim and the muscular atrioventricular septum.

ping atrial and ventricular musculatures which exist because of the differential attachments of the leaflets of the mitral and tricuspid valves. This is the muscular AV septum (Fig. 2), continuous antero-superiorly with the fibrous tissues making up the so-called central fibrous body. This fibrous component is composed of the rightward margin of the area of fibrous continuity between the leaflets of the mitral and aortic valves together with the membranous septum, the latter divided by the attachment of the septal leaflet of the tricuspid valve into atrioventricular and interventricular components (Fig. 3).

This complex arrangement of the atrial septum, coupled with the structure of the venoatrial connections, means that the walls of the

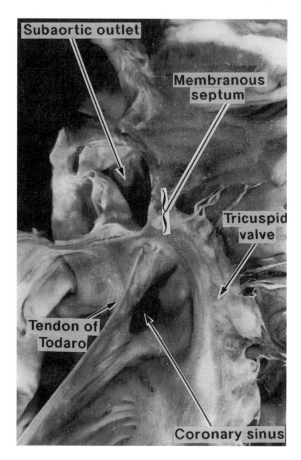

Figure 3. This dissection, made by removing the right coronary sinus of the aorta, shows the intimate relationship of the apex of the triangle of Koch to the subaortic outflow tract.

right atrium form a series of muscular bands which surround a number of holes. The holes are the orifices of the superior and inferior caval veins and the coronary sinus, the floor of the oval fossa, the wide mouth of the right atrial appendage, and the orifice of the tricuspid valve. Some of the musculature surrounding and separating these holes is arranged in prominent bundles. These are the terminal crest, marking the junction of appendage and venous component, the rims of the oval fossa, and the vestibule of the tricuspid valve. The terminal crest has other important components and relations. Extending laterally from the crest into the appendage are the prominent pectinate muscles, with one being particularly obvious, the so-called septum spurium. In many hearts, fibrous webs arise from the crest and guard the orifices of the inferior caval vein and coronary sinus—the eustachian and thebesian valves. From the junction of these webs, a fibrous strand runs into the sinus septum in the majority of hearts, burying itself in the musculature and extending forward to insert into the central fibrous body. This is the tendon of Todaro. In most hearts, there is also a diverticulum inferiorly between the terminal crest, the orifice of the coronary sinus and the vestibule of the tricuspid valve. This is the so-called post-eusta-

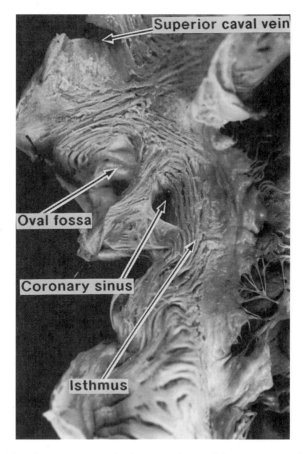

Figure 4. This dissection reveals the typical parallel orientation of myocardial fibers in the prominent muscle bundles of the right atrium.

chian sinus. Careful stripping of the endocardium from the inner wall of the right atrium shows a markedly parallel alignment of the atrial musculature in all these prominent bundles (Fig. 4).

When the walls of the right atrium are removed, together with the septal components, the extent of the AV junctions can then be appreciated. Careful dissection shows that the septal AV junction is confined to the area of the muscular AV septum (Fig. 5). Even the posterior part of this area is probably not a true septum, since an extensive epicardial tissue plane extends forward beneath the mouth of the coronary sinus, carrying the artery to the AV node, which takes origin from the dominant coronary artery. Removal of the floor of the coronary sinus reveals that this tissue plane is related directly to the diverging posterior margins of the walls of the right and left ventricles. More anteriorly, the muscular AV septum becomes confluent with the fibrous membranous septum, both of these septa separating the cavity of the right atrium from the extensive posterior diverticulum of the subaortic outflow tract (Fig. 3). Beyond the fibrous septum, the right atrial musculature is contiguous with the supraventricular crest of the right ventricle. It is the anterior extent of the membranous septum, therefore, which marks the border between the septum and the right parietal AV junction.[5]

The Specialized Atrioventricular Junctional Area

Following the meeting of the German Pathological Society in 1910, the distinguished pathologists of that time proposed a series of criteria for recognizing histologically specialized myocardial cells.[7,8] They suggested that the cells should be histologically discrete, should be capable of being followed from section to section and, to be considered tracts, should be insulated from their nonspecialized neighbors by fibrous sheaths. It has yet to be shown that these excellent suggestions are lacking. Because of this, they are the yardstick we use when defining histologically specialized myocardium.[3] On this basis, we describe the histologically specialized AV conduction axis as possessing transitional cells, a compact AV node, the penetrating AV bundle (of His), a nonbranching segment, and the branching AV bundle with its bundle branches (Fig. 6). The compact node is a relatively small half-oval of densely packed cells set against the sloping atrial septal aspect of the central fibrous body (Fig. 7a). Transitional cells are attenuated atrial myocardial cells, usually separated by fibroareolar spaces, which approach the node from the vestibule of the tricuspid valve, the sinus

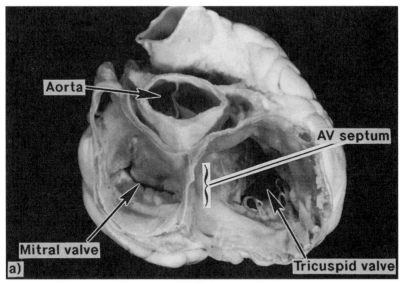

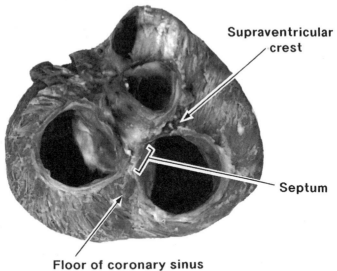

Figure 5. These dissections, made by removing in (**b**) the atrial musculature, shows the limited nature of the true atrioventricular septum. The so-called "anterior septum" is the superventricular crest of the right ventricle, while the "posterior septum" is the floor of the coronary sinus overlapping the diverging walls of the right and left ventricles.

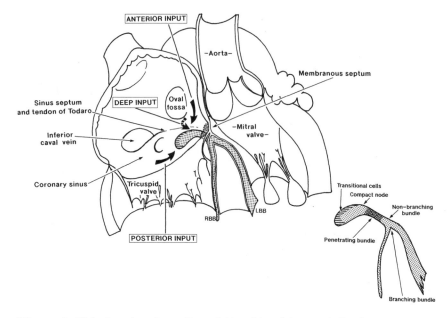

Figure 6. This drawing shows the relationship of the specialized components of the atrioventricular junctions relative to the anatomic structure of the junctions themselves.

septum, the anterior rim of the oval fossa, and the left atrial aspect of the septum (Fig. 7). The extent of the transitional cells is very limited. They, and the compact node, are located very much at the apex of the triangle of Koch, this being the area delimited by the tendon of Todaro, the septal attachment of the tricuspid valve and the orifice of the coronary sinus (Fig. 3). The larger part of the atrial musculature entering the triangle to give rise to the transitional cells, although made up of well-oriented atrial fibers (Fig. 4), is histologically nonspecialized when examined at light microscopic level, the muscle bundles being made up of ordinary atrial myocytes. There are no insulated tracts running through these areas to encroach upon the histologically specialized tissues.

At the apex of the triangle of Koch, most of the fibers running down from the oval fossa cross over the compact AV node, which is buried beneath the right atrial surface. The specialized cells group together and enter the substance of the central fibrous body. Then, as soon as they are enclosed within the fibrous tissue, the axis formed, by definition, becomes the penetrating bundle (of His, Fig. 7b). By virtue of the

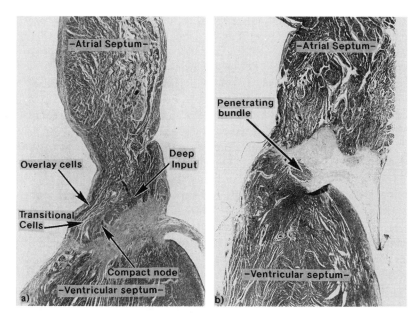

Figure 7. These sections show the histologic arrangement of (**a**) the atrioventricular node and (**b**) the penetrating atrioventricular bundle of His.

location of the central fibrous body separating right atrium from left ventricular outflow tract, the axis has only a short course to run through the fibrous tissue before it reaches the crest of the muscular ventricular septum. This penetration occurs in the triangle between the noncoronary and right coronary leaflets of the aortic valve. Having passed through the fibrous septum to reach the muscular septum, the bundle then runs a nonbranching course of variable length before dividing to form the right and left bundle branches. The fibers of the left bundle branch, insulated from the septal myocardium, fan out on the smooth left ventricular septal surface, while the right bundle branch, again an insulated structure, penetrates back through the musculature of the septum to surface beneath the medial papillary muscle of the right ventricle.

Functional Correlates

Most attempts to correlate structure and function in the AV node have been made in animal hearts. In this respect, it should be realized that there are important, but subtle, differences between the precise location of the conduction axis and its relationship to the septal structures between humans, rabbits, and dogs. It has been the failure to recognize these differences which has underscored, in part, some of the apparent controversies concerning the structure of the AV node.[2,3] It should also be appreciated that, when we performed our own study correlating structure and function in the rabbit node, we were unaware of the full significance of Tawara's initial account.[1]

In his superb monograph, Tawara described for the first time the AV node, or "knoten", and clarified its relationship to the penetrating AV bundle. In this respect, it should also be noted that as distinguished an anatomist as Sir Arthur Keith had experienced difficulty in replicating the initial findings of His the Younger.[9] Only when guided by the descriptions of Tawara was Keith able to confirm the existence of the penetrating AV bundle.[10] Tawara had proposed that, using morphological criteria, the best guide to the transition from AV node to penetrating bundle was the point at which the axis of conduction tissue became engulfed by the central fibrous body, the fibrous tissue then insulating the axis from atrial electrical events. This remains an entirely satisfactory criterion, and one which we now endorse.[3] Unfortunately, when conducting our earlier study on anatomical-electrophysiological correlations in the rabbit heart,[11] we had been unaware of this sensible proposal. Thus, much of what we described, at that time, as the AV node should now be considered, using Tawara's criterion, to represent the penetrating AV bundle. We would now redefine, therefore, our so-called "closed AV node" as the penetrating AV bundle (Fig. 8). It is then, perhaps, significant that we found that only a small proportion of AV delay occurring within this enclosed component of the conduction axis. Nine-tenths of our observed incremental delay was detected in areas occupied by transitional cells, which were confluent inferiorly and superiorly with pathways of atrial myocardial cells approaching the nodal area from the terminal crest and the rims of the oval fossa.

These findings are pertinent to at least two areas of ongoing controversy. The first concerns the location of the so-called slow pathway into the AV node, and its relationship to the histologically specialized area. All the circumstantial evidence from the presumed sites of clinical ablation indicates that, at the site of destruction of tissue, the pathway of conduction is composed of ordinary working atrial myocardium. We are now aware of at least four instances of histological studies which confirm these assumptions. The first account was published by Bharati and her colleagues.[12] The second example, as yet unpublished, was shown to us by Drs. Lesh and Ursell from the University of California

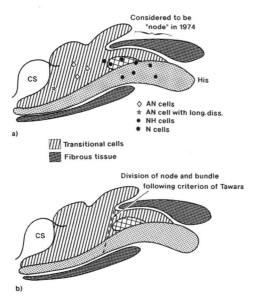

Figure 8. As shown in these diagrams, what we originally described as "closed AV node" in the rabbit (**a**) should now, following the criterion of Tawara, be considered to represent the penetrating atrioventricular bundle of His (**b**).

in San Francisco. The third and fourth cases have been studied in our laboratory (Fig. 9), although they have yet to be published in detail. All cases show unequivocally that the lesion which abolished conduction through the slow pathway was located within the ordinary atrial myocardium of the vestibule of the tricuspid valve, specifically in the so-called "isthmus" (Fig. 9). We had also previously studied cases in which stimulation studies of recipient hearts after cardiac transplantation revealed dual pathways in most cases, but with no obvious histological differences within the histologically specialized conduction tissues.[13] Subsequent studies, again in our laboratory, have shown subtle changes in the overall orientation of the myocardial fibers within the prominent muscular bands of the right atrial wall.[14] Taken together, therefore, we conclude that it is the geometric arrangement of atrial myocardial fibers which determines the potential for "slow" and "fast" conduction into the AV node, perhaps coupled with changes in the array of cellular connections between the atrial myocardial cells, or modulations produced by neural influences. We see no evidence whatsoever which supports the concept that histologically specialized pathways are involved in these electrical events. We anticipate that similar influ-

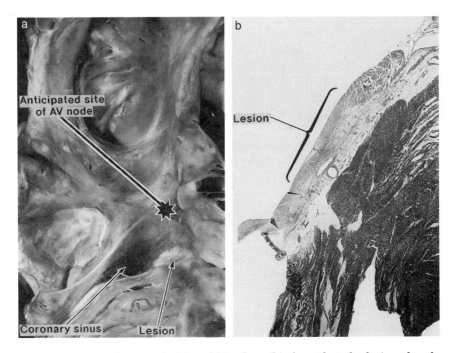

Figure 9. This photograph (**a**) and histology (**b**) show that the lesion placed successfully to ablate the slow pathway onto the atrioventricular node does **not** involve the histologically specialized tissue.

ences of myocardial geometry may underscore the potential for flutter or fibrillation within the atrial walls.

Our initial attempted electrophysiological-anatomical correlates are also significant to the controversy concerning the arrangement of the canine AV node. In a recent polemic, Racker proposed[2] that contemporary accounts of the AV node were at variance not only with her own findings, but also with those of Tawara. We have difficulty in accepting this contention. Stimulated by her account, we reexamined the conduction system of the dog, and reevaluated the original description of Tawara.[1] In both instances, our reexamination confirmed the excellence of the initial criterion suggested by Tawara, namely that node becomes bundle when the conduction axis is surrounded by fibrous tissue and insulated from the atrial myocardium. This is a critical distinction to make when seeking to evaluate the claims of Racker.[2] When her illustrations are studied in detail, it is our opinion that her so-called "distal AV node" is insulated entirely within the fibrous tissue. Hence, following the criterion of Tawara, it should be described as part of the penetrating AV bundle. Recognition of this feature reconciles the account of Racker not only with our own findings, but also with the original description of Tawara.[7]

Conclusions

In a well-researched recent account, Moulton[15] reviewed earlier descriptions of the histological arrangement of the specialized conduction tissues, emphasizing apparent contradictions which still exist between different investigators. In our opinion, despite the excellence of this review, Moulton[15] failed to give full credit to the monumental monograph of Tawara.[1] Equally significantly, he did not discuss the excellent criteria established by Monckeberg and Aschoff for recognition of myocardial histological specialization.[7,8] Moulton could also, perhaps, have asked his own pathologist to prepare serial histological sections through the AV junctional area. He could then check for himself the validity of the apparently different schools of thought. He would then, perhaps, come to recognize that the function of a given myocardial cell cannot be predicted from its histological appearance, not even when studied with the electron microscope.[16] It remains our belief that the initial account of the histologically specialized AV conduction axis given by Tawara[1] was entirely accurate. In essence, this account was endorsed by the study of Hecht and colleagues,[17] is in keeping with the extensive writings of Lev and Bharati,[18] and is supported by the review of the working group of the European Society of Cardiology.[4] When evaluated in the light of the criterion concerning the distinction of node and bundle (see above), it is also consistent with the published illustrations, albeit not the authorial interpretation, of Racker.[2] The significant point from all these studies for the present discussion is that the areas ablated by cardiologists to treat AV nodal reentry and atrial flutter are unequivocally composed of ordinary, histologically nonspecialized, working atrial myocardium. It is very likely the orderly geometric arrangement of the myocardial fibers, perhaps conditioned by intercellular connections, which produces enhanced conduction through these areas.

Acknowledgements: We are indebted to our clinical colleagues who have continued to encourage us to make our correlative studies—particularly Dr. Wyn Davies of St Mary's Hospital, Imperial College School of Medicine, London, England, and Dr. Janet McComb of Freeman Hospital, Newcastle-upon-Tyne, England.

References

1. Tawara S. Das Reizleitungssystem des Säugetierherzens. Eine Anatom-isch-Histologische Studie über das Atrioventrikularbündel und die Pur-kinjeschen Fäden. Jena, Gustav Fischer, 1906.

2. Racker DK. Atrioventricular node and input pathways: a correlated gross anatomical and histological study of the canine atrioventricular junctional region. Anat Rec 1989;26:336–354.

3. Ho SY, Kilpatrick L, Kanai T, et al. The architecture of the atrioventricular conduction axis in dogs and humans: its significance to ablation of the atrioventricular nodal approaches. J Cardiovasc Electrophysiol 1995;6: 26–39.

4. Anderson RH, Becker AE, Brechenmacher C, et al. The human atrioventricular junctional area: a morphological study of the A-V node and bundle. Eur J Cardiol 1975;3:11–25.

5. Dean JW, Ho SY, Rowland E, et al. Clinical anatomy of the atrioventricular junctions. J Am Coll Cardiol 1994;24:1725–1731.

6. Guiraudon GM. Editorial comment. Anatomy of atrioventricular attach-ments, connections and junction: in media stat virtus. J Am Coll Cardiol 1994;24:1732–1734.

7. Aschoff L. Referat uber die Herzstorungen in ihren Beziehungen zu den Spezifischen Muskelsystem des Herzens. Verh Dtsch Pathol Ges 1910;14: 3–35.

8. Monckeberg JG. Beitrage zur normalen und pathologischen Anatomie des Herzens. Verh Dtsch Pathol Ges 1910;14:64–71.

9. Keith A. An Autobiography. New York: Philosophical Library; 1950: 254–259.

10. Keith A. The auriculo-ventricular bundle of His. Lancet 1906;1:623–625.

11. Anderson RH, Janse MJ, van Capelle FJL, et al. A combined morphologic and electrophysiologic study of the atrioventricular node of the rabbit heart. Circ Res 1974;35:909–920.

12. Bharati S, Lev M. Pathological observations of radiofrequency catheter ablation of cardiac tissue. In: Shoei K, Huang S. eds. Radiofrequency Cathe-ter Ablation of Cardiac Arrhythmias: Basic Concepts and Clinical Applica-tions. Armonk, NY: Futura Publishing Co; 1994:41–81.

13. Ho SY, McComb JM, Scott CD, et al. Morphology of the cardiac conduction system in patients with electrophysiologically proven dual atrioventricular nodal pathways. J Cardiovasc Electrophysiol 1993;4:504–512.

14. Sanchez-Quintana D, Anderson RH, Ho SY. Architecture of the atrial mus-culature in the triangle of Koch. Submitted for publication, 1996.

15. Moulton KP. Selective ablation of the slow atrioventricular nodal pathway: evolving concepts in atrioventricular junctional anatomy and physiology. In: Shoei K, Huang S, eds. Radiofrequency Catheter Ablation of Cardiac Arrhythmias: Basic Concepts and Clinical Applications. Armonk, NY: Fu-tura Publishing Co; 1994:205–228.

16. Tranum-Jensen J, Janse MJ. Fine structural identification of individual cells subjected to microelectrode recording in perfused cardiac prepara-tions. J Mol Cell Cardiol 1982;14:233–247.

17. Hecht HH, Kossmann CE, Childers RW, et al. Atrioventricular and intraventricular conduction: revised nomenclature and concepts. Am J Cardiol 1973;31:232–244.

18. Lev M, Bharati S. Anatomy of the conduction system in normal and congenitally abnormal hearts. In: Roberts NK, Gelband H, eds. Cardiac Arrhythmias in the Neonate, Infant and Child. New York: Appleton-Century-Crofts; 1977:29–54.

CHAPTER 5

Atrioventricular Nodal Function in Atrial Fibrillation:

What Is the Optimum Ventricular Rate?

S. Bertil Olsson, Jonas Carlson, Magnus Holm,
Ann-Marie Nilsson

Introduction

When atrioventricular (AV) conduction is unaffected by any drug, atrial fibrillation (AF) almost always causes an irregular and rapid ventricular response. The mechanisms behind the irregularity have attracted much interest over the years. Studies of intra-atrial[1-3] and intranodal[4] conduction during AF, and computerbased analysis of interrelation between RR intervals during AF,[5-7] have contributed to an understanding of the ventricular response during AF.

Although it has been recognized for some time that an increased ventricular rate caused by AF may lead to cardiac enlargement and heart failure, it was not until recently that the concept of tachycardiomyopathy in pharmacologically treated patients with AF was emphasized.[8-10] The importance of normalizing the ventricular rate has also been stressed although well-defined target heart rate levels are seldom given.

The present chapter aims to: (1) describe the mechanisms underlying the variable and irregular ventricular response during AF; (2) briefly discuss the mechanisms likely to be responsible for tachycardiomyopathy in AF; and (3) suggest clinical goals for treatment of the rapid and irregular ventricular activation in patients with AF.

From *Nonpharmacological Management of Atrial Fibrillation*, edited by F.D. Murgatroyd and A.J. Camm. © 1997, Futura Publishing Co., Inc., Armonk, NY.

AV Nodal Conduction during Atrial Fibrillation

Although the distribution of RR intervals during AF seems to be largely unpredictable within certain limits of the naked eye, careful analyses of a large number of RR intervals from ambulatory ECG recordings reveal a distinct and intraindividual highly reproducible pattern.[5,6] Thus, when the distribution of RR intervals is studied at narrow and well-defined average heart rate levels, e.g., at a distinct balance between the vagal and the sympathetic nervous discharge, a characteristic and highly reproducible RR distribution pattern appears (Fig. 1). Provided that the RR distribution can be studied over a wide range of average heart rate levels, a bimodal RR distribution can be found in a majority of patients, suggesting two separate RR populations, each having a slightly skewed pattern (a lambda distribution). When the RR distribution is studied over a range of heart rate levels, two mechanisms appear responsible for the variability of the average heart rate. The first and quantitatively most important mechanism is a successive change of the relation between the number of RR intervals belonging to the different RR populations. The second mechanism is a succesive change of the cycle length content of each entire RR population. These changes can be identified in a three-dimensional graph of the relation between average heart rate, individual RR interval length, and relative RR distribution pattern (Fig. 2). The transition from the dominance of one RR population to a dominance of the other takes place at average heart rate levels between 80 and 120 bpm.[5,6] Interestingly, atrial incisions far away from the AV node cause a marked redistribution of the RR pattern in any individual.[7] Thus, patients who initially have a bimodal RR distribution pattern may exhibit a unimodal pattern after atrial incision and vice versa.

We suggested earlier that the bimodal RR distribution pattern is caused by the conduction of the impulse from the atrium via two anatomically distinctly separated routes—from the interatrial septum and from the terminal part of the crista terminalis between the ostium of the coronary sinus and the tricuspid valve, respectively.[5,7]

The fact that atrial incisions rearrange the RR distribution[7] suggests a nonrandom input of fibrillatory wavelets to these two separate entrances to the node. This interpretation has recently obtained support from independent studies, each illustrating that intra-atrial conduction during AF is not a random process.[1-3] Instead, the instances of excitation of closely adjacent areas are well correlated[3] and the impulse

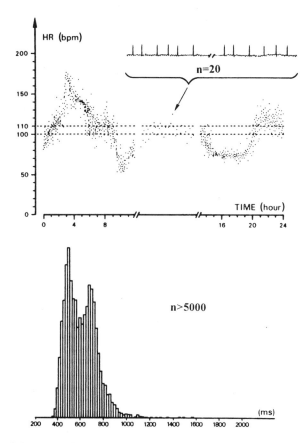

Figure 1. Schematic illustration of the method used for studying distribution of RR intervals at different levels of autonomic nervous balance. After recording ambulatory ECG for 24 hours, each QRS complex is identified and all RR intervals are calculated. The recording is then divided into consecutive segments of 20 QRS complexes each and the average heart rate is calculated for each segment. All individual RR intervals within segments with the same average heart rate are thereafter pooled and presented in a histogram.

directions of consecutive excitation fronts are often unchanged.[1,2] Although there is no available report concerning the interrelationship between time and direction of atrial excitation at different perinodal positions, the studies mentioned above indicate a likely temporal association between fibrillatory wavelets reaching the different entrances to the AV node.

There is sometimes a trimodal distribution pattern of the RR inter-

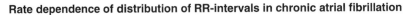

Rate dependence of distribution of RR-intervals in chronic atrial fibrillation

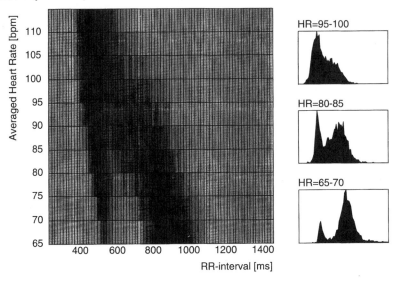

Figure 2. Example of distribution of RR intervals at different levels of autonomic balance in an individual with a marked separation between two RR populations—one "slow" and one "fast". Note that an increased heart rate is achieved by two mechanisms—increasing abundance of RR intervals of the "fast" RR population as well as a successive dislodgement of the entire RR population towards shorter RR values. Three individual histograms from different heart rate levels are presented. The distribution of RR intervals over all studied heart rate levels is presented in the "three-dimensional" figure.

vals during AF in heart-rate-stratified analysis of RR distribution.[5] When the third RR population appears only at low heart rates, the electrocardiographic picture is often compatible with AF, third degree AV block, and nodal escape rhythm. In other instances however, three RR populations may appear at higher heart rate levels. The possible input from a left atrial extention of the AV node[4] may be an explanation for this finding.

Figure 3 gives an example of the atrial myocardial conduction around the AV node during AF, using a temporal and spatial averaging technique.[11] This figure illustrates an impulse direction which is largely towards the AV node, not only from the anterior part of the septum, but also from the atrial tissue between the coronary sinus ostium and tricuspid valve. The conduction pattern is compatible with an AV conduction from both of the suggested atrionodal entrances. In-

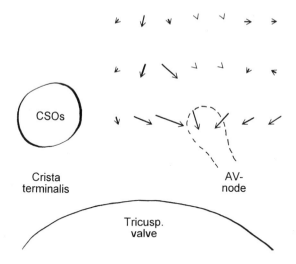

Figure 3. Atrial excitation over the interatrial septum above and around the AV node in a patient with atrial fibrillation. The pooled data from an 8 sec recording is presented, using a temporal averaging technique. The direction of the arrows indicates the dominant direction of conduction of all excitation waves reaching the different part of the recording area during the 8 sec. The length of an arrow indicates the significance of the averaged impulse direction. Note that impulses are mainly traveling towards the AV node. During these 8 sec, the node is reached by 22 impulses from the crista terminalis, having a cycle length of 317 ± 95 ms (mean $\pm$ SD), while 41 impulses with a cycle length of 188 ± 67 ms approach the node from the anterior part of the interatrial septum. CSOs = coronary sinus ostium.

terestingly, the cycle length differs between impulses reaching the AV node from different directions.

Once the excitation wave has entered the AV node, the signal is influenced by complex electrophysiological phenomena. Thus, in addition to decremental conduction, cancellation, augmentation, and echo phenomena influence the advancement of the excitation wave.[4] The atrial rate during AF is several times higher than that of the ventricles. Therefore, when the excitation of the node occurs exclusively and consequently via one of the two atrionodal routes, the possibility for reentry into the atrial myocardium via the other route is evident, a mechanism which may assist in the perpetuation of the arrhythmia,[7] although this mechanism remains to be clarified.

In summary, the ventricular response during AF is influenced by electrophysiological as well as anatomical phenomena not only in the AV node but also within the atria. These factors yield a specific conduction pattern which can be deducted from analysis of distribution of large RR interval data. The possible contribution of AV nodal reentry on the perpetuation of the arrhythmia still remains to be verified.

Effect of Ventricular Rate and Regularity on Myocardial Function

Myocardial oxygen consumption increases linearly with increased heart rate,[12] explaining the development of the so-called tachycardiomyopathy[8] in patients with AF and high ventricular rates. Thus, a heart rate increase from resting conditions to the order of 150/min by atrial pacing is accompanied by a doubling of the myocardial oxygen consumption.[12] It is well documented that not only patients with rapid and regular tachyarrhythmias, but also patients with AF in combination with advanced signs of left ventricular failure, may completely recover after normalization of the ventricular rate.[13]

The origin of the tachycardiomyopathy in patients with AF is more complicated than in patients with regular tachycardias. A variability of the cardiac cycle influences the force of contraction.[14] The augmentation of contraction by postextrasystolic potentiation is accompanied by a marked increase of myocardial oxygen consumption.[15] Studies of augmentation of contraction and myocardial oxygen demand at postextrasystolic potentiation have been done at so-called paired pulse stimulation,[16] i.e., when every spontaneous or basic paced beat is followed by a second stimulus close to the refractory period, thereby causing a consequent bigeminy rhythm. Thus, when a consequent paired stimulation is applied, the left ventricular contraction is augmented with a mean ejection fraction increase from 0.48 to 0.62,[15] however at the expense of a threefold increase of the myocardial oxygen consumption per effective heart beat. In AF, the variability of the cardiac cycle may differ widely although most patients have a coefficient of variation of consecutive RR intervals between 20% and 40%.[17] Obviously, the maximal irregularity of the ventricular rhythm imposes a high metabolic demand which far exceeds that which the irregularity of the ventricular response in AF may induce. It cannot be excluded, however, that the irregular ventricular response seen in AF may contribute to the development of left ventricular dilatation and cardiac failure in some of these patients via the mechanism of an increased myocardial oxygen demand.

What Is the Optimum Ventricular Rate in Atrial Fibrillation?

As pointed out earlier, the ventricular rate during AF is modulated by the autonomous nervous system. Mostly, the ventricular rate is too high without medication. The goal of the treatment is to adjust the ventricular rate to optimum levels with respect to circulatory demands and symptoms.

Thus, the ventricular rate should not be accompanied by symptoms of too low or too high a rate at any moment. These demands imply that the resting ventricular rate should be adjusted to a level which is not too low. Obvious symptoms of a resting heart rate that is too low are dizziness and syncope.[18] Fatigue as a consequence of heart failure associated with too low a ventricular rate is another possible symptom. Long-term neurological symptoms possibly caused by intermittent long pauses have been much debated. A recent publication including a control group failed to illustrate any beneficial effect of pacemaker treatment on this indication, however.[19]

The highest ventricular rate during AF is induced by the same mechanism which increases the sinus rhythm to high levels, i.e., sympathetic stimulation in association with withdrawal of vagal tone. The principles for optimization of increased ventricular rate during AF also follow the same rules as if the patient is in sinus rhythm. Thus, underlying or associated diseases demand a limitation of ventricular rate increase to a level which is lower in such patients than in patients without these prerequisites. The symptoms of a ventricular rate that is too high include palpitations and cardiac failure. Syncope may occur as the result of too high a ventricular rate at the onset of the arrhythmia in patients with paroxysmal AF.

The adjustment of ventricular rate should be done, having the individual's specific demands in mind. It is often difficult to reach optimal ventricular rates during rest as well as during exercise. Thus, a drug adjustment of inadequate resting ventricular rate often causes suboptimal ventricular rates at exercise and vice versa. In addition to the patient's history and resting ECG, conventional or simplified exercise ECG tests and ambulatory ECG monitoring are useful tools to reach optimum ventricular rates without undesirable side effects.

Summary and Conclusions

The AV node has two anatomically well-defined entrances from the atria—identical to the locations of the pathways of AV nodal reentrant tachycardia. There is evidence of a gross temporal relation between the excitation of these atrionodal routes during AF. The ventricular response during AF therefore appears as two populations of RR intervals, usually partially overlapping, but sometimes almost completely separated and sometimes completely overlapping. An increased average heart rate is caused by two mechanisms—a successive transfer from the RR population with longer individual RR intervals to that with shorter intervals as well as a change of the entire RR population towards shorter values, illustrating a homogeneous autonomic influence on the involved structures.

The tachycardiomyopathy in AF has been explained as the consequence of high average ventricular rate but the ventricular irregularity may also contribute since it causes an increased myocardial oxygen demand.

The ventricular rate should be adjusted in AF to adequate levels both during rest and during physical or mental stress, a goal that implies individual targets and is often difficult to reach by pharmacological means. Neither the lowest nor the highest heart rate during AF should be accompanied by symptoms which are rate-related. Resting ECG, exercise tests, and ambulatory ECG monitoring may be useful tools in these attempts.

References

1. Gerstenfeld EP, Sahakian AV, Swiryn S. Evidence for transient linking of atrial excitation during atrial fibrillation in man. Circulation 1992;86: 375–382.
2. Holm M, Blomström P, Brandt J, et al. Determination of preferable directions of impulse propagation during atrial fibrillation by time averaging of multiple electrogram vectors. In: Olsson SB, Allessie MA, Campbell RWF, eds. Atrial Fibrillation: Mechanisms and Therapeutic Strategies. Armonk, NY: Futura Publishing Co; 1994:67–80.
3. Botteron GW, Smith JM. Quantitative assessment of the spatial organization of atrial fibrillation in the intact human heart. Circulation 1996;93: 513–518.
4. Janse MJ. The role of the atrioventricular node in atrial fibrillation. In: Olsson SB, Allessie MA, Campbell RWF, eds. Atrial Fibrillation: Mechanisms and Therapeutic Strategies. Armonk, NY: Futura Publishing Co; 1994:127–140.
5. Olsson SB, Cau N, Dohnal M, Talwar KK. Noninvasive support for and characterisation of multiple intranodal pathways in patients with mitral valve disease and atrial fibrillation. Eur Heart J 1986;7:320–333.
6. Cai N, Dohnal M, Olsson SB. Methodological aspects on the use of heart rate stratified RR interval histograms in the analysis of AV-conduction during atrial fibrillation. Cardiovasc Research 1987;21(6):445–462.

7. Olsson SB, Naisheng C, Dohnal M, William-Olsson G. Effects of crista terminalis myotomy on the AV-nodal function in atrial fibrillation. In: Attuel P, Coumel P, Janse MJ, eds. The Atrium in Health and Disease. Mt. Kisco, NY: Futura Publishing Co; 1989:249–269.

8. Rosenquist M, Lee M, Moulinier A, et al. Long-term follow-up of patients undergoing AV-junctional ablation. J Am Coll Cardiol 1990;16:1467–1474.

9. Hinz G, Siostrzonek P, Kreiner G, Gössinger H. Improvement in left ventricular systolic function after successful radiofrequency His bundle ablation for refractory chronic atrial fibrillation and recurrent atrial flutter. Am J Cardio 1992;69:489–492.

10. Wellens HJJ, Rodriguez LM, Smeets LRM, et al. Tachycardiomyopathy in patients with supraventricular tachycardia with emphasis on atrial fibrillation. In: Olsson SB, Allessie MA, Campbell RWF, eds. Atrial Fibrillation: Mechanisms and Therapeutic Strategies. Armonk, NY: Futura Publishing Co; 1994:333–342.

11. Holm M, Johansson R, Olsson B, et al. A new method for analysis of atrial activation during fibrillation by temporal averaging of multiple discrete excitation vectors. IEEE Trans Biomed Eng 1996;43(2):198–210.

12. Holmberg S. Coronary circulation at rest and during pacing-induced tachycardia: studies on patients with and without coronary heart disease. Thesis, Elanders Boktryckeri AB, Göteborg, Sweden 1971.

13. Grogan M, Smith HC, Gersh BJ, Wood DL. Left ventricular dysfunction due to atrial fibrillation in patients initially believed to have idiopathic dilated cardiomyopathy. Am J Cardiol 1992;69:1570–1573.

14. Hoffman BF, Bindler G, Suckling EE. Post-extrasystolic potentiation of contraction in cardiac muscle. Am J Physiol 1956;185:95.

15. Geschwind H, Huet Y, Laine JF, Teisseire B, Dhainaut JF, Laurent D. Coût énergétique de la potentialisation post-extrasystolique chez l'homme. Arch Mal Coeur 1984;77:747–753.

16. Paired Pulse Stimulation of the Heart. Cranefield, PF Hoffman BF. New York: The Rockefeller University Press; 1968.

17. Khalsa A, Olsson B, Henriksson BÅ. Effect of oral verapamil on ventricular irregularity in long-standing atrial fibrillation. Acta Med Scand 1979;205:39–47.

18. Pollak A, Falk RH. Pacemaker therapy in patients with atrial fibrillation. Am Heart J 1993;125:824–830.

19. Saxon LA, Albert BH, Uretz EF, Denes P. Permanent pacemaker placement in chronic atrial fibrillation associated with intermittent AV block and cerebral symtoms. PACE 1990;13:724–729.

CHAPTER 6

Drugs and the Ventricular Rate in Atrial Fibrillation:

Efficacy, Limitations, and Risks

Hein J.J. Wellens

Atrial fibrillation (AF) is an arrhythmia resulting in loss of atrial contribution to ventricular filling, an inappropriately rapid and irregular ventricular rate, and an increased incidence of thromboembolic complications.

The loss of an appropriately timed atrial contraction and the rapid and irregular ventricular rate may lead to impaired cardiac function, which ultimately may result in a dilated cardiomyopathy. As early as 1949, Philips and Levine[1] realized that AF without other evidence of heart disease might result in heart failure. It is obvious, therefore, that one should attempt to restore and secure sinus rhythm in the patient suffering from AF. Unfortunately, this is not be possible in a large number of patients and, in these cases, chronic AF has to be accepted. Therapy should aim at the maintenance of an adequate ventricular rate in rest and during normal activities, prevention of inappropriate exertional tachycardia, and protection against thromboembolic complications.

The purpose of this chapter is to review our current pharmacological approach to ventricular rate control during persistent atrial fbrillation.

Determinants of the Ventricular Rate during Atrial Fibrillation

AF is an arrhythmia during which the atria have a totally irregular rhythm with a rate ranging from 350 to 600 beats per minute (bpm).

From *Nonpharmacological Management of Atrial Fibrillation*, edited by F.D. Murgatroyd and A.J. Camm. © 1997, Futura Publishing Co., Inc., Armonk, NY.

Under those circumstances the ventricular rate is determined by the properties of the atrioventricular (AV) conduction system. In the presence of a normally functioning conduction system, the ventricular rhythm will be totally irregular with a mean rate between 100 bpm to 160 bpm. The ventricular rate will be determined by the refractory period of the AV conduction system, with the AV node having the highest refractory period of the different components of the conduction system (AV node, His bundle, and bundle branches). The refractory period will shorten during adrenergic stimulation and lengthen during vagal stimulation. A factor playing a role in the ventricular rate during AF is the phenomenon of concealed conduction: prolongation of AV nodal refractoriness by partial penetration of impulses in the AV node,[2] with an inverse relation between the atrial rate during AF and the ventricular response.[3]

In discussing the use of drug therapy in controlling the ventricular rate during chronic AF, one should concentrate therefore on the effect of those drugs on the refractory period of the AV conduction system and on changes promoting concealed conduction in the AV node.

The Optimal Ventricular Rate in Atrial Fibrillation

There is only limited information on the optimal ventricular rate during AF. Rawles[4] suggested that in rest the optimal heart rate might be higher during AF than during sinus rhythm. This has also been observed during exercise.[5] It is likely that both in rest and during exercise the behavior of the heart rate will also depend on the presence or absence of additional cardiac abnormalities apart from the arrhythmia.[6] That was recently shown by Van den Berg et al.[7] in patients with chronic AF and different degrees of impaired functional capacity. They found that in patients with a diminished peak VO_2 (≤ 20 ml/min/kg) the ventricular rate rose rapidly at low exercise levels. However, the maximal attainable ventricular rate during exercise was much lower in these patients as compared to those having a peak VO_2 of >20 ml/min/kg.

Drug Therapy for Ventricular Rate Control during Atrial Fibrillation

As discussed, an inappropriate rise in ventricular rate during AF will affect cardiac function both in rest and during exercise. When drugs are used under these circumstances, three situations have to be recognized: (1) control of the ventricular rate during AF in the untreated patient presenting with the arrhythmia; (2) maintenance of an adequate heart rate during rest and normal daily activities; and (3) prevention of inappropriate exertional tachycardia.

Digitalis

Digitalis should be discussed first because historically it was the first pharmacological intervention in the treatment of AF.[8] Primarily as a result of its vagal effect, digitalis prolongs AV nodal conduction time and increases the refractory period of the AV node thereby slowing the ventricular rate during AF. Digitalis also shortens the refractory period of the atrium resulting in an increase in atrial rate during AF. This enhances concealed conduction in the AV node leading to slowing of the ventricular rate.[9] An attractive aspect of digitalis is the positive inotropic effect of the drug making it especially useful to treat or to prevent the development of impaired cardiac function in the patient with AF. While digitalis is an effective drug for ventricular rate control in rest, it has little effect on controlling heart rate during daily activities and vigorous exercise. This was already observed by Blumgart in 1924[10] and later confirmed by others in patients in whom adequate doses of digitalis were documented by measuring the serum concentration[11,12]. The explanation for the absence of adequate rate control with exertion is given by the fact that the predominant effect of digitalis is neurally (vagally) mediated.

It takes a few hours before digoxin, the most commonly used digitalis preparation, starts to slow the ventricular rate, and it is therefore not the drug of choice when acute control of the heart rate is required.

Too much digitalis will produce toxicity which may become manifest as complete AV block or accelerated AV junctional or ventricular rhythms. A regular bradycardia or tachycardia in a patient with AF and taking digitalis should immediately raise the suspicion of digitalis intoxication.[13]

Beta-Blocking Agents

The administration of beta-adrenergic blocking agents results in lengthening of the refractory period of the AV node and an increase in AV nodal conduction time. Beta-blockade, at least as shown for metoprolol,[14] reduces the fibrillatory rate in AF and therefore does not promote concealed conduction in the AV node. When given intravenously, beta-blocking drugs result in rapid control of the ventricular rate during AF. However, the negative inotropic effect of these drugs may induce heart failure and should be a reason not to use them before the presence and severity of underlying heart disease is evaluated. Esmolol, an intravenous beta-blocker with a short half-life time (of approximately 10 minutes) induces short-term control of the ventricular rate and has the advantage of rapid dissipation of unwanted effects. Administration of this drug will give an idea about the effect of a beta-blocking drug and how this is tolerated by the patient.

Chronic use of a beta-blocking agent is primarily prescribed for rate control during exercise. Several studies[15,16] have shown heart rate reduction at all levels of exercise. This does not imply that exercise level and duration increase after beta-blockade in patients with AF. This might not only be related to the dose of the beta-blocking agent, but also to the functional capacity of the patient. Paradoxically, in patients with markedly impaired cardiac function and a dilated "tachy" cardiomyopathy, beta-blockade may result in increased exercise capacity.[17]

Calcium Channel Blockers

The calcium channel blocking drugs verapamil and diltiazem increase the refractory period of the AV node and prolong AV nodal conduction time. No information is available on the effect on the fibrillatory rate and on concealed conduction in the AV node. Both drugs, when given intravenously, rapidly control the ventricular rate during AF. Their negative inotropic effect is partially offset by their vasodilating properties. Verapamil and diltiazem are both used for ventricular rate control during exercise and most studies report a modest improvement in exercise capacity.[18-20]

Other Drugs

Both sotalol and amiodarone are used for ventricular rate control in chronic AF. Sotalol works because of its beta-blocking properties. It is not very likely that the class III antiarrhythmic properties will lengthen the refractory period of the AV node. No studies are available in which the efficacy of sotalol for ventricular rate control in AF is compared with that of "ordinary" beta-blocking agents.

Amiodarone is effective in controlling heart rate both in rest and during exercise.[21] This is not surprising in view of the lengthening effect of the drug on the refractory period of the AV conduction system. Long-term administration of the drug is, however, limited by its side effects.

Another drug that has been evaluated in patients with chronic AF (and heart failure) has been the angiotensin converting enzyme inhibitor lisinopril.[22] It was shown that the drug improved exercise duration and peak VO_2, while the ventricular rate diminished, but not significantly.

Practical Considerations and Future Developments

The selection of the type and dose of drug(s) in the control of the ventricular rate during AF should be individualized (Table 1). Many factors play a role, such as complaints, type and severity of underlying heart disease, presence of heart failure, age, profession, etc. In the elderly patient, who engages in a minimal amount of exercise, treatment with digitalis only is frequently possible. However, the younger patient with much greater physical needs usually requires a combination of digitalis with either a calcium channel blocker or a beta-blocking drug. Confirmation of correct dosing of the different drugs requires exercise testing and 24-hour ECG recordings.

It is not known at this time if other modes of rate control in chronic AF such as His bundle ablation and "physiologic" pacing or modification of AV nodal conduction by radiofrequency (RF) ablation of part of the

Table 1

Effects of Different Drugs on Ventricular Rate During Atrial Fibrillation in Rest and During Exercise and on Exercise Tolerance

	Control Ventricular Rate		
	Rest	*Exercise*	*Exercise Tolerance*
Digitalis	+	−	No improvement
Beta-blocker	+	+	No improvement
Calcium channel blocker	+	+	Modest improvement
Amiodarone	+	+	Modest improvement

AV node[23] will be preferred in the future. In selected cases where heart rate control was not possible by drug therapy, such an approach has been shown to be beneficial.[24] However, the crucial question that should be addressed in the coming years is: "What is the best treatment for the individual patient?". Will it become possible to select the patient who should be treated pharmacologically or nonpharmacologically?

Another important issue is the amount of effort one should place on trying to keep the patient in sinus rhythm by repeated cardioversion versus accepting AF striving for appropriate ventricular rate control by pharmacological or nonpharmacological means. This problem is currently being investigated in Germany (the PIAF study), the Netherlands (the RACE study), and in the USA (the AFFIRM study). By looking at mortality, morbidity, quality of life, and costs, these studies will provide us with more information on how to use drugs in patients with chronic AF.

References

1. Philips E, Levine SA. Auricular fibrillation without other evidence of heart disease: a cause for reversible heart failure. Am J Med 1949;7:478–489.
2. Moe GK, Abildskow JA. Observations on the ventricular dysrhythmia associated with atrial fibrillation in the dog heart. Circ Res 1964;14:447–460.
3. Chorro FJ, Kirchhof CJHG, Brugada J, et al. Ventricular response during irregular atrial pacing and atrial fibrillation. Am J Physiol 1990;259: H1015–H1021.
4. Rawles JM. What is meant by a "controlled" ventricular rate in atrial fibrillation? Brit Heart J 1990;63:157–161.
5. Gosselink ATM, Crijns HJGM, Van den Berg MP, et al. Functional capacity before and after cardioversion of atrial fibrillation: a controlled study. Brit Heart J 1994;72:161–166.
6. Atwood JE, Myers J, Sullivan M, et al. Maximal exercise testing and gas exchange in patients with chronic atrial fibrillation. J Am Coll Cardiol 1988;11:508–513.
7. Van den Berg MP, Crijns HJGM, Gosselink ATM, et al. Chronotropic response to exercise in patients with atrial fibrillation: relation to functional state. Brit Heart J 1993;70:150–153.
8. MacKenzie J. Diseases of the Heart. 3rd edition. London: Oxford Medical; 1914:211–236.
9. Meijler FL. An "account" of digitalis and atrial fibrillation. J Am Coll Cardiol 1985;5:60A-68A.
10. Blumgart H. The reaction to exercise of the heart affected by auricular fibrillation. Heart 1924;11:49–56.
11. Redfors A. Digoxin dosage and ventricular rate at rest and exercise in patients with atrial fibrillation. Acta Med Scand 1971;190:321–333.
12. Beasly R, Smith DA, McHaffie DJ. Exercise heart rates at different serum digoxin concentrations in patients with atrial fbrillation. Brit Med J 1985; 290:9–11.

13. Wellens HJJ, Conover M. The ECG in Emergency Decision Making. Philadelphia: WB Saunders Co; 1991:139–159.
14. Van den Berg MP, De Langen CDJ, Crijns HJGM, et al. Effect of metoprolol on atrial fibrillatory rate, atrioventricular nodal concealed conduction and ventricular response during atrial fibrillation in pigs. J Cardiovasc Pharm 1994;23:846–851.
15. Di Bianco R, Morganroth J, Freitag RJ. Effect of nadolol on the spontaneous and exercise provoked heart rate in patients with chronic atrial fbrillation receiving stable doses of digoxin. Am Heart J 1984;108:1121–1127.
16. Atwood JE, Sullivan M, Forbes S. Effects of beta-adrenergic blockade on exercise performance in patients with chronic atrial fibrillation. J Am Coll Cardiol 1987;10:314–320.
17. Van den Berg MP, Van Veldhuisen DJ, Crijns HJGM, et al. Reversion of tachycardiomyopathy after beta-blocker. Lancet 1993;341:1667.
18. Lang R, Klein H, Segni E. Verapamil improves exercise capacity in chronic atrial fbrillation: double-blind cross over study. Am Heart J 1983:105:820–824.
19. Roth A, Harrison E, Mitani G, et al. Efficacy and safety of medium and high-dose diltiazem alone and in combination with digoxin for control of heart rate at rest and during exercise in patients with chronic atrial fibrillation. Circulation 1986;73:316–324.
20. Lundstrom T, Ryden L. Ventricular rate control and exercise performance in chronic atrial fibrillation: effects of diltiazem and verapamil. J Am Coll Cardiol 1990;16:86–90.
21. Perelman MS, McKenna WJ, Rowland E, et al. A comparison of bepredil with amiodarone in the treatment of established atrial fbrillation. Brit Heart J 1987;58:339–344.
22. Van den Berg MP, Crijns HJGM, Van Veldhuisen DJ, et al. Effects of lisinopril in patients with heart failure and chronic atrial fbrillation. J Card Fail 1995;5:355–363.
23. Williamson BD, Man KC, Daoud E, et al. Radiofrequency catheter ablation modifcation of atrioventricular conduction to control the ventricular rate during atrial fibrillation. N Engl J Med 1994;331:910–917.
24. Rodriguez LM, Smeets JLRM, Xie B, et al. Improvement in left ventricular function by ablation of atrioventricular nodal conduction in selected patients with lone atrial fbrillation. Am J Cardiol 1993;72:1137–1141.

PART III

Controlling the Ventricular Rate Without Drugs

CHAPTER 7

Atrioventricular Nodal Ablation for Atrial Fibrillation:

Do Patients Feel Better?

Adam P. Fitzpatrick

Introduction

Atrioventricular junctional (AVJ) ablation for chronic and paroxysmal atrial fibrillation (AF) is a treatment of growing importance. While it involves a skilled procedure and subsequent lifelong cardiac pacing, many patients benefit greatly from such treatment. For patients with impaired left ventricular (LV) function, there is the prospect that AVJ ablation may improve LV function and reduce heart failure, and trials are under way to address this issue.

Background

In the last few years, all regular tachyarrhythmias have been approached by catheter ablative techniques.[1-3] Success has been variable, but in many cases, especially with supraventricular tachycardias, a cure can be expected in over 90% of patients. The management of AF, in contrast, still presents a major problem. The options for treatment are all palliative, and despite major research efforts, will likely remain so for the foreseeable future.

Catheter ablation for AF is focussed on palliation by disconnection of the fibrillating atria from the ventricles by complete AV junctional ablation,[4,5] or the much newer approach of direct atrial ablation.[6] The latter approach is new and experimental, and aims to emulate the sur-

From *Nonpharmacological Management of Atrial Fibrillation*, edited by F.D. Murgatroyd and A.J. Camm. © 1997, Futura Publishing Co., Inc., Armonk, NY.

gical "maze" procedure.[7] Presently, using conventional ablation catheter technology, these procedures are immensely time consuming,
largely empirical and involve a great deal of X-ray exposure. New catheter technology advances, with the ability to fashion linear endomural
lesions in right and left atria, should facilitate this approach. For now,
however, catheter ablation for AF means destroying the normal AV
conduction system and committing patients to lifelong artificial ventricular (and, in paroxysmal AF, dual chamber) pacing.

At first, such an approach to the problem seems aggressive. It is
often perceived that patients with chronic (>6 months duration) AF,
can be well controlled with relatively simple medication, e.g., digoxin.
However, a detailed history often reveals marked exercise intolerance.
This is because patients with AF often have good control of ventricular
rate reponse at rest with cardiac glycosides, yet have poor control of
ventricular rate on gentle exercise.[8] Often, a second drug is needed to
control ventricular rate, or multiple drugs are needed. This often results in worsening of symptoms due to drug side effects. In the recent
APT (Ablate and Pace Trial),[9] of patients with chronic AF undergoing
AV junctional ablation and pacing, health status questioning prior to
treatment revealed much worse functional capacity than had been expected for an unselected group of patients with chronic AF.

Atrial Fibrillation and Ventricular Function

Tachycardia-induced cardiomyopathy as a potential cause of heart
failure has received increasing attention during the past few years. The
chronic high heart rates of AF combined with the irregularity of the
rhythm may lead to impairment of LV function. This may be completely
reversible in some patients.[10,11] Clinical recognition of this syndrome
may be difficult because it can easily be confused with idiopathic dilated
cardiomyopathy,[12] but it was suspected as long ago as 1913.[13]

Recently, interest has refocused on the improvement of ventricular
function with control of AF. This is largely due to the safe treatment
of patients with medically refractory AF, initially in the 1980s by direct
current high-voltage discharge,[14,15] and in the last few years by radiofrequency ablation.[16] Packer et al. provided an important report in 1986
on a series of eight patients with supraventricular tachycardias other
than AF, in whom tachycardia-induced cardiomyopathy was reversed
when the tachycardia was controlled by closed-chest ablation which
either destroyed the tachycardic focus or interrupted conduction
through the AV junction.[17] Several groups have now reported that AF

patients with ventricular dysfunction may experience a similar improvement in ventricular function following AV junctional ablation. Lemery et al. provided a case report in 1987.[18] Rosenqvist et al. reported in 1990 that four out of five patients with ejection fractions <35% prior to ablation showed significant increases in ejection fraction at long-term follow-up.[19] Mean ejection fraction for the five patients was 27% at baseline versus 45% at follow-up. A report by Fitzpatrick et al., of 107 patients who received AV nodal ablations for paroxysmal or chronic AF, found that 19 patients suffered episodes of congestive heart failure prior to ablation, and only eight patients following ablation.[20]

Quality of Life and Outcomes after AVJ Ablation in Patients with AF

Because there is experimental and clinical evidence of improvement in LV function after AVJ ablation, this would be expected to translate into improved functional capacity, a reduction in consumption of health care, and possibly an improved prognosis. A number of studies have addressed these issues in varying depth. Generally, the studies found an improvement, but more comprehensive data were needed.

A study was therefore undertaken to address patient well-being and activity status, access to health care, and morbidity and mortality after AVJ ablation. One hundred and seven patients underwent radiofrequency AVJ ablation and permanent pacing for paroxysmal or established medically refractory AF between 1989 and 1994, at the University of California, San Francisco. We conducted telephone interviews with all patients who were alive at follow-up and assessed quality of life (scored as 1 = poor, to 5 = excellent), limitation of various daily activities (1 = very limited, to 3 = not limited), and health care consumption before and after the procedure. Doctor visits, emergency room and hospital admissions, pacemaker follow-up visits, number of antiarrhythmic drug trials and anticoagulation, new stroke, heart failure episode or death, and maintenance of a dual chamber pacing mode were noted before and after the procedure. The telephone interviews were all conducted by a premedical student with an interest in the study, but no special understanding of the procedure or the complex issues being addressed; we thereby hoped to avoid bias of questioning.

Ninety patients were alive and provided information, of whom 55 were female, with a mean age of 60 ± 16 years, after a mean follow-up of 2.3 ± 1.2 years. The mean LV ejection fraction (LVEF) was 51 ± 11%. Seventeen patients out of the 107 in the series had died. These were six females and 11 males, with a mean age of 69 ± 13 years, whose fate was confirmed a mean of 2.8 ± 1 years after ablation. Fifty-four patients who were alive at follow-up (33 female, age 61 ± 16 years, LVEF = 51 ± 10%, Group I) had chronic AF at the time of ablation, and 46 (22 female, 59 ± 12 years, LVEF = 51±11%, Group II) had paroxysmal episodes.

Among the 90 survivors, the quality of life index (Fig. 1) improved significantly from 1.9 ± 1.2 to 3.6 ± 1.1 (P<0.001). Overall, activities of daily living became significantly easier, with improvement in the score from 2 ± 0.4 to 2.4 ± 0.3 (P<0.001). Including pacemaker follow-up visits (3.6 ± 4 per patient per year), patients visited the doctor significantly less frequently each year after treatment (5.06 ± 7 visits) than before (10 ± 13 visits, P<0.03). Annual emergency room visits (3.1 ± 8 vs. 0.2 ± 0.62, P<0.03) and hospital admissions (2.8 ± 6.8 vs. 0.17 ± 0.54, P<0.03) fell significantly. Concurrent or serial antiar-

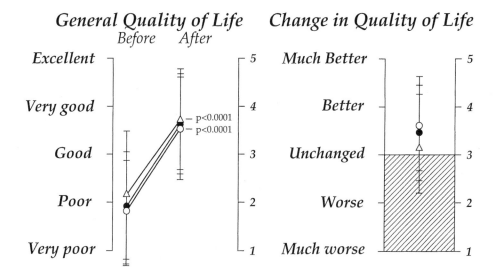

Figure 1. Change in quality of life after AV junctional ablation and permanent pacing for chronic atrial fibrillation, as assessed by numeric scoring from a telephone questionnaire of patients.

rhythmic drug trials prior to ablation were 6.2 ± 4 per patient, and these fell significantly to 0.46 ± 1.5 during follow-up ($P<0.001$). Congestive heart failure episodes occurred in 19 patients prior to, and in 8 patients after treatment.

We anticipated that the effect of AVJ ablation and pacing on patients with established AF might be different from patients with paroxysmal AF who were still predominantly in sinus rhythm. Therefore, the impact of the procedure on the measured parameters was assessed separately.

In both established and paroxysmal AF, quality of life improved. In Group 1 (patients with established AF), quality of life scores after treatment rose from 1.8 ± 1.14 to 3.5 ± 1.1 ($P<0.0001$), and in Group 2 (patients with paroxysmal AF), quality of life scores similarly rose from 2.1 ± 1.3 to 3.7 ± 1.1 ($P<0.0001$). Whether AF was established or paroxysmal, the frequency of intermittent symptoms index significantly improved, from 2.45 ± 0.63 to 1.26 ± 0.52 ($P<0.0001$) in Group 1 patients, and from 2.53 ± 0.6 to 1.25 ± 0.5 ($P<0.0001$) in Group 2 patients.

Patients' specific activities of daily living became significantly easier (Fig. 2). The pooled score of all activities rose from 1.9 ± 0.6 to 2.39 ± 0.5 ($P<0.001$) in Group 1. Vigorous exercise capacity increased significantly from 1.46 ± 0.66 to 2 ± 0.8 ($P<0.0001$). Moderate exercise capacity increased significantly from 1.85 ± 0.83 to 2.4 ± 0.8 ($P<0.0001$). Carrying groceries became significantly easier (2.0 ± 0.8 to 2.46 ± 0.75, $P<0.0001$), climbing stairs improved (1.8 ± 0.76 to 2.1 ± 0.7, $P<0.005$), walking was significantly easier (1.9 ± 0.76 to 2.56 ± 0.7, $P<0.0001$), and bathing and dressing were also easier (2.53 ± 0.7 to 2.84 ± 0.42, $P<0.005$). In Group 2, patients with paroxysmal AF, activities of daily living were not significantly improved. The pooled score of all activities was 2.2 ± 0.57 before and 2.35 ± 0.5 after (P = ns). Vigorous exercise capacity improved from 1.6 ± 0.6 before and 1.9 ± 0.8 after (P = ns). Moderate exercise capacity (2.1 ± 0.9 before vs. 2.3 ± 0.8 after, P = ns), carrying groceries (2.3 ± 0.8 to 2.36 ± 0.8, P = ns), climbing stairs (2.2 ± 0.78 to 2.27 ± 0.78, P = ns), walking (2.19 ± 0.78 to 2.5 ± 0.7, P = ns), and bathing and dressing (2.8 ± 0.48 to 2.75 ± 0.5, P = ns) were unchanged after treatment. These findings were consistent with expected activity impact for patients with intermittent symptoms who were predominantly in AF. However, it is interesting to speculate on the mechanism of improved functional capacity in patients with established AF. This might have been entirely due to heart rate control, with exercise heart rates determined by the

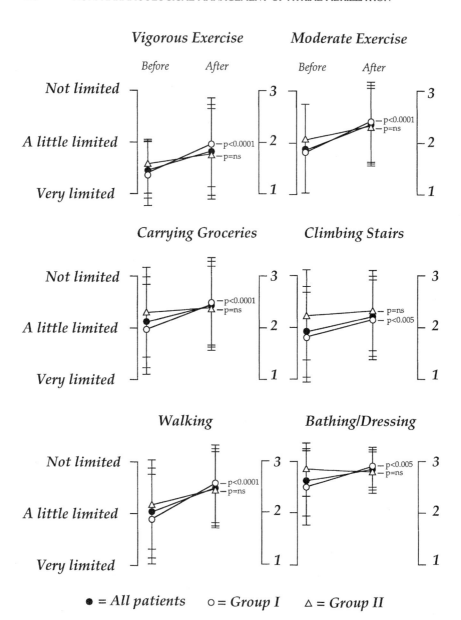

Figure 2. Change in activities of daily living after AV junctional ablation and pacing for chronic atrial fibrillation, as assessed by telephone questionnaire (mean ± SD).

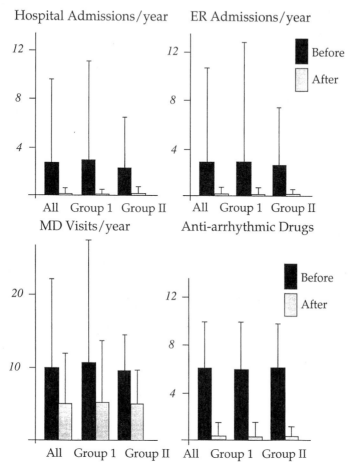

Figure 3. Change in consumption of health care resources after AV junctional ablation and permanent pacing for chronic atrial fibrillation (mean ± SD).

pacemaker, but it is interesting to speculate that an improvement in LV function might have occurred.

Consumption of health care resources (Fig. 3) in patients with established and paroxysmal AF was markedly reduced by ablation and pacing. Hospital admissions, either direct or via the emergency room, decreased from 3.3 ± 8.2 to 0.13 ± 0.49 (*P*<0.03) in Group 1, and from 2.27 ± 4.1 to 0.2 ± 0.6 (*P*<0.005) in Group 2. Accident and emergency room visits for AF, not leading to hospital admission, decreased significantly, from 3.4 ± 9.8 to 0.16 ± 0.65 per year (*P*<0.03), in Group 1, and from 2.7 ± 5.3 to 0.25 ± 0.56 per year in Group 2 ($P<0.005$). Outpatient doctor visits, including pacemaker follow-up (3.36 ± 4.1 per year), decreased to 5.2 ± 7.9 from 11 ± 16.7 per year ($P<0.03$) in Group 1 patients, and to 4.8 ± 5.1 visits from 8 ± 5.5 visits ($P<0.03$) in Group 2, which had 3.3 ± 48.7 pacemaker follow-up visits per year. Antiarrhythmic drugs used decreased significantly from 6.12 ± 4.4 prior to ablation to 0.43 ± 1.8 ($P<0.0001$) during follow-up in Group 1, and from 6.3 ± 3.5 prior to ablation to 0.5 ± 0.8 during follow-up in Group 2 ($P<0.0001$).

Significant events that were recorded for Group 1 included congestive heart failure episodes in 12 patients prior to treatment, and in four patients afterward, and eight strokes prior to treatment and two afterward. In Group 2, congestive heart failure episodes were documented in seven patients prior to treatment, and in four patients afterward; four incidences of stroke occurred prior to treatment and one during follow-up.

Patients with established AF were treated with a ventricular pacing mode. Eight patients received VVI, and 46, VVIR pacemakers, with pacing rate on exercise modulated by a biosensor. In patients with paroxysmal AF, 36 patients were treated with a dual chamber pacing mode without atrial tracking or with upper-rate limited atrial tracking (where DDD pacemakers had been implanted). At follow-up, 28 of 36 patients remained in a dual chamber mode, and eight patients had required reprogramming to ventricular rate-responsive pacing only. When DDD pacing was used (13 patients), the upper tracking rate was limited, usually to approximately 90 beats per minute. This prevented tracking of rapid AF, but potentially limited exercise in sinus rhythm because of development of Wenckebach or 2:1 AV block. At follow-up, two patients had been programmed to DDIR to prevent tracking of AF but afford rate-responsiveness and AV synchrony during exercise, and two patients had been upgraded to DDDR. In eight patients in whom DDDR pacemakers were used, tracking of AF was constrained by programming a low upper atrial-tracking rate, while at faster rates AV synchrony was maintained by programming a faster sensor-determined upper rate. In two of these patients, tracking of AF was limited by a "conditional ventricular tracking limit" (Intermedics Relay™, Intermedics, Inc., Angleton, Texas). This limited atrial tracking to a maximum of 35 beats above the programmed backup pacing rate in the absence of sensor activity. Sensor activity would indicate an appropriate rate increase with exercise, rather than atrial tachycardia at rest. Overall, 28 out of 36 patients initially treated with dual chamber pacemakers remained in a dual chamber mode at follow-up. Sixteen patients required pacing system revisions during follow-up. This was for a hardware failure in eight patients (generator power failure = 4, lead failure = 4), and for upgrade (4) or downgrade (4) to a more appropriate pacing mode in the other eight patients.

During follow-up, three patients died of carcinoma, three of stroke, six of congestive heart failure, two of acute myocardial infarction, and one of multisystem failure after heart transplantation. Two patients died suddenly. Baseline LV function was significantly worse in patients who died (ejection fraction 38 ± 13%) than in survivors (51 ± 11%, $P<0.05$).

From the results of this study, we concluded that there was evidence that AVJ ablation and pacing was beneficial in terms of quality of life and health care costs, whether AF was established or not. Ability to perform daily activities was only improved where AF was established. It appeared that heart failure episodes, in particular, were diminished after such treatment, but this could not be confirmed with this study design. Additionally, there was concern about the numbers of deaths, although most were either unrelated to the underlying heart disease, or were due to progression of underlying heart disease. Of great concern are the two patients who died suddenly, where a pacemaker malfunction or cardiac damage due to the ablation might have been the cause. Evidence from another center,[21] however, suggests a similar rate of sudden death in patients treated by direct current ablation, and patients treated medically. Therefore, this rate of sudden death of 1% to 2% might be expected in a population with AF, many of whom have quite severe underlying heart disease. Additonally, the very discrete nature of myocardial lesions made with radiofrequency energy suggests that extensive scarring and possible arrhythmogenic ventricular damage as a result of the ablation itself is quite unlikely.

This evidence suggests that patients with AF who are treated by radiofrequency AVJ ablation benefit greatly from the procedure whether AF is permanent or paroxysmal. The health care cost savings would appear to be potentially great. However, this study calls for further prospective randomized studies to confirm its findings, since all data were collected retrospectively. Radiofrequency catheter ablation of the AV junction with subsequent permanent pacing is effective for medically refractory paroxysmal or chronic AF. Quality of life, daily activity, and health care costs are significantly improved. A dual chamber pacing mode continues to be used in the majority of patients so-treated.

References

1. Jackman WM, Xunzhang W, Friday KJ, et al. Catheter ablation of accessory atrioventricular pathways (Wolff-Parkinson-White syndrome) by radiofrequency energy. New Eng J Med 1991;324:1605–1611.

2. Calkins H, Sousa J, El-Atassi R, et al. Diagnosis and cure of Wolff-Parkinson-White syndrome or paroxysmal supraventricular tachycardias during a single electrophysiologic test. New Eng J Med 1991;324:1612–1618.

3. Feld GK, Fleck RP, Chen PS, et al. Radiofrequency catheter ablation for the treatment of human type I atrial flutter: identification of a critical zone in the reentrant circuit by endocardial mapping techniques. Circulation 1992;86:1233–1237.

4. Olgin JE, Scheinman MM. Comparison of high-energy direct current and radiofrequency catheter ablation of the atrioventricular junction. J Am Coll Cardiol 1993;21:557–564.

5. Rosenqvist M, Lee MA, Moulinier L, et al. Long-term follow-up of patients after transcatheter direct current ablation of the atrioventricular junction. J Am Coll Cardiol 1990;16:1467–1474.

6. Haïssaguerre M, Marcus FI, Fischer B, Clementy J. Radiofrequency catheter ablation in unusual mechanisms of atrial fibrillation: report of three cases. J Cardiovasc Electrophysiol 1994;5:743–751.

7. Feinberg MS, Waggoner AD, Kater KM, et al. Restoration of atrial function after the maze procedure for patients with atrial fibrillation: assessment by Doppler echocardiography. Circulation 1994;90:285–292.

8. Rawles JM, Metcalfe MJ, Jennings K. Time of occurrence, duration and ventricular rate of atrial fibrillation: the effect of digoxin. Br Heart J 1990; 63:225–227.

9. Jensen D. Ablate and Pace Trial (APT). Personal communication.

10. McLaren CJ, Gersh BJ, Sugrue DD, et al. Tachycardia-induced myocardial dysfunction: a reversible phenomenon? Br Heart J 1985;53:323–327.

11. Packer DL, Bardy GH, Worley SJ, et al. Tachycardia-induced cardiomyopathy: a reversible form of left ventricular dysfunction. Am J Cardiol 1986; 57:563–570.

12. Grogan M, Smith HC, Gersh B, et al. Left ventricular dysfunction due to atrial fibrillation in patients initially believed to have idiopathic dilated cardiomyopathy. Am J Cardiol 1992;69:1570–1573.

13. Gossage AM, Hicks JA. On auricular fibrillation. Q J Med 1913;6:435–440.

14. Gallagher JJ, Svenson RH, Kasell JH, et al. Catheter technique for closed-chest ablation of the atrioventricular conduction system. N Engl J Med 1982;306:194–200.

15. Scheinman MM, Morady F, Hess DS, et al. Catheter-induced ablation of the atrioventricular junction to control refractory supraventricular arrhythmias. JAMA 1982;248:851–855.

16. Huang SK, Bharati S, Graham AR, et al. Closed-chest catheter desiccation of the atrioventricular junction using radiofrequency energy: a new method of catheter ablation. J Am Coll Cardiol 1987;9:349–358.

17. Packer DL, Bardy GH, Worley SJ, et al. Tachycardia-induced cardiomyopathy: a reversible form of left ventricular dysfunction. Am J Cardiol 1986; 57:563–570.

18. Lemery R, Brugada P, Cheriex E, et al. Reversibility of tachycardia-induced left ventricular dysfunction after closed-chest ablation of the atrioventricular junction for atrial fibrillation. Am J Cardiol 1987;60:1406–1408.
19. Rosenqvist M, Lee MA, Moulinier L, et al. Long-term follow-up of patients after transcatheter direct current ablation of the atrioventricular junction. J Am Coll Cardiol 1990;16:1467–1474.
20. Fitzpatrick AP, Kourouyan HD, Siu A, et al. Quality of life and outcomes after radiofrequency His-bundle catheter ablation and permanent pacemaker implantation. Am Heart J 1996;131:499–507.
21. Windecker S, Plumb VJ, Epstein AE, Kay GN. Does AV nodal ablation impair long-term survival compared with medical treatment of atrial fibrillation? J Am Coll Cardiol 1994;1A:84A. Abstract.

CHAPTER 8

Atrioventricular Nodal Modification for Atrial Fibrillation:

What Does it Really Do?

Panagiotis Th. Panotopoulos, Calambur Narasimhan, Zalmen Blanck, Mohammad R. Jazayeri, Masood Akhtar

Introduction

Atrial fibrillation (AF) is the most frequent chronic sustained tachyarrhythmia, with a prevalence from 0.2% to 0.9% in different age groups in the general population.[1] Control of the ventricular response (VR) has been one of the therapeutic targets in patients in whom maintenance of sinus rhythm cannot be achieved. Pharmacological treatment is generally used as the approach of first choice in this setting. Although usually successful, the pharmacological approach is limited by a number of potential problems. Difficulty in achieving adequate control of the ventricular rate during activity without overly suppressing it at rest, frequent need for drugs with negative inotropic effect in patients with severe left ventricular systolic dysfunction, and other systemic and proarrhythmic effects of drugs are some of these problems.

These limitations led to the development of nonpharmacological ways of controlling the VR in patients with refractory AF. Atrioventricular (AV) nodal ablation[2,3] and implantation of a permanent pacemaker has been used for this purpose. The use of radiofrequency (RF) energy has been shown to be a safe and effective way of inducing complete AV block.[4,5] In such patients, clinical improvement defined as resolution of symptoms and improvement in exercise tolerance has been documented, associated frequently with an increase in the left ventricular

From *Nonpharmacological Management of Atrial Fibrillation*, edited by A.J. Camm and F.D. Murgatroyd. © 1997, Futura Publishing Co., Inc., Armonk, NY.

ejection fraction.[6,7] The major disadvantage of such an approach is obviously the lifelong dependence on a permanent pacemaker.

Recent reports have suggested an alternative ablative approach: application of RF energy to the posterior or midseptal part of the tricuspid annulus seems to offer control of the ventricular response in a significant percentage of patients with AF, with small risk for creating complete heart block.[8-13] In this chapter, we will review the available data on this therapeutic approach and discuss the techniques used and its applicability in clinical practice.

Clinical Data

The effect of AV nodal modification on the ventricular response in patients with AF has been addressed by six published series so far. In four series, patients with chronic or paroxysmal AF were included. In two, the effect of AV nodal modification was studied on induced AF. The results of these series are summarized in Table 1.

Williamson et al.[8] studied 19 patients with AF and uncontrolled ventricular rates despite the use of medications. Application of the RF energy was done with anatomic criteria, in a manner similar to that which is followed in patients with "slow pathway" ablation for AV nodal reentry tachycardia (AVNRT).[14] The posterior and, in case of no success, the mid part of the tricuspid annulus was targeted. An average ventricular rate of less than 120/min during isoproterenol infusion was used as the endpoint. The procedure was successful in 14 (74%) of the patients and the results achieved were maintained over 8 months of follow-up, in all but one patient who required a second procedure. Four patients (21%) had inadvertent complete heart block (CHB) during the procedure, requiring implantation of a permanent pacemaker. In an attempt to explain the effect of their procedure the authors suggested that ablation of the posterior atrionodal inputs to the AV node was responsible for the slowing of the ventricular rate. Alternatively, partial damage to the compact node could be responsible for the slowing of the VR and, in the cases of more severe damage, of the CHB, despite the seemingly identical location between the successful RF applications and those which resulted in AV block.[8]

Feld et al.[9] studied 10 patients with AF and symptomatic, rapid ventricular response. RF energy was delivered initially midway between the His bundle and the coronary sinus os on the tricuspid valve annulus. Decrease of the VR below 100/min was used as an endpoint. If this was not achieved, RF energy was delivered at more posterior

Table 1
AV Node Modification for Atrial Fibrillation

Study	n	Mean Age (y)	Success	Mean Rate Before AVNM	Mean Rate After AVNM	P Value	Mean Number of RF Applications	AV Block
Williamson, 1994a	19	62 ± 15	14 (74%)	92 ± 20b	66 ± 11b	<0.001	11 ± 5	4 (21%)
Feld, 1994a	10	62 ± 10	7 (70%)	128 ± 11b	83 ± 10b	<0.01	17 ± 12	0
Della Bella, 1995c	14	55.1 ± 11.5	12 (86%)	NR	60–95	NR	8.7 ± 3.5	2 (14%)
				157 ± 38d	67 ± 10d	NR		
Lüderitz, 1996e	10	62 ± 11	9 (90%)	NR	NR	NR	9.9 ± 8.3	0
Blanck, 1995f	18	34 ± 8	13 (72%)	526 ± 93g 114	612 ± 107g 98	<0.0001	5 ± 4	0
Kreiner, 1996f	30	50 ± 12	NR	449 ± 98g 133	515 ± 129g 116	<0.001	3 ± 2	0

a = chronic AF; b = successful procedures, only; c = 2 patients with AF, 6 patients with SR, 6 patients with atrial flutter/atrial tachycardia; d, 2 patients with AF; e = 4 patients with chronic and 6 patients with paroxysmal AF; f = induced AF; g = cycle length; y = years; AVNM = AV node modification; RF = radiofrequency; NR = not reported.

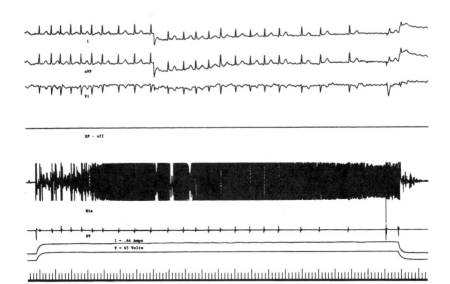

Figure 1. Surface ECG leads, right ventricular endocardial, current and voltage recording from a patient with AF undergoing AV nodal modification for rate control. Note the abrupt decrease in ventricular rate during RF energy application. (Modified with permission from Feld et al.[9])

sites (Fig. 1). A rate below 120/min after administration of 1 mg of atropine IV was used as a criterion of a successful response. Seven patients had a successful procedure result and remained symptom free over a 14-month follow-up period. In two patients in whom the initial procedure was unsuccessful, AV nodal ablation was done and the remaining patient had successful DC cardioversion after a month of amiodarone loading. The authors' interpretation of their data was that elimination of the slow pathway with its short refractory period was responsible for the slowing of the VR in the patients with a successful procedure.[9] Like Williamson et al.,[8] these authors also considered as an alternative possibility that damage to the compact node could be responsible for the observed results. In both studies, the effect of the modification procedure on the electrophysiological properties of the AV node could not be assessed because of the presence of chronic AF.

Della Bella et al. studied 14 patients with symptomatic, paroxysmal AF, atrial flutter, or atrial tachycardia.[10] None of them had dual AV nodal physiology. A high frequency potential in the low posterior septum was targeted[15] when the modification procedure was done in a rhythm other than AF (12 patients). In the latter case an anatomic approach was used (2 patients). Prolongation of the shortest achievable cycle length with 1 : 1 AV conduction during high right atrial pacing (pre-Wenckebach cycle length) to above 500 ms in patients with sinus rhythm, and VR slowing in those with AF, were the endpoints of the procedure. CHB occurred inadvertently in two patients, one with atrial flutter and one with AF, during the procedure. During 6 months of follow-up, recurrence of AF was documented in 11 patients, with a ventricular rate of 75–78/min. The investigators concluded that the "slow pathway" is an atrial input to the AV node, with distinct conducting properties and that ablation of this input leads to slowing of the VR in AF. Although they did not assess the properties of the AV node systematically after each RF application, they suggested that the modification procedure was a "quantitative" one, with a gradual effect on the AV node, that built up as a result of several consecutive applications. They also suggested that the presence of different atrial inputs to the AV node, perhaps located in the left atrium, could account for the procedure failures.[10]

Finally, in a short report by Lüderitz, 10 patients with chronic or paroxysmal AF and rapid VR had a modification procedure. A successful permanent effect was achieved in nine patients and no AV block was induced accidentally.[11]

In two more published reports (Fig. 2), the effect of the AV node modification on the ventricular rate during AF was studied, in patients with AVNRT. None of the patients had clinical AF and the effects of the procedure were studied on the ventricular rate of AF induced by burst pacing. The study done by Blanck et al.[12] was designed to assess the effect of elimination of dual antegrade AV nodal physiology on the ventricular response of induced AF. In this study, which was done under autonomic blockade, elimination of dual pathway physiology had a sensitivity of 77%, a specificity of 80%, and a positive predictive value of 91% for slowing of the ventricular response during AF.

The anatomic approach was used for the procedure and no inadvertent CHB occurred (Fig. 3). Slowing of the VR during AF was also noted in some patients without dual AV node physiology at baseline. The authors suggested that during AF the VR is determined by the electrophysiological properties of the slow pathway and that complete elimination of the dual AV node physiology would result in a slower ventricular rate.[12]

A similar report by Kreiner et al.[13] included 30 patients with dual AV node physiology, inducible AVNRT at baseline, and no history of AF. Potentials similar to the ones described by Jackman[15] or Haïssaguerre,[16] and in their absence, anatomic landmarks, were targeted,

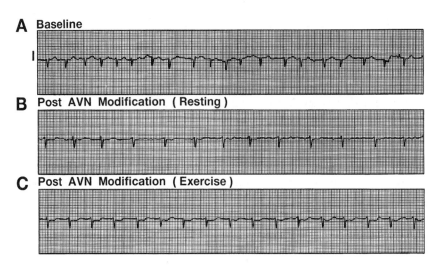

Figure 2. Effect of AV nodal modification on the ventricular rate in a patient with AF. **Panel A**: resting rate at baseline. **Panel B**: resting rate after AV nodal modification. **Panel C**: rate during exercise, after AV nodal modification. Note that the resting rate before the modification is faster than the exercise rate after the procedure.

with the endpoints of the complete elimination of the dual AV node physiology or the inability for 1:1 AV conduction along the slow pathway. The investigators confirmed the results of the previous studies, but they suggested that the effect of the procedure may not offer sufficient rate control in patients with short fast pathway pre-Wenckebach cycle length. In the presence of longer fast pathway pre-Wenckebach cycle length, fast antegrade conduction along the AV node would depend more on a potentiating, through summation,[17] effect of conduction along the slow pathway.[13]

Despite the different methodologies and patient populations involved, in the above studies the success rate in reducing VR during AF was in the range of 70–90%.[8-11] Over a period of follow-up that ranged from 6 to 14 months, the patients with a successful procedure had persistently reduced ventricular rates compared to those before the procedure and had resolution of the symptoms related to rapid ventricular response. In one study, despite the stability over time of the mean resting, "ambulatory" and minimal ventricular rate, the maximal ventricular rate increased by 25%. The authors attributed this increase to the improved exercise capacity of the patients with a successful procedure.[8]

The incidence of CHB during the procedure was small but definite.

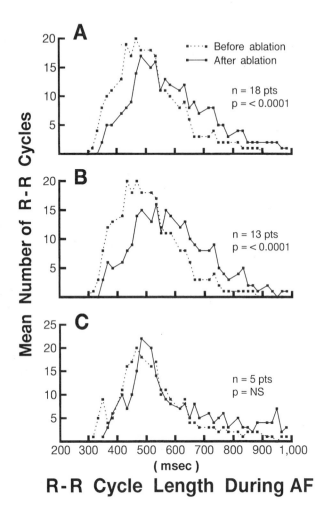

Figure 3. Graphs showing frequency distribution of the ventricular cycle lengths during AF before and after ablation. For each ventricular (RR) cycle length, the mean number of RR cycles is shown before and after a selective slow pathway ablation. The frequency distribution curves are shown for: (**A**) all 18 patients; (**B**) the 13 patients who had statistical slowing of the ventricular rate; and (**C**) the 5 patients who did not have a slowing of the ventricular response. Only the data in the groups of patients in A and B show a significant change in the RR response to AF after ablation. (Reprinted with permission from Blanck et al.[12])

It is of note that all episodes of inadvertent CHB occurred during AF. None occurred with application of the RF energy during sinus rhythm, a fact consistent with the data from the use of RF energy for AV nodal modification in the setting of AVNRT, in which the incidence of AV block is less than 1%.[18] In addition, the relatively high incidence in one center, during the first of the reported series,[8] perhaps had to do with low threshold for acceptance of the AV block as the end result, since in the case of failure of the AV nodal modification procedure, AV nodal ablation would essentially be the procedure of choice.

Defining Controlled Ventricular Response

In patients with persistent AF, control of the ventricular response is one of the major therapeutic targets. Nevertheless, the question of what the optimal range of ventricular rates is, in patients with AF, has not been addressed adequately. A higher VR compensates partially for the reduction in cardiac output attributed to the loss of contractile atrial function. Frequently, however, VR is higher than what would be needed for maximization of the cardiac output, leading instead to hemodynamic compromise.[19] In addition, high ventricular rates can lead to tachycardia-induced cardiomyopathy[20] and, finally, irrespective of the hemodynamic consequences or its effect on exercise tolerance, a rapid and irregular ventricular response can be responsible for a variety of symptoms. The issue is complicated more by the need to assess these parameters both at rest and during exercise. In everyday practice, "common sense" approaches to the problem are being used, with reliance on patient symptomatology and exercise tolerance, as well as on the individual physician's idea of what is an appropriate resting heart rate.

Determinants of Ventricular Response in AF

A conceptually simple model that would explain the effect of AV nodal modification on the VR in AF would be based on the conventional views on the structure and function of the AV node: it consists of multiple fibers with a wide spectrum of refractoriness and conducting properties, the more anterior fibers being faster, with a longer refractory period, the more posterior ones conducting slower, with a shorter refractory period. During AF, the AV node receives input at a very fast rate from the atria. At that rate, the rate of conduction through the node will be determined by the posterior fibers (i.e., the "slow" pathway), because of their shorter refractory period. Elimination of the posterior fibers should therefore slow the ventricular rate. Leaving, on the other hand, the fast AV nodal pathway unaffected would allow not only "normal" AV conduction at rest, but also acceleration of the ventricular rate during exercise, thus maintaining the "chronotropic competence" of the AV node.

Consistent with this schematic view are prior observations about the electrophysiological determinants of the ventricular rate during AF. The AV nodal effective refractory period (ERP) and the pre-Wenckebach cycle length have been the variables that correlate most closely with both the mean rate and the minimum relative risk (RR).[21,22]

AV node modification results in prolongation of both parameters,[23] and prolongation of both the mean and the minimum RR cycles should be expected (Figs. 4 and 5). On the contrary, attempts to modify the

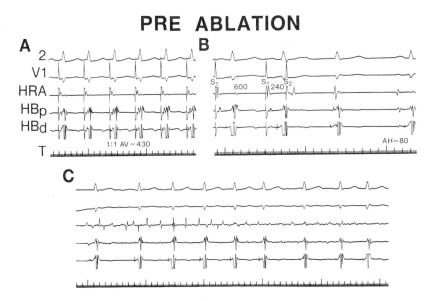

Figure 4. Tracings showing ventricular response to AF (**Panel A**) before elimination of dual pathway physiology. The shortest 1:1 AV conduction and the AV nodal ERP are 430 ms and <240 ms, respectively (**Panels A and B**). Compare with Figure 5. Tracings from top to bottom are ECG (leads 2 and V_1), high right atrium (HRA), proximal (HBp) and distal (HBd) His bundle recordings, and time (T) lines. (Modified with permission from Blanck et al.[12])

POST ABLATION

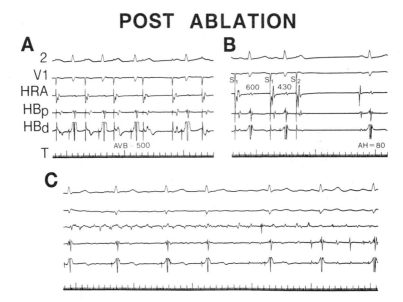

Figure 5. Tracings showing ventricular response to AF (**Panel C**) after elimination of dual pathway physiology. Same patient as in Figure 4. The shortest 1:1 AV conduction and the AV nodal ERP are now 500 ms and 430 ms, respectively (**Panels A and B**). Tracings from top to bottom are ECG (leads 2 and V_1), high right atrium, proximal and distal His bundle recordings, and time lines. (Modified with permission from Blanck et al.[12])

AV node and slow the VR in patients with AF, with application of RF current anteriorly in the tricuspid annulus, resulted in success only in one third of the patients, the incidence of CHB was high, and only one third of those who had an initial response had a long-lasting effect.[24] It is of note that none of the electrophysiological parameters correlated with the VR in AF changes as a result of "fast" pathway ablation.[23]

The Role of the "Slow" Pathway

The slowing of the VR in patients with AF by ablating the "slow" AV nodal pathway raises the issue of the possible role that the "slow" AV nodal pathway may have in such patients. Available data indicate that in the presence of dual physiology at baseline, its complete elimination will lead to comparatively lower VR.[12] This is consistent with observations that complete elimination of the dual AV nodal physiology leads to greater prolongation of the AV nodal ERP and the pre-Wenckebach cycle length.[23] However, absence of demonstrable dual AV nodal physiology does not predict failure of the procedure. In accordance with this are the results of the study by Della Bella et al.[10] and Blanck et al.[12] despite the small numbers of patients studied, as well as the wide discrepancy between the reported prevalence of dual AV nodal physiology in various groups of patients[25] and the apparent success of the AV node modification procedure in patients with AF.[8-11] Comparison of patients with and without dual AV nodal physiology showed that the VR during induced AF adhered to the above mentioned electrophysiological parameters and did not relate directly to the presence or absence of dual physiology per se (Fig. 6).[26]

Our difficulty in precisely defining the mechanism by which AV node modification reduces the ventricular rate in patients with AF reflects our limited knowledge about the structure and the function of the AV node and the perinodal atrial structures. Both the concept of the ability of the AV node to conduct in the conventional way and the concept of the presence of two discrete antegrade pathways, with properties as described above, have been challenged. The AV node as a structure with its ability to conduct described by the classic concepts of AV nodal refractoriness and concealed conduction is supported by a number of clinical and experimental data.[27,28] More recently, the validity of this model has been challenged by observations from right ventricular (RV) pacing and extrastimulation during AF.[29] Specifically, it was noted that RV pacing at cycle lengths considerably longer than the shortest RR cycles of "undisturbed" AF would lead to total elimination of antegrade conduction.[30] In addition, introduction of single premature ventricular complexes (PVCs) in patients with AF, would result in a histogram of return cycle lengths similar to that of the RR intervals during AF.[31] The alternative hypothesis that emerged was that the AV node does not conduct, but instead behaves as a pacemaker/oscillator which is being electrotonically modulated by input from the atria or the ventricles. During AF, "translation of fibrillatory impulses into successful antegrade conduction is caused by discontinuous, electrotonically mediated propagation within the AV node."[31] (This hypothesis has not become widely accepted, however.)[32-34]

The concept of the AV node with discrete fast and slow antegrade pathways is also a rather simplistic one. Evidence exists for the presence of multiple pathways,[23] the anatomical substrates of which are atrionodal connections rather than discrete intranodal pathways.[35] In this context, the posterior/midtricuspid annulus is the location of a preferential atrial input to the AV node. Whether the patients who failed

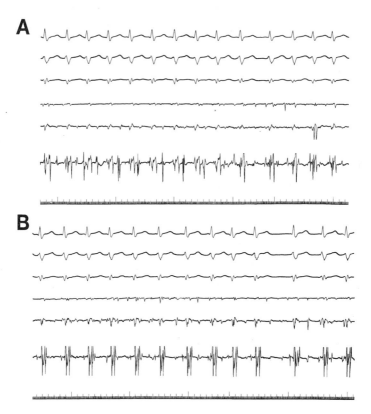

Figure 6. Tracings showing no significant change in the ventricular response to AF in a patient before (**A**) and after (**B**) successful AV nodal modification for AVNRT. Tracings from top to bottom are ECG (leads I, II and V_1), high right atrium, proximal and distal His bundle recordings, and time lines. Although the AVNRT was noninducible after the procedure, dual pathway physiology persisted. In this patient, the shortest 1:1 AV conduction and the AV nodal ERP were the same before and after the ablation (not shown). (Modified with permission from Blanck et al.[12])

AV nodal modification have preferential inputs/conduction through so far unexplored areas (i.e., left sided) remains to be seen.

Conclusion

Available data indicate that AV nodal modification can offer control of the VR in patients with AF in whom a pharmacological approach has failed or has not been tolerated. The procedure can be done during sinus rhythm or during AF. In the former case, targeting "slow pathway" potentials or following the anatomic approach have both been utilized successfully, with prolongation of the AV nodal ERP and the pre-Wenckebach cycle length as endpoints. When the procedure is being done during AF, the anatomic approach has been used with success, but may result in AV block in up to 20% of the patients.

Whether this method can be used earlier in the management of AF and whether the effect achieved is a long-lasting one, remains to be seen. Although successful application of this technique obviates the need for AV nodal ablation and permanent pacemaker implantation, inadvertent CHB can occur. The risk is apparently higher when the procedure is being done during AF rather than during SR and the patient should be prepared to accept this.

References

1. Kannel WB, Wolf PA. Epidemiology of atrial fibrillation. In: Falk RH, Podrid PJ, eds. Atrial Fibrillation: Mechanisms and Management. Raven Press, 1992.
2. Gallagher JJ, Svenson RH, Kasell JH, et al. Catheter technique for closed-chest ablation of the atrioventricular conduction system. N Engl J Med 1982;306:194–200.
3. Scheinman MM, Morady F, Hess DS, Gonzalez R. Catheter-induced ablation of the atrioventricular junction to control refractory supraventricular arrhythmias. JAMA 1982;248:851–855.
4. Jackman WM, Wang X, Friday KJ, et al. Catheter ablation of atrioventricular junction using radiofrequency current in 17 patients: comparison of standard and large tip electrodes. Circulation 1991;83:1562–1576.
5. Yeung-Lai-Wah J, Alison J, Lonergan L, et al. High success rate of atrioventricular node ablation with radiofrequency energy. J Am Coll Cardiol 1991; 18:1753–1758.
6. Twidale N, Sutton K, Bartlett L, et al. Effects on cardiac performance of atrioventricular node catheter ablation using radiofrequency current for drug-refractory atrial arrhythmias. PACE 1993;16:1275–1284.
7. Kay GN, Bubien RS, Epstein AE, Plumb VJ. Effect of catheter ablation of atrioventricular junction on quality of life and exercise tolerance in paroxysmal atrial fibrillation. Am J Cardiol 1988;62:741–744.
8. Williamson BD, Man KC, Daoud E, et al. Radiofrequency catheter modification of atrioventricular conduction to control the ventricular rate during atrial fibrillation. N Engl J Med 1994;331:910–917.
9. Feld GK, Fleck RP, Fujimura O, et al. Control of rapid ventricular response by radiofrequency catheter modification of the atrioventricular node in patients with medically refractory atrial fibrillation. Circulation 1994;90:2299–2307.
10. Della Bella P, Carbucicchio C, Tondo C, Riva S. Modulation of atrioventric-

ular conduction by ablation of the "slow" atrioventricular node pathway in patients with drug-refractory atrial fibrillation or flutter. J Am Coll Cardiol 1995;25:39–46.

11. Lüderitz B, Pfeiffer D, Tebbenjohanns J, Jung W. Nonpharmacologic strategies for treating atrial fibrillation. Am J Cardiol 1996;77:45A-52A.

12. Blanck Z, Dhala AA, Sra J, et al. Characterization of atrioventricular nodal behavior and ventricular response during atrial fibrillation before and after a selective slow-pathway ablation. Circulation 1995;91:1086–1094.

13. Kreiner G, Heinz G, Siostrzonek P, Gössinger HD. Effect of slow pathway ablation on ventricular rate during atrial fibrillation: dependence on electrophysiological properties of the fast pathway. Circulation 1996;93: 277–283.

14. Jazayeri MR, Hempe SL, Sra JS, et al. Selective transcatheter ablation of the fast and slow pathways using radiofrequency energy in patients with atrioventricular nodal reentrant tachycardia. Circulation 1992;85: 1318–1328.

15. Jackman WM, Beckman KJ, McClelland JH, et al. Treatment of supraventricular tachycardia due to atrioventricular nodal reentry by radiofrequency catheter ablation of slow-pathway conduction. N Engl J Med 1992; 327:313–318.

16. Haïssaguerre M, Fiorenzo G, Fischer B, et al. Elimination of atrioventricular nodal reentrant tachycardia using discrete slow potentials to guide application of radiofrequency energy. Circulation 1992;85:2162–2175.

17. Zipes DP, Mendez C, Moe GK. Evidence for summation and voltage dependency in rabbit atrioventricular nodal fibers. Circ Res 1973;32:170–177.

18. Kalbfleisch SJ, Morady F. Catheter ablation of atrioventricular nodal reentrant tachycardia. In: Zipes DP, Jalife J, eds. Cardiac Electrophysiology: From Cell to Bedside. 2nd ed. Philadelphia: WB Saunders; 1995.

19. Rawles J. What is meant by a "controlled" ventricular rate in atrial fibrillation? Br Heart J 1990;63:157–161.

20. Peters KG, Kienzle MG. Severe cardiomyopathy due to severe chronic rapid atrial fibrillation: complete recovery after reversion to sinus rhythm. Am J Med 1988;85:242–244.

21. Toivonen L, Kadish A, Kou W, Morady F. Determinants of the ventricular rate in atrial fibrillation. J Am Coll Cardiol 1990;16:1194–2000.

22. Rowland E, Curry P, Fox K, Krikler D. Relation between atrioventricular pathways and ventricular response during atrial fibrillation and flutter. Br Heart J 1981;45:83–87.

23. Jazayeri MR, Sra JS, Deshpande SS, et al. Electrophysiologic spectrum of atrioventricular nodal behavior in patients with atrioventricular nodal reentrant tachycardia undergoing selective fast or slow pathway ablation. J Cardiovasc Electrophysiol 1993;4:99–111.

24. Duckeck W, Engelstein ED, Kuck K-H. Radiofrequency current therapy in atrial tachyarrhythmias: modulation versus ablation of atrioventricular nodal conduction. PACE 1993;16:629–636.

25. Denes P, Wu D, Dhingra RC, et al. Dual atrioventricular nodal pathways: a common electrophysiologic response. Br Heart J 1975;37:1069–1076.

26. Brugada P, Roy D, Weiss J, et al. Dual atrio-ventricular nodal pathways and atrial fibrillation. PACE 1984;7:240–247.

27. Langendorf R, Pick A, Katz LN. Ventricular response in atrial fibrillation:

role of concealed conduction in the AV junction. Circulation 1965;332: 69–75.

28. Moe GK, Abildskov JA. Observations on the ventricular dysrhythmia associated with atrial fibrillation in the dog heart. Circ Res 1964;14:447–460.
29. Meijler FL, Fisch C. Does the atrioventricular node conduct? Br Heart J 1989;61:309–315.
30. Wittcampf FHM, De Jongste MJL, Lie HI, Meijler FL. Effect of right ventricular pacing on ventricular rhythm during atrial fibrillation. J Am Coll Cardiol 1988;11:539–545.
31. Wittcampf FHM, De Jongste MJL, Meijler FL. Competitive anterograde and retrograde atrioventricular junctional activation in atrial fibrillation. J Cardiovasc Electrophysiol 1990;1:448–456.
32. Dreifus LS, Mazgalev T. "Atrial paralysis": does it explain the irregular ventricular rate during atrial fibrillation? J Am Coll Cardiol 1988;11: 546–547.
33. Watanabe Y, Watanabe M. Impulse formation and conduction of excitation in the atrioventricular node. J Cardiovasc Electrophysiol 1994;5:517–531.
34. Vereckei A, Vera Z, Pride HP, Zipes DP. Atrioventricular nodal conduction rather than automaticity determines the ventricular rate during atrial fibrillation and atrial flutter. J Cardiovasc Electrophysiol 1992;3:534–543.
35. McGuire MA, Janse MJ, Ross DL. "AV nodal" reentry. II. AV nodal, AV junctional or atrionodal reentry? J Cardiovasc Electrophysiol 1993;4: 573–586.

CHAPTER 9

Pacemaker Selection after Atrioventricular Nodal Ablation

David L. Hayes

When direct current (DC) or radiofrequency (RF) ablation of the atrioventricular (AV) node is successfully performed for control of a refractory paroxysmal or chronic supraventricular rhythm disorder, a permanent pacemaker is obviously required. RF ablation of the AV node is being performed in increasing numbers. It is estimated that in 1993, permanent pacemaker implantation following AV nodal ablation accounted for 2,802 implants or 2.5% of the total implants performed.[1] Unpublished data compiled by industry from a variety of sources estimate that in 1995 there were more than 7,000 AV nodal ablations performed for the control of atrial fibrillation (AF) and an estimated 15,500 AV nodal ablations worldwide. (Springer MG. Personal communication. April, 1996.) AV node modification is performed much less frequently, but complete AV block may occur as a complication of this procedure.[2] Whether the AV block is desirable or a complication of a selective ablation, permanent pacing is still required.

Despite the frequency with which AV nodal ablation is performed, there is limited data available regarding pacemaker selection in this group of patients. This chapter will examine pertinent existing literature, recommendations for pacemaker selection in the post-AV nodal ablation patient and special implant considerations.

Existing Postablation Follow-Up Series

Several series of patients receiving permanent pacemakers after AV nodal ablation have been reported. The purpose of these follow-up studies was to determine the efficacy of various pacing modes in the

From *Nonpharmacological Management of Atrial Fibrillation*, edited by F.D. Murgatroyd and A.J. Camm. © 1997, Futura Publishing Co., Inc., Armonk, NY.

postablation patient population as well as complications associated with specific pacing modes.

Rajamannan and colleagues[3] assessed pacing modes and complications in 78 consecutive patients undergoing AV node ablation. The ablation was performed for paroxysmal AF in 14 patients, chronic AF/flutter in 44 patients, or some other supraventricular rhythm disturbance in 20 patients. At the time of hospital discharge, seven different pacing modes had been used in this group of patients (Fig. 1). Single chamber ventricular pacing, VVI or VVIR, was used in 48 patients. A dual chamber pacing mode was utilized in the remaining 30 patients. Late complications included recurrent AV nodal conduction in two patients with chronic AF and one patient with recurrent syncope in whom pacemaker function was normal. Initial pacing modes were compared to pacing modes at last follow-up with a mean follow-up of 12.3 months (range, 0 to 89 months).

At follow-up, 56 patients (72%) were paced in a single chamber mode, and 22 (28%) dual chamber, with 11 (14%) patients requiring a change in pacing mode. Reasons for a change in pacing mode included: development of chronotropic incompetence, development of chronic AF and pacemaker syndrome. Mode changes are detailed in Figure 1.

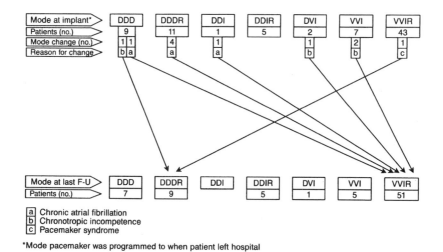

Figure 1. Distribution of pacing modes following AV nodal ablation at the time of pacemaker implantation and at last follow-up. The reasons for mode change included: (**a**) development of chronic AF; (**b**) chronotropic incompetence; and (**c**) pacemaker syndrome. (From Gross et al.[4]).

The authors concluded that the frequent use of VVIR pacing in this population reflected the predominance of chronic AF/flutter as the rhythm requiring ablation. For patients not in chronic AF at the time of AV node ablation, DDDR pacing provides the greatest flexibility for future pacing needs.

Gross et al.[4] analyzed a group of 17 patients that received DDDR pacemakers following ablation. Sixteen of the 17 patients were in normal sinus rhythm (NSR) at the time of pacemaker implantation. During a mean follow-up of 12.5 months (± 12.3 months), 7 of the 17 patients were exclusively in NSR, and 2 of the 17 were exclusively in AF. NSR was detected during 60% of total follow-up visits. One patient that was transiently programmed to VVIR mode developed pacemaker syndrome when she returned to NSR. The authors conclude that a substantial number of patients were predominantly in NSR and that nearly all patients had periods of NSR. They were unable to make any definitive comments regarding long-term efficacy of DDDR pacing in this group of patients or whether DDDR pacing has an effect on the maintenance of NSR.

In a larger series of 228 patients, Wolfe and colleagues[5] assessed long-term outcome of DDDR pacing after AV nodal ablation in patients with paroxysmal AF. Of the 228 patients, 163 underwent ablation for paroxysmal AF and 65 for chronic AF. DDDR pacemakers were placed in 48% of the patients with paroxysmal AF. During a mean follow-up of 13.2 ± 12.9 months, 13 of the 78 patients developed chronic AF and required reprogramming to the VVIR pacing mode. The probability of maintaining DDDR pacing was 0.85 at 1 year and 0.67 at 2 years (Kaplan-Meier analysis). The authors concluded that there is a progressive increase in the number of patients with paroxysmal AF that subsequently develop chronic AF and therefore a decrease in the proportion who can be maintained in the DDDR pacing mode.

Pacemaker utilization was also included in another report from the same institution looking at the role of RF ablation in the management of supraventricular arrhythmias in 760 consecutive patients.[6] Of the 112 patients that required pacing after AV nodal ablation for AF and/or flutter, 62 patients with paroxysmal atrial arrhythmias received DDDR pacemakers and 57 patients, presumably with chronic AF and/or flutter, received VVIR pacing systems. During follow-up, there were no complications specifically related to pacing mode.

A follow-up series was also described by Sadoul et al.[7] Seventy-five patients with drug-refractory atrial flutter and/or AF were paced following AV nodal ablation. Pacing modes were VVIR in 53 (71%), VVI in 12 (16%), DDDR in 5 (6.6%), and DDD in 5 (6.6%). Of the rate-adaptive pacing systems used, 80% were activity sensors and 20% were minute ventilation sensors. At a mean follow-up of 25 months, there were 24 patients (28%) that had not had a recurrence of AF or flutter. Eight of these patients developed pacemaker syndrome and 3 of the 8 were upgraded to DDDR pacing. This led the authors to conclude that in patients with paroxysmal AF or flutter, a dual chamber rate responsive pacemaker with a reliable fallback mechanism should be utilized.

Jensen and colleagues followed 50 patients that underwent RF ablation of the AV node.[8] They reported on 41 patients that received permanent pacemakers including 30 paced VVIR, 6 paced VVI, and 5 paced DDDR. During a mean follow-up of 17 months, 5 patients required pacing mode changes. One patient developed pacemaker syndrome and was upgraded from VVI to DDDR. Details are not provided for 2 patients upgraded from VVIR to DDDR, another patient that was changed from VVI to VVIR, and a final patient that was reprogrammed from DDDR to VVIR. When quality of life was assessed in the 41 surviving patients, 36 reported improvement, 2 were unchanged, and 3 were worse. These subjective outcomes did not specifically reflect the response to pacing but reflected the entire ablation experience and comparison to preablation quality of life.

In the discussion of their results, they state that patients currently undergoing ablation and pacemaker implantation would more often receive dual chamber pacemakers with the capability of mode switching than did patients during the 1990–1992 study recruitment. They recommend VVIR pacing in chronic AF and in patients that do not have self-limiting attacks of AF and require DC cardioversion. DDDR pacing with mode-switching capability is recommended in patients with self-limiting episodes of AF.

More specific recommendations for pacing modes after AV nodal ablation emerged from a series of patients reported by Bernard et al.[9] They retrospectively reviewed 192 patients undergoing AV nodal ablation for various supraventricular arrhythmias. They conclude that rate-adaptive pacing is essential with the exception of those patients ablated for AV node reentry who develop inadvertent high-grade AV block. In this small subset of patients, they believe DDD pacing is adequate. They recommend VVIR pacing for those with atrial flutter, permanent AF, poorly controlled AF, and paroxysmal AF in patients >70 years old and/or male sex, and/or associated advanced cardiac disease. They consider DDDR pacing the mode of choice in sinus node dysfunction and/or in patients <60 years of age, and/or females, and/or with idiopathic arrhythmias, and/or when retrograde ventriculoatrial (VA) conduction persists. They recommend that the DDDR pacemaker chosen have some algorithm for management of endless loop tachycardia in those patients with intact VA conduction. These recommendations appear to be based on comparison of patients with and without chronic arrhythmias at 4 years of follow-up. The mean age of patients with chronic rhythm disturbances was 62 years, 64% were male, and 78% had associated advanced cardiac disease. Fourteen of 28 patients assessed had intact VA conduction. By comparison, the group remaining in NSR had a mean age of 57 years, were 73% female, only 3 patients had associated cardiac disease, and only 2 of 11 patients assessed had intact VA conduction.

In a report of three patients with refractory multifocal atrial tachycardia, DDDR pacing with mode switching was utilized.[10] A mean follow-up of only 4 months was reported, but pacing remained successful at that point and no antiarrhythmic medications had been required.

Emerging Prospective Data

A registry of ablation patients that were prospectively followed, Ablate and Pace Trial (APT), should provide information regarding this group of patients. (Ellenbogen KA, Jensen DN. Personal communication. April, 1996.) The trial recruited patients from twenty US centers and includes 160 patients with data collected at baseline, 3 months, and 12 months. This trial will provide additional information regarding 12-month follow-up of ablated patients, including pacing mode at baseline and follow-up, and reasons for mode changes.

Another trial is underway which may definitively answer many of remaining questions regarding pacing after AV nodal ablation. The "Atrial Pacing (Periablation) in Paroxysmal Atrial Fibrillation Trial" ((PA)³ Trial) is a multicenter Canadian trial that has been designed to determine the effect of atrial-based pacing on the frequency of recurrent paroxysmal atrial rhythm disturbances. Patients identified for ablation receive a DDDR pacemaker 3 months prior to AV nodal ablation. During this 3-month period, they are randomized to either atrial pacing or no pacing. After the AV nodal ablation, they are randomized to either DDDR or VDD pacing mode and then they cross over to the other pacing mode at 6 months. The pacemakers used are capable of mode switching and they also count the number of mode-switch events, allowing the investigators to determine the frequency with which the paroxysmal rhythm disturbance has recurred. (Gillis AM. Personal communication. April, 1996.)

Special Considerations in Implantation Technique

Several issues merit discussion regarding permanent pacemaker implantation in the postablation patient. First, should the pacemaker be implanted before or after the ablation? A temporary pacemaker is usually placed at the beginning of the ablation. There are several published series of patients with a preexistent pacemaker who subsequently underwent AV nodal ablation.[11-15] Potential concerns of AV nodal ablation in the patient with an existing permanent pacemaker include: transient electrical interference with pacemaker function; transient alteration in sensing and/or pacing thresholds; and dislodgement of acutely placed pacing leads by the temporary catheters used for the ablation procedure. There is general agreement that the pacemaker programmer should be available during the ablation procedure, pacemaker telemetry may be helpful in detecting interference, and the pacemaker should be interrogated following the procedure.

Another more complex issue is how to proceed with the patient with a paroxysmal rhythm disturbance that is in the pathological rhythm at the time of pacemaker implantation. Reported options are: cardioversion to normal sinus rhythm allowing implantation of a dual chamber pacemaker, implantation of a single chamber ventricular pacing system, or blindly placing the atrial lead. Because of potential long-term advantages of dual chamber pacing for the patient in whom normal sinus rhythm remains the dominant rhythm, extra effort at the time of implant to allow atrial lead placement is warranted. Most of the experience in this situation is anecdotal. Cardioversion prior to atrial lead placement can be done quickly and safely in most patients. Alternatively, blindly placing an atrial lead during AF is done without knowing whether pacing and/or sensing thresholds are adequate. Reports of this technique are largely anecdotal.

In the future, dual-site atrial pacing may also be a consideration for this group of patients. Small series of patients have been described that have received pacemakers configured to allow simultaneous dual-site atrial pacing for the purpose of decreasing the frequency of paroxysmal AF.[16-19] The proposed mechanism of this technique is beyond the scope of this paper. Early applications of dual-site atrial pacing have met with some success. If this technique is proven beneficial in controlling paroxysmal AF, then some ablation procedures may be obviated. Alternatively, dual-site atrial pacing could be adjunctive in the ablated patient. Pacing the postablation patient with paroxysmal AF with a

DDDR pacemaker configured to dual-site atrial pacing may be advantageous.

Recommendations for Pacemaker Selection

When prescribing a permanent pacemaker for the postablation patient the following factors should be considered: dominant atrial rhythm (chronic vs. paroxysmal rhythm disturbance); atrial rhythm at the time of pacemaker implantation; potential for long-term maintenance of normal sinus rhythm; and cost.

Of the studies described above, none are individually decisive as to the optimal pacing mode following AV nodal ablation. However, several of the studies do reach similar conclusions as does an excellent prior review of the subject.[20] Until the more definitive trials are available, existing studies, as well as conventional wisdom, suggest the following: the pacemaker of choice following AV nodal ablation for chronic AF is VVIR, while the pacemaker of choice following AV nodal ablation for paroxysmal supraventricular rhythm disorders is usually DDDR. Qualifications exist in recommending DDDR pacing following AV nodal ablation. First, the long-term efficacy of dual chamber pacing has not been proven and longer follow-up in larger groups of patients is necessary.

Whether dual chamber pacing results in lower morbidity[21] and/or mortality in this group of patients, as it appears to in the nonablated pacing population, is unknown. Some insight into this question may emerge from an ongoing prospective trial of pacing modes in patients with atrioventricular block (UK PACE). (Camm AJ. Personal communication. March, 1996.)

Consideration should be given to the clinical description of the type and frequency of AF or flutter of the patient to be paced. Suttorp[22] developed a helpful classification of types and frequency of attacks of AF or atrial flutter (Table 1). Although this classification will not determine the appropriate pacing mode, except those classified as chronic/incessant, it may help guide the clinician.

If dual chamber pacing is selected following AV nodal ablation, there is general agreement that the device should have the capability of some form of mode switching.

Mode switching refers to the ability of the pacemaker to automatically change from one mode to another in response to an inappropriately rapid atrial rhythm. Automatic Mode Switching, AMS™ was introduced by Telectronics, Inc. (Englewood, CO).[23] With AMS™, when functioning

Table 1
Types and Frequency of Attacks of Atrial Fibrillation or Atrial Flutter

Types	Modes of Onset and Duration
Paroxysmal AF or Afl	Sporadic, recurrent or frequent
Recent onset	Lasting 24 hours
Long-standing	Lasting 24-hours–6 months
Transient AF or Afl	Acute, during intercurrent trigger/disease
Chronic AF or Afl	Sustained/permanent lasting >6 months
Frequency	
Sporadic (infrequent)	Monthly or less
Recurrent	Weekly
Frequent	Almost daily, up to weekly
Incessant	Daily, covering >12 hours/day

AF = atrial fibrillation; Afl = atrial flutter.
Adapted and reproduced with permission from: Suttorp MJ. Paroxysmal atrial fibrillation and atrial flutter: current concepts and new strategies. State University Groningen: The Netherlands, p 7. Thesis.

in the DDDR mode, the algorithm would automatically reprogram the pacemaker to the VVIR mode if the pacemaker met specific criteria for what it considered a pathological atrial rhythm. In the DDD or DDDR pacing modes, if a supraventricular rhythm disturbance occurs and the pathological atrial rhythm is sensed by the pacemaker, rapid ventricular pacing may occur. Any pacing mode that eliminates tracking of the pathological rhythm, i.e., DDI, DDIR, DVI, DVIR, also eliminates the ability to track normal sinus rhythm which is usually the predominant rhythm. Mode switching avoids this limitation.

Although the original mode switch was from DDDR to VVIR, there are now other mode switch combinations (Table 2).[22-25]

The original AMS® was successful but there were some clinical problems associated with the algorithm, in that the mode-switching criteria were too easily fulfilled, resulting in frequent mode switching. Refinement of subsequent algorithms has made this a very successful feature.

Since the introduction of mode switching, multiple variations of this feature have been developed. One algorithm functions by measuring intervals between atrial events.[26] The pacemaker utilizes a counter that considers a short interval as one that is shorter than the programmed mode-switching rate, and a long interval as one that is longer than the programmed mode-switching rate. When the counter accrues

Table 2
Available Mode-Switching Combinations

- DDDR to DDIR
- DDDR to VVIR
- DDD to DDIR
- DDD to VVI
- VDDR to VVIR
- VDD to VVIR
- VDD to VVI

a specified number of short intervals, the pacemaker reprograms to the VVIR mode and remains in this mode until a specified number of long intervals has occurred and altered the counter, and mode switching reverts.

Another device mode-switches when the mean atrial rate exceeds approximately 180 bpm. Once the mode switch has occurred, the ventricular rate is gradually changed to the sensor-indicated rate. When the mean atrial rate drops below approximately 180 bpm or five consecutive atrial paced events occur, the pacemaker switches back to the programmed atrial tracking mode.[25]

An alternative algorithm provides automatic mode switching from DDDR to VVIR when detected atrial activity exceeds the upper rate limit (URL).[27] Like AMS™, the objective of this feature is to limit the time that the paced ventricular rate is at the URL in response to pathological atrial arrhythmias.

Albeit a significant variation from classic mode switching, yet another method is available to avoid inappropriate tracking of atrial rhythm disturbances by comparing the tracking rate and the sensor-indicated rate.[28] With this feature, the maximum pacing rate in the DDDR or VDDR pacing modes is limited to 35 bpm above the programmed pacing rate (but never less than 80 bpm) in the absence of sensor-driven signals indicating exercise. When exercise is occurring, this interim limit is overridden and the programmed maximum pacing rate is in effect.

One publication specifically assessed the efficacy of mode switching in patients paced following ablation of the AV node for paroxysmal AF.[29] In this relatively small study, 12 patients received a DDDR pacemaker with a mode-switching algorithm based on the heart rate as a whole and on the beat-to-beat changes in atrial rate. If the changes in atrial rate are gradual, they are identified as physiological and do not result in mode switching. If the changes in atrial rate are rapid, mode switching will occur even if the absolute rate is not particularly high. This is different from several of the other algorithms described in that the pathological atrial rhythm is not required to exceed the upper rate limit prior to mode switching.

In this study, an intrapatient comparison was made between the DDDR mode without mode switching programmed "on" and DDDR/DDIR with mode switching activated. Ventricular tracking of AF occurred in 35% of total beats at rest and 24% of total beats during exercise when mode switching was not activated. With mode switching, ventricular tracking of AF occurred in 4% of total beats at rest and 2% of total beats during exercise.

In most countries, it is difficult to disassociate the issue of cost from pacemaker selection. Cost analyses are difficult for many reasons. Pacemaker hardware costs vary significantly among different parts of the world and even within different geographic areas of the same country. Also, because there are no conclusive studies showing DDDR efficacy in ablated patients, or studies demonstrating significant mode-related complications with VVIR pacing, no cost analysis has been done in this group of patients. There are prior cost analyses of single versus dual chamber pacing in the general pacing population which demonstrate that more than initial hardware costs must be taken into account when comparing single and dual chamber pacing. For example, a larger number of initial single chamber pacemakers will obviously lower the initial costs. However, if several of these patients require rehospitalization and reoperation to upgrade to a dual chamber pacing system for pacemaker syndrome, the overall costs are altered significantly.

In several of the studies discussed previously in this chapter, there were patients that initially received single chamber pacemakers that later required an upgrade to a dual chamber system. Therefore, despite the higher initial cost and despite the lack of unequivocal proof of long-term efficacy of dual chamber pacing in the ablated patient, the potential clinical benefits offered by the flexibility of DDDR pacemakers cannot be denied.

Summary

Following AV nodal ablation, a rate-adaptive pacemaker should be used in the majority of patients. The only patients that might not require rate adaptation are those ablated for a rapid nodal pathway. Even in this group, the long-term flexibility of a pacemaker with rate-adaptive capabilities is probably desirable.

In the absence of data from a prospective study in which post-AV nodal ablation patients are randomized to DDDR versus VVIR, the optimal pacing mode must be decided on the basis of the patient's clinical features and existing retrospective literature.

The patient with chronic AF/flutter is best served with a VVIR pacemaker. DDDR pacing offers the greatest flexibility in the patient with a paroxysmal supraventricular rhythm disturbance in whom normal sinus rhythm is the dominant rhythm. The DDDR device chosen should have the capability of some type of mode switching to accommodate the patient when the paroxysmal atrial rhythm disturbance recurs.

If the patient arrives for pacemaker implantation in the atrial rhythm disturbance, it seems reasonable to attempt restoration of normal sinus rhythm by cardioversion and proceed with DDDR pacemaker placement. This again assumes that normal sinus rhythm is the dominant rhythm. Placement of an atrial lead blindly during the atrial rhythm disturbance has been performed. The data supporting this technique are too limited to advocate its practice at this time.

The APT Trial and the PA^3 Trial should allow more definitive guidelines for pacemaker selection following AV nodal ablation. Until this information is available, an approach has been suggested using DDDR devices with mode-switching capability in patients ablated for paroxysmal atrial rhythm disturbances and VVIR devices for those with chronic atrial rhythm disturbances.

References

1. Bernstein AD, Parsonnet V. Survey of cardiac pacing and defibrillation in the United States in 1993. Am J Cardiol 1996;78:178–196.
2. Brignole M, Menozzi C. Control of rapid heart rate in patients with atrial fibrillation: drugs or ablation? PACE 1996;19:348–356.
3. Rajamannan NM, Neubauer SA, Hayes DL, et al. Permanent pacing following AV nodal ablation. PACE 1994;17:770. Abstract.
4. Gross JN, Roth JA, Ben-Zur UM, et al. DDDR pacing post AV node ablation: a reasonable strategy or an exercise in futility? PACE 1994;17:769. Abstract.
5. Wolfe DA, McLaughlin S, Windecker S, et al. DDDR pacing following AV Nodal ablation: long-term outcome in patients with paroxysmal atrial fibrillation. PACE 1994;17:862. Abstract.
6. Kay GN, Epstein AE, Dailey SM, et al. Role of radiofrequency ablation in the management of supraventricular arrhythmias: experience in 760 consecutive patients. J Cardiovasc Electrophysiol 1993;4:371–389.
7. Sadoul N, Dodinot B, de Chillou C, et al. Pacemaker selection after atrioventricular node ablation. PACE 1994;17:770. Abstract.

8. Jensen SM, Bergfeldt L, Rosenqvist M. Long-term follow-up of patients treated by radiofrequency ablation of the atrioventricular junction. PACE 1995;18:1609–1614.

9. Bernard V, Clementy J, Gencel L, et al. Choix du mode de stimulation apres ablation du faisceau de His. Arch Mal Coeur 1994;87:1581–1587.

10. Tucker KJ, Law J, Rodriques MJ. Treatment of refractory recurrent multifocal atrial tachycardia with atrioventricular junction ablation and permanent pacing. J Invas Cardiol 1995;7:207–212.

11. Chin MC, Rosenqvist M, Lee MA, et al. The effect of radiofrequency catheter ablation on permanent pacemakers: an experimental study. PACE 1990;13:23–29.

12. Pfeiffer D, Tebbenjohanns J, Jung W, et al. Pacemaker function during radiofrequency ablation. PACE 1993;16:882. Abstract.

13. Chang AC, McAreavey D, Tripodi D, et al. Radiofrequency catheter atrioventricular node ablation in patients with permanent cardiac pacing systems. PACE 1994;17:65–69.

14. Ellenbogen KA, Wood MA, Stambler BS, et al. Effects of radiofrequency ablation on implanted pacing systems. PACE 1994;17:770. Abstract.

15. van Gelder BM, Bracke FALE, El Gamal MIH. Upper rate pacing after radiofrequency catheter ablation in a minute ventilation rate adaptive DDD pacemaker. PACE 1994;17:1437–1440.

16. Daubert C, Mabo P, Berder V, et al. Atrial tachyarrhythmias associated with high degree interatrial conduction block: prevention by permanent atrial resynchronisation. Eur J Cardiac Pacing Electrophysiol 1994;1: 35–44.

17. Prakash A, Saksena S, Giogberidze I, et al. Arrhythmia recurrence patterns during atrial pacing. JACC 1996;27:74A. Abstract.

18. Daubert C, Gras D, Leclercq C, et al. Biatrial synchronous pacing: a new approach for prevention of drug refractory atrial flutter. Circulation 1995; 92:532. Abstract.

19. Sopher SM, Murgatroyd FD, Slade AKB, et al. Dual site atrial pacing promotes sinus rhythm in paroxysmal atrial fibrillation. Circulation 1995;92: 532. Abstract.

20. van Hemel NM. The interplay between radiofrequency catheter ablation of arrhythmias and cardiac pacing. In: van Hemel NM, Wittkampf FHM, Ector H, eds. Developments in Cardiovascular Medicine, Vol. 175: The Pacemaker Clinic of the 90's. Essentials in Brady-Pacing. Dordrecht, The Netherlands: Kluwer Academic Publishers; 1995:199–214.

21. Andersen HR, Thuesen L, Bagger JP, et al. Prospective randomised trial of atrial versus ventricular pacing in sick-sinus syndrome. Lancet 1994; 344:1523–1528.

22. Suttorp MJ. Paroxysmal atrial fibrillation and atrial flutter: current concepts and new strategies. State University Groningen: The Netherlands; pg.7. Thesis.

23. Meta™ DDDR 1250H Multiprogrammable Minute Ventilation, Rate Responsive Pulse Generator with Telemetry. Physician's Manual. Telectronics Pacing Systems, Englewood, CO, 1991.

24. VIGOR™ DDD Model 950/955. Physician's Manual. Cardiac Pacemakers, Inc, St. Paul, MN, 1994.

25. THERA® DR 7940/41/42/50/51/52 Product Information Manual. Medtronic®, Inc, Minneapolis, MN, 1994.
26. META™ DDDR 1254. User's Guide. Telectronics Pacing Systems, Englewood, CO, 1993.
27. VIGOR™ DR Model 1230/1235. Physician's Manual. Cardiac Pacemakers, Inc, St. Paul, MN, 1995.
28. Relay™ 293–03 and 293–04 Cardiac Pulse Generator. Physician's Manual. Intermedics, Inc, Angleton, TX, 1992.
29. Brignole M, Gianfranchi L, Menozzi C, et al. A new pacemaker for paroxysmal atrial fibrillation treated with radiofrequency ablation of the AV junction. PACE 17;1994:1889–1894.

CHAPTER 10

Ventricular Pacing for Rate Control in Atrial Fibrillation

Chu-Pak Lau

Introduction

The hallmark of atrial fibrillation (AF) is an irregularly irregular ventricular response. Although restoration of sinus rhythm is theoretically the most ideal therapy, in many patients ventricular rate control remains the mainstay of treatment. Patients with long-standing AF have a reduced chance of conversion to sinus rhythm by either chemical or electrical means.[1] Even with the use of the more efficacious transvenous atrial defibrillation, advanced age and long-standing AF are unfavorable prognostic factors for successful defibrillation, probably due to pathological changes in the atria.[2] In addition, long-term maintenance of sinus rhythm is difficult, and the use of medication may be associated with proarrhythmogenic side effects.[3] There is also a general reluctance in hospital general medical practice to restore sinus rhythm, and rate control has been used in the majority of patients presenting with AF.[4] In patients with paroxysmal AF in which maintenance of sinus rhythm is the treatment of choice, additional rate control therapy is often required for breakthrough episodes.[5]

Thus, for the majority of patients with both paroxysmal and chronic AF, ventricular rate control is either the sole or an adjunctive therapy. Conventional drug therapy such as digoxin does not control ventricular rate during exercise, and patients with paroxysmal AF who are on digoxin have paradoxically longer episodes of AF without an effect on the ventricular rate during a recurrence.[5] Although beta-blockers and calcium channel blockers may be more effective to control ventricular response during exercise, their use is often associated with depressed cardiopulmonary performance. Indeed, oxygen transport kinetics

From *Nonpharmacological Management of Atrial Fibrillation*, edited by F.D. Murgatroyd and A.J. Camm. © 1997, Futura Publishing Co., Inc., Armonk, NY.

which reflects daily activities is depressed in AF and further reduced with beta-blockers.[6] As a result, nonpharmacological therapy to control ventricular response for AF is an attractive alternative.

Hemodynamic Considerations

The adverse hemodynamic consequences of AF are: (1) ineffectively contracting atrium; (2) an irregular ventricular response; and (3) inappropriate ventricular rate.

Resting Hemodynamics

The above issues have been investigated in open chest, heart-blocked dogs.[7,8] In an early study,[7] it was reported that irregular ventricular response might increase cardiac output compared with a regular rhythm in the presence of sympathetic blockade. This was postulated to be due to prolongation of effective left ventricular filling time during fast AF, as some of the early ventricular responses did not induce an effective stroke output. In addition, a positive inotropic effect following a closely coupled beat may further augment stroke volume. A subsequent study has used dogs with an intact autonomic nervous system.[8] At a ventricular pacing interval of 400 ms, the occurrence of AF was associated with a significant reduction of cardiac output of about 20% due to ineffective atrial contraction. However, ventricular irregularity itself significantly reduced cardiac output, both during AF and during atrioventricular (AV) synchronous pacing. Ventricular irregularity alone becomes unimportant during AV dissociation or when the AV interval is abnormal. The induction of mitral valve regurgitation by irregularity in ventricular rhythm was considered to reduce cardiac output. In a recent study of 10 patients with paroxysmal AF undergoing radiofrequency AV nodal ablation, ventricular irregularity was also found to result in a reduction in cardiac output.[9]

In the presence of intact AV conduction, however, the increase in ventricular rate during AF counteracts some of the harmful effects of ineffective atrial contraction and ventricular irregularity. A number of studies have addressed the hemodynamics of AF compared to sinus rhythm, but there has been a general lack of consistency in the results. The limitations of these studies included the heterogeneity of the populations studied, especially the presence or absence of ischemic and rheumatic heart diseases. Furthermore, the comparisons were made with sinus rhythm restored by cardioversion, and the results were necessarily influenced by the use of anesthetic agents and the time taken for atrial function to recover. In addition, the relevance of these hemodynamic changes after electrical conversion to those occurring at the onset of AF is questionable.

The effect of induced AF on cardiac hemodynamics has recently been investigated in 10 patients without structural heart disease.[10] AF was electrically induced and cardiac hemodynamics were compared to atrial and ventricular pacing at a rate identical to AF. Compared with sinus rhythm, the onset of AF was associated with a reduction in systolic blood pressure. However, there were no consistent changes in cardiac output at the onset of AF compared with sinus rhythm, but cardiac output was lower compared with regular atrial pacing at rates similar to those of induced AF (Fig. 1).

Compared with sinus rhythm or rate-matched atrial pacing, AF was associated with an elevated pulmonary arterial and wedge pressure. As in an animal study,[8] the hemodynamic changes during AF were similar to those seen during regular ventricular pacing with AV dissociation at an equivalent rate, although the latter was associated with a lower systolic blood pressure and higher right atrial pressure due to persistent (ventriculoatrial) VA conduction. Myocardial lactate extraction was similar during sinus rhythm, atrial pacing, and AF, but tended to be higher during regular ventricular pacing.

Exercise Hemodynamics

During exercise, cardiac output increases about three times compared with rest, and most of this increase is mediated by an increase in rate rather than by maintenance of AV synchrony.[11] Thus, the loss of effective atrial contraction during AF becomes less important during exercise. An inappropriate chronotropic response occurs in AF,[12] especially when metabolic reserve is used as a standard for rate response. Figure 2 shows the pattern of chronotropic response in patients with AF, with some patients exhibiting an exaggerated, some reduced, and the majority of patients, an irregular response with respect to metabolic reserve. The relative incidence of these chronotropic response patterns and the influence on exercise capacity are probably dependent on the population of patients studied. For instance, chronotropic incompetence probably occurs in most patients after AV nodal ablation. In pacemaker patients without prior AV nodal ablation, a 74% response of hyperchronotropicity at some stages of exercise was reported,[12] whereas chrono-

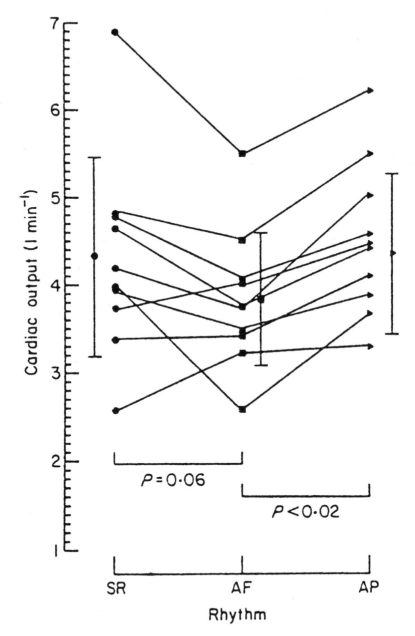

Figure 1. Individual values of cardiac output in 10 patients during sinus rhythm (SR), rate matched atrial pacing (AP) and during AF. (Reproduced with permission from Lau et al.[10])

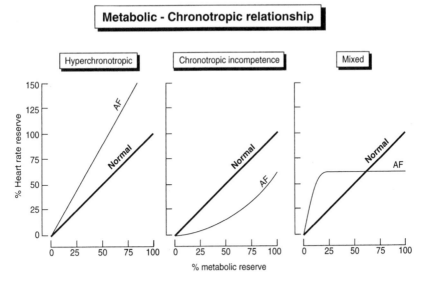

Figure 2. Pattern of chronotropic response to exercise as a function of metabolic reserve.

tropic incompetence was observed during early stages of exercise in 21% of patients. The variable patterns of chronotropic response and presence of underlying cardiac diseases probably determine the exercise capacity in patients with AF. Thus, previous studies have reported a variable influence of AF on exercise cardiopulmonary function, ranging from severely impaired to almost normal exercise capacity in patients with lone AF. Using an age and sex matched control, however, we have shown that cardiopulmonary exercise capacity in lone AF was reduced.[6] In addition, the ineffective atrial contraction played a significant role in impairing early oxygen transport to the tissues during exercise, which may contribute to impaired daily activities and symptoms in patients with AF.[6] The role of rate irregularity alone on exercise remains to be investigated.

Thus, at rest, the loss of effective atrial contraction in AF reduced stroke volume by 20%, although this may be compensated by an increase in resting heart rate. In patients with persistent AF and normal left ventricular function, improvement in regularity seems to be the goal of therapy. An increase in ventricular rate may not be important in patients with normal structural heart disease and may be considered as a "compensatory" response, but it may be detrimental in these patients. During exercise, the loss of an effectively contracting atrium becomes less important; the maintenance of an appropriate chrono-tropic response is the most important goal of pacing therapy during AF.

Pacing Methods for Rate Control

During atrial flutter, ventricular rate can be difficult to control due to 2:1 AV conduction. In a patient with persistent flutter and tachycardia-induced cardiomyopathy, a specially designed atrial pacemaker with rapid atrial pacing capability (600 bpm) was used to artificially induce and maintain AF (Table 1).[13] The induced AF was hemodynamically much better tolerated than atrial flutter. Although an interesting concept, treatment of similar patients can now be effected by either radiofrequency ablation of the AV node or the flutter itself.

AF developed in a substantial proportion of dual chamber paced patients with either sinoatrial disease or heart block. A rapid ventricular response will occur if AF is tracked in the conventional DDD mode. A number of pacemaker algorithms are now implemented in dual chamber devices which either change to a nonatrial tracking mode (auto-

Table 1
Pacing Methods for Rate Control in Atrial Fibrillation

Methods	Principle
Atrial pacing	1. To induce and maintain AF in rapidly conducting atrial flutter. 2. ? Pacing to terminate AF.
Automatic mode/rate conversion	Control ventricular response in dual chamber paced patients during AF by changing to a different pacemaker mode or a reduced upper rate.
Rate adaptive pacing	Increase ventricular rate in slow AF.
Intercalated ventricular pacing	Induction of compensatory pause by ventricular pacing for each conducted AF beat, thus prolonging diastole and control rate and regularity.
Overdrive ventricular pacing	Ventricular rate stabilization by right ventricular pacing at a rate faster than the mean AF rate which abolishes short cycles during AF.

matic mode conversion) or a reduced upper tracking rate (automatic rate conversion).[14] In patients with slow AF at rest and during exercise, the use of an implanted sensor to increase ventricular rate will improve cardiac hemodynamics, exercise capacity, and quality of life over constant rate ventricular pacing.[15] However, in patients with relatively fast AF, the concept of bradycardia support ventricular pacing will not control the spontaneous rapid ventricular rate response. Two recently available ventricular pacing techniques have been studied to control both the rate and regularity of AF.

Intercalated Ventricular Pacing (IVP)

It is a well-known clinical observation that randomly occurring ventricular ectopic contractions can prolong the compensatory pause during AF. In 1965, Langendorf suggested that this effect was due to concealed AV conduction.[16] With the development of techniques of cardiac pacing and electrophysiological studies, it becomes possible to artificially introduce a ventricular stimulus after a sensed conducted beat at desired coupling intervals. The effects on the regularity, pulse rate control, and cardiac hemodynamics during a pacing protocol in which a regularly introduced ventricular stimulus was effected for every conducted beat during AF were investigated (Fig. 3).[17] Successful intercalation was achieved in all patients, although to varying extent (mean 86 ± 14%, range 64 to 100%). The best interval for IVP was achieved at 232 ± 28 ms, which was slightly longer than the ventricular effective refractory period (217 ± 21 ms). Shortening of the coupling interval by more than 20 ms resulted in failure of successful intercalation and rate control, but lengthening of this interval by 50 ms did not reduce the efficacy of IVP (Fig. 4). IVP effectively reduced the pulse rate from 137 ± 26 bpm to 75 ± 14 bpm ($P<0.001$) and the rhythm regularized.

Hemodynamic Effects

Compared with AF, there was an increase in systolic arterial pressure and a decrease in diastolic pressure, but no change in mean blood pressure after pacing. Variabilities in pulse-to-pulse systolic and diastolic pressures were also reduced (from 23 ± 6 mm Hg to 17 ± 7 mm Hg, $P<0.01$ and from 10 ± 2 mm Hg to 6 ± 2 mm Hg, $P<0.001$, respectively).

A small reduction in cardiac output during IVP compared with AF

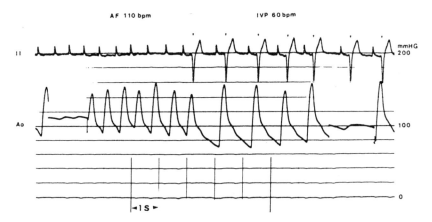

Figure 3. Selected ECG and arterial pressure recordings from a patient with lone AF. AF with a mean ventricular rate of 110 bpm is shown on the left. Intercalated ventricular paced beats (IVP, arrows) were then introduced after every conducted beat in AF at a coupling interval of 320 ms. This resulted in fusion of the arterial pulses between the conducted and paced beat, with resultant pulse rate reduction to 60 bpm. Note the regularization in the pulses, and increase of the pulse pressure. Ao = femoral arterial pressure; II = lead II of electrocardiogram. (Reproduced with permission from Lau et al.[17])

as a result of a reduction in heart rate (from 3.7 ± 0.7 L/min to 3.3 ± 0.8 L/min, $P<0.001$). However, in five patients with a rate of ≥150 beats/min during AF, cardiac output was either unchanged (three patients) or higher (two patients) during pacing, indicating an increased effectiveness at high heart rate. In addition, the mean stroke volume was considerably higher during pacing and myocardial extraction state was not affected during IVP. In five patients with mitral stenosis, IVP resulted in an increase in cardiac output and a reduction of transmitral valvular gradient.

Figure 4. Pulse rate and the percent of patients achieving successful intercalation as a function of the coupling interval. Increasing the coupling interval from the best interval for up to 50 ms did not significantly affect the pulse rate or the effectiveness of coupling, although shortening of the coupling interval by 10 ms to 20 ms significantly affected both parameters. P values were derived by paired comparisons with the corresponding values achieved at best coupling interval. IVP = intercalated ventricular paced beats. (Reproduced with permission from Wittkampf et al.[18])

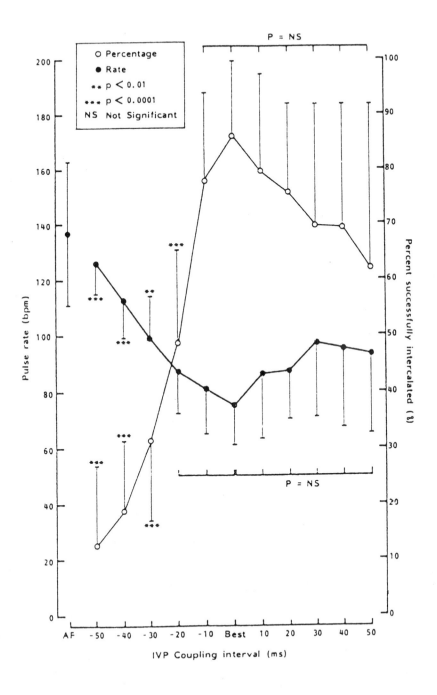

Mechanism of Pulse Rate Control by IVP

Because the paced beat did not result in an effective pulse, the major contribution to the reduction in pulse rate was determined by the coupling interval (mean 232 ms) used in achieving IVP. The mean cycle length of AF was a function of the concealed antegrade AV conduction consequent on rapid atrial stimulation of the AV node. If concealed retrograde penetration was induced by pacing, the mean postpacing -R interval should be a reflection of both concealed antegrade and retrograde conduction. A difference of 82 ± 44 ms between the means of RR and postpacing -R intervals was found, which is a representation of the extent of induced concealed VA conduction.

Applications and Limitations

This technique allows rapid rate control and regularizes RR intervals during AF. It may be useful in patients with rapid AF who require immediate rate control for hemodynamic reasons, e.g., after cardiac surgery with epicardial pacing wire in situ, while giving time for antiarrhythmic agents to act.

The potential risk of inducing ventricular arrhythmia cannot be excluded, although the range of IVP interval is wide and extends beyond the ventricular effective refractory period. The usefulness of this algorithm during exercise remains to be investigated.

Overdrive Ventricular Pacing

It was observed that regular right ventricular pacing not only abolished the long RR cycle during AF, but also unexpectedly eliminated the shorter cycles.[18,19] In 13 patients with AF who had implanted VVI pacemakers, it was observed that >95% of right ventricular capture was effected at a pacing cycle length longer than the shortest RR but slightly above the mean RR interval (Fig. 5). Based on this concept, two different ventricular stabilization algorithms have been proposed to regularize ventricular response (Fig. 6).

Ventricular Rate Stabilization Algorithms

In 10 patients with AF implanted pacemakers, Wittkampf et al.[19] reported an algorithm to regularize the RR interval during AF. Follow-

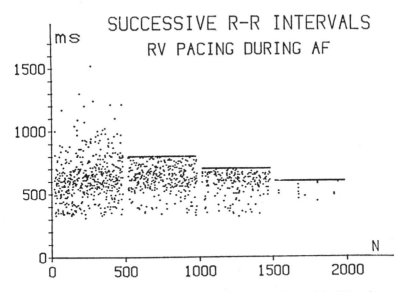

Figure 5. Four episodes of 500 RR intervals in a patient with AF and normal AV conduction and paced at pacing intervals of 2000, 800, 700, and 600 ms, respectively. Pacing at 600 ms abolished most of the short cycles below 500 ms. (Reproduced with permission from Wittkampf et al.[19])

ing each sensed beat, the pacemaker decreases its pacing interval by 10 ms, but the pacing interval will increase by 1 ms after a paced beat. As a result, the pacing rate will always adjust itself in such a way that 9% of all R waves are conducted and that the remaining 91% are paced. When the sense-to-pace ratio is 1:9, the pacing interval will decrease by 10 ms and increase by 9 ms, resulting in an overall 1 ms decrease of the pacing interval every 10 beats and a decrease in the number of conducted R waves. With a ratio of 1:11, the result will be an increase of the pacing interval by 1 ms every 12 beats and an increase in the number of conducted R waves, so stabilization will occur at a ratio of 1:10. The same results can be obtained with steps of 100 ms and 10 ms respectively, but then the fluctuations in pacing interval are 10 times faster than with 10 ms and 1 ms. An increase of 1 ms per beat will cause a change from 100 bpm to 70 bpm in 3 minutes at 100% pacing. The pacing rate algorithm has to be protected by setting lower and upper rate limits, to avoid high rate pacing. At rest the mean value of RR interval instability was reduced from 21% without pacing to 1.5% during the stabilization pacing algorithm (at 93%)[19]. At the cost of a 2%

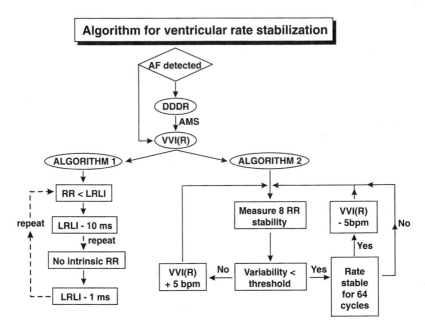

Figure 6. Two algorithms for ventricular rate stabilization pacing. In algorithm 1 (Vitatron BV, Dieren, the Netherlands), a ratio of paced to conducted beats can be set by using an interval increment and decrement function on a beat-to-beat basis. In algorithm 2 (Telectronics Pacing Systems, Englewood, CO), an average rate was calculated for every 8 cycles, and a rate regularization threshold is used to determine whether the pacing rate should increase or not.

increase in mean heart rate, a threefold reduction of the RR instability results.

Using an average of eight RR intervals to assess variability, Greenhut et al.[20] reported an algorithm which increases the ventricular rate by 5 bpm for a programmable variability threshold. Variability threshold is defined as the mean absolute difference between eight consecutive RR intervals and expressed as a percentage of the mean pacing cycle length. If the RR variability was less than the programmed variability threshold for 64–128 RR intervals, the pacing rate was increased by 5 bpm. A variability threshold of 10% was reported as a trade-off between the magnitude of rate increase and the regularity achieved.

Hemodynamic Effects

Preliminary evaluation of ventricular rate stabilization algorithms in pacemaker patients has been studied.[21] In patients with rapid AF, a threshold variability of 5%, 10%, or 20% was tested, and cardiac output was invasively measured. At a variability threshold of 5%, cardiac output was significantly higher compared with spontaneous AF, although the pulmonary wedge pressure was unchanged. Pacing at 10% and 20% variability thresholds further improved the RR coefficient of variability. However, although effective acutely, this algorithm did not affect the acute symptomatology and patient well-being in a randomized study over backup ventricular pacing mode.[21]

We have studied the changes in the pacing interval required to achieve rate regularization during different daily activities and exercise.[22] Pacing intervals to achieve 95% right ventricular capture were shortest during standing compared to either supine position or sitting, and further reduction was required during exercise. However, to achieve about 90% to 95% complete right ventricular pacing, the mean pacing interval was significantly longer than the minimum RR interval and slightly shorter than the mean RR interval in all postures. In a randomized comparison of 15 patients with AF paced with overdrive pacing versus the VVI mode, it was shown that rate regularity was significantly improved, and the maximum oxygen consumption was significantly better than intrinsic AF alone. However, the ability to regularize shorter RR intervals was reduced during exercise.

Mechanism of Overdrive Ventricular Pacing

The induction of concealed VA conduction was generally recognized to be the principle of ventricular rate slowing.[16] However, an electronically modulated automatic nodal pacemaker was postulated as the alternative explanation.[18] During right ventricular pacing, retrogradely conducted and well-organized impulses could depolarize and reset such a pacemaker focus. However, the patient population studied with implanted pacemakers has relatively long RR cycle lengths, and 13 patients were on antiarrhythmic agents. In a more recent study in open chest dogs,[23] RR intervals shorter than 120 ms were less successfully suppressed by overdrive ventricular pacing, which did not support the occurrence of an electrotonically modulated pacemaker at least at high rate setting.

Clinical Applications and Limitations

Ventricular rate regularity algorithm represents a simple means by which rate regularization can be achieved in AF. This algorithm can be incorporated in simple VVIR devices for patients with AF, and in a

DDDR device as an adjunct to automatic mode switching to the VVIR mode (Fig. 6). However, this algorithm suffers from the limitation that the mean pacing rate was actually increased compared with the spontaneous rhythm, which may increase the level of myocardial oxygen consumption. In addition, the success during rapid AF was further reduced unless a higher pacing rate was used. Furthermore, the utility of this technique in the general population of patients with AF without a pacemaker is unknown. The clinical usefulness of this principle and the long-term effect on left ventricular function remain to be evaluated.

Conclusion

A significant proportion of patients with AF will require ventricular rate control. The goals of rate control are enhancement of regularity and normalization of chronotropic response. Ventricular pacing using either paired or I overdrive pacing significantly regularizes RR intervals in AF, and may be an adjunct to patients with chronic or paroxysmal AF with implanted pacemakers. However, especially with overdrive ventricular pacing, this technique does not reduce the rapid rate response associated with AF.

References

1. Kwbac G, Malowany L. Functional capacity of patients with atrial fibrillation and controlled heart rate before and after cardioversion. Can J Cardiol 1992;8:941–946.
2. Lok NS, Lau CP. Hemodynamic effects and clinical predictors of low energy transvenous atrial defibrillation. PACE 1997. In press.
3. Coplen SE, Antmann EM, Berlin JA, et al. Efficacy and safety of quinidine therapy for maintenance of sinus rhythm after cardioversion: a meta-analysis of randomized controlled trials. Circulation 1990;82:1106–1116.
4. Lok NS, Lau CP. Presentation and management of patients admitted with atrial fibrillation: a review of 291 cases in a regional hospital. Int J Cardiol 1995;48:271–278.
5. Rawles JM, Metcalfe MJ, Jennings K. Time of occurrence, duration and ventricular rate of paroxysmal atrial fibrillation: the effect of digoxin. Br Heart J 1990;63:225–227.
6. Lok NS, Lau CP. Oxygen uptake kinetics and cardiopulmonary performance of lone atrial fibrillation and the effects of sotalol. Chest 1997. In press.
7. Millar K, Eich RH, Burgess JM, Abildskov JA. Enhancement of cardiac output by irregular rhythm. Circulation 1969;39:III-146. Abstract.
8. Naito M, David D, Michelson EL, et al. The hemodynamic consequences

of cardiac arrhythmias: evaluation of the relative roles of abnormal atrioventricular sequencing, irregularity of ventricular rhythm and atrial fibrillation in a canine model. Am Heart J 1983; 284–291.

9. Clark DM, Plumb VJ, Kay GN. The hemodynamics of atrial fibrillation: the independent effect of an irregular RR interval. Circulation 1995;92: I–141. Abstract.

10. Lau CP, Leung WH, Wong CK, Cheng CH. Haemodynamics of induced AF: a comparative assessment with sinus rhythm, atrial and ventricular pacing. Eur Heart J 1990;11:219–224.

11. Karlof I. Haemodynamic effect of atrial triggered versus fixed rate pacing at rest and during exercise in complete heart block. Acta Med Scand 1975; 197:195–206.

12. Corbelli R, Masterson M, Wilkoff BL. Chronotropic response to exercise in patients with atrial fibrillation. PACE 1990;13:179–187.

13. Moreira DAR, Shepard RB, Waldo AL. Chronic rapid atrial pacing to maintain atrial fibrillation: use to permit control of ventricular rate in order to treat tachycardia induced cardiomyopathy. PACE 1989;12:761–775.

14. Lau CP, Tai YT, Fong PC, et al. The use of implantable sensors for the control of pacemaker mediated tachycardias: a comparative evaluation between minute ventilation sensing and acceleration sensing dual chamber rate adaptive pacemakers. PACE 1992;15:34–44.

15. Lau CP, Butrous GS, Ward DE, Camm AJ. Comparative assessment of exercise performance of six different rate adaptive right ventricular cardiac pacemakers. Am J Cardiol 1989;63:833–839.

16. Langendorf R, Pick A, Katz LN. Ventricular response in atrial fibrillation: role of concealed conduction in the AV junction. Circulation 1965;32:69–75.

17. Lau CP, Leung WH, Wong CK, et al. A new pacing method for rapid regularization and rate control in atrial fibrillation. Am J Cardiol 1990;65: 1198–1203.

18. Wittkampf FHM, de Jongste MJL, Lie HI, Meijler FL. Effect of right ventricular pacing on ventricular rhythm during atrial fibrillation. J Am Coll Cardiol 1988;11:539–545.

19. Wittkampf FHM, de Jongste MJL. Rate stabilization by right ventricular pacing in patients with atrial fibrillation. PACE 1986;9:1147–1153.

20. Greenhut S, Dawson A, Steinhaus B. Effectiveness of a ventricular rate stabilization algorithm during atrial fibrillation in dogs. PACE 1995;18: 810. Abstract.

21. Fraser J, Greenhut S, Steinhaus B, et al. Acute effectiveness of ventricular rate stabilization in pacemaker patients with atrial fibrillation. PACE 1996;19:720. Abstract.

22. Jiang ZY, Lau CP, Tang MO. Effect of right ventricular rate adaptive pacing on rate regularity in atrial fibrillation. PACE 1996;19:698. Abstract.

23. Vereckei A, Vera Z, Pride HP, Zipes D. Atrioventricular nodal conduction rather than automaticity determines the ventricular rate during atrial fibrillation and atrial flutter. J Cardiovasc Electrophysiol 1992;3:534–543.

CHAPTER 11

Current Trials in the Management of Atrial Fibrillation:

Atrial Pacing Trial and Investigation of Rhythm Management Trial

D. George Wyse

Much of the excitement engendered by new knowledge is tempered by the realization that there is much to be done before the promise of such knowledge is widely applied. The use of powerful antiarrhythmic drugs to suppress ventricular premature depolarizations (VPDs) after recent myocardial infarction prior to the results of the Cardiac Arrhythmia Suppression Trial,[1] is an example of the pitfalls which can arise through application of knowledge that has been incompletely evaluated. As cost has become an increasingly important consideration in the selection of therapeutic strategies, the imperative to practice "evidence-based" medicine has become more acute. The premier evidence for such an approach comes from well-executed randomized clinical trials and, in that regard, scrutiny of the management of atrial fibrillation (AF) is no exception.

This chapter will describe two areas where randomized clinical trials in the management of AF are developing. It will do so by outlining two trials that are currently in progress. Therefore, it will be largely descriptive and there will be a dearth of data. Brief reference will also be made to other related trials known to the author which are in the planning stage or have just begun. The two randomized trials to be described here are quite different in scope and purpose. Accordingly, the chapter will have two distinct sections: an atrial pacing trial and an investigation of maintaining sinus rhythm versus heart control alone.

From *Nonpharmacological Management of Atrial Fibrillation*, edited by F.D. Murgatroyd and A.J. Camm. © 1997, Futura Publishing Co., Inc., Armonk, NY.

Atrial Pacing Trial

There is considerable interest in the role of pacing the atria to control AF, maintain rhythm, and thereby preserve atrioventricular (AV) synchrony. Other chapters will focus on the details of optimal atrial pacing. The major clinical basis for such an approach is largely based on recent trials such as one in which patients with sick sinus syndrome were randomized to AAI or VVI pacing.[2] In that trial, there was much less AF and fewer thromboembolic events in those randomized to AAI pacing. The rationale for considering atrial pacing to control AF includes the possibility that atrial pacing could alter the substrate for AF and/or it could suppress triggers of AF. The substrate may be altered by decreasing dispersion of atrial repolarization during episodes of relative bradycardia. Furthermore, maintenance of AV synchrony may help prevent stretch-induced shortening of the atrial effective refractory period. The characteristic shortening of atrial effective refractory period as a key factor in the notion that "atrial fibrillation begets atrial fibrillation" is well-known.[3] With respect to triggers, atrial pacing at higher than customary rates ($\geq$70 pulses per minute) and restoration of brisk rate responsiveness with exercise may reduce the frequency of atrial premature beats that often initiates AF.

In 1994, a group of Canadian electrophysiology centers initiated a study to examine the role of atrial pacing in control of paroxysmal AF. The study is entitled, "Atrial Pacing (Periablation) in Paroxysmal Atrial Fibrillation" ((PA)[3] Trial). The two phases of the study will be outlined below.

The primary endpoint in both phases is the time to onset of the first episode of sustained AF. The secondary endpoints include the frequency of paroxysmal AF in phase 1 and the frequency and duration of AF in phase 2. In addition, there are two major substudies which will examine: (1) quality of life and functional capacity, using standardized questionnaires and the 6-minute walk test; and (2) heart chamber size, using echocardiography. The hypothesis for the primary endpoint is the null hypothesis, and the sample size calculated for that endpoint is 50 patients in each arm of the study.

In order to be included in the study, subjects must have had three or more episodes of paroxysmal AF in the past year. At least one of these episodes must be documented by an ECG to last continuously for 5 minutes or more. The subject must also have documented resistance or intolerance to medical therapy of a sufficient nature such that ablation of the AV node has been proposed as definitive therapy. For the echocardiography substudy, a two-dimensional echocardiogram must have been done within 6 months of enrollment. The exclusion criteria include: age less than 18 years, life expectancy less than 1 year, chronic and persistent AF, isolated atrial flutter, reversible causes for AF, and inability to comply with follow-up. The study and its consent form have been approved by each center's Institutional Review Board.

A schema for the main study is outlined in Figure 1. After qualification and consent, a mode-switching, multimodal, dual chamber pacemaker with extensive telemetry capability (Medtronic Thera®DR) is implanted. There are two phases in the study. In the first phase, the patients are randomly assigned to rate-responsive atrial pacing (DDIR) at a low rate of 70 pulses per minute or "no atrial pacing" (DDI, rate 30 pulses per minute). The DDI mode of atrial pacing was selected to allow utilization of the device's telemetry to track episodes of AF. The duration of phase 1 is 3 months but no data accrue toward the primary and other endpoints for the first 2 weeks. The purpose of the 2-week run-in phase is to permit maturation of the newly implanted pacemaker leads and temporary use of antiarrhythmic drugs if there is an exacerbation of paroxysmal AF. Antiarrhythmic drug use is discouraged in phase 1 but their use is tracked as a secondary endpoint. Early crossover from DDI/30 to DDIR/70 is possible after documentation of the primary endpoint and when the patient is experiencing intolerable paroxysmal AF. The primary endpoint (first recurrence of paroxysmal AF which is continuous for ≥5 minutes) is tracked by the device's telemetry, and telemetry reliability is verified by 24-hour ambulatory electro-

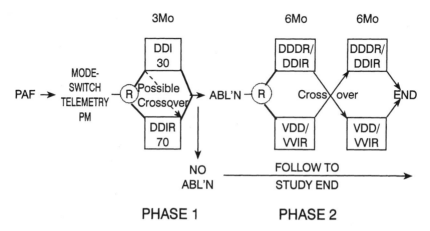

Figure 1. Schematic overview of the protocol of the "Atrial Pacing (Periablation) in Paroxysmal Atrial Fibrillation" study ((PA)[3] Trial).

cardiography. At the end of phase 1, a decision is made concerning whether or not AV node ablation is still needed. If ablation is not needed, the patient is followed and seen every 2 months until the end of the study.

When ablation of the AV node is done, the subject enters phase 2 of the study and is randomized to the DDDR mode (low rate 70 pulses per minute) with mode switching to the DDIR mode when paroxysmal AF occurs; or, to the VDD mode (low rate 50 pulses per minute) with mode switching to the VVIR mode. As in phase 1, events do not accrue toward the primary and other endpoints until 2 weeks after the ablation to permit any transient changes related to the ablation to subside. Data collection is the same as in phase 1 and subjects are seen every 2 months. Antiarrhythmic drug use or change is permitted in this phase after occurrence of a primary endpoint but usage is tracked as a secondary endpoint. At the end of the first 6 months of phase 2, subjects are crossed-over to the alternate mode of pacing and followed for another 6 months to the end of the study. In this schema, the total duration of each subject's participation is 16 months. Quality of life, functional capacity, and echocardiographic substudy data are collected at enrollment, the end of phase 1, cross-over in phase 2, and at the end of the study.

The PA[3] Trial began enrollment in late 1994 and by January 1997 a total of 86 subjects had been randomized into phase 1. It was initially anticipated that the 18 participating centers might take 3 years to recruit the calculated sample size of 100 subjects. In that case the final study results would not be available until late 1998 or early 1999. However, enrollment is proceeding ahead of target and the final results should be available sooner than that.

The other pacing trial taking place in Canada which may provide some secondary data with respect to atrial pacing and AF is the Canadian Trial of Physiologic Pacing (CTOPP). Enrollment of the calculated sample size of 2,540 subjects in CTOPP was completed as of February 1, 1996. The follow-up phase after the last patient was recruited is approximately 18 months and, therefore, results of CTOPP should be anticipated in late 1997 or early 1998.

Trial of Maintenance of Rhythm versus Heart Rate Control

Planning for this National Heart, Lung and Blood Institute (NHLBI) sponsored study began in 1992 and the background is summarized in a publication from the NHLBI Working Group on Atrial Fibrillation.[4] Briefly, the results of recent trials documenting the efficacy of warfarin for stroke reduction, coupled with the emergence of catheter ablation of the AV node and pacing as a definitive therapy for heart rate control, juxtaposed to the inefficacy and potential risks of antiarrhythmic drug therapy to maintain rhythm, have framed the research question of this trial.

The trial is entitled "Atrial Fibrillation Follow-up: Investigation of Rhythm Management" (AFFIRM). A manuscript describing the protocol is currently undergoing peer review for publication. Thus, although it is possible to verbally describe the protocol, only the briefest outline can be provided here. The primary endpoint is total mortality and the sample size of 2,650 patients in each arm is based on the null hypothesis. There are two secondary composite endpoints: mortality plus disabling stroke plus nonfatal cardiac arrest with permanent anoxic encephalopathy; and, the last endpoint plus major bleeds plus other nonfatal cardiac arrests. Assessment of quality of life, cognitive function, functional capacity, and cost are also planned in both arms.

The AFFIRM investigators wished to include patients who have AF that was likely to recur and that in itself was capable of causing morbidity or mortality. Therefore, the working definition for inclusions is: "important atrial fibrillation for which a physician would prescribe long-term therapy". The AFFIRM investigators also wished to enroll a high-risk study population because they thought that, at the end of the study, generalization of the results from a high-risk population to a low-risk population was safer than the converse. Accordingly, subjects must be 65 years of age or older unless they have at least one clinical risk factor for stroke. There are a number of exclusion criteria which are generally aimed at excluding those with reversible causes of AF, those who are not eligible for both therapy strategies, those with conditions potentially confounding for the endpoints, and subjects who are anticipated to be problematic with respect to compliance or follow-up.

Subjects with qualifying AF who consent to particiapate are randomized to one of the two strategies. Treating physicians are then allowed to select initial therapy from a list of approved drugs. When two drug trials have been deemed unsuccessful because of intolerance or inefficacy, the investigator and treating physician have the option to continue pharmacological trials or proceed to approved "innovative therapies". It is in this manner that innovative therapies such as those described elsewhere in this book will be incorporated into AFFIRM.

Guidelines for antithrombotic therapy with warfarin are provided which permit substitution with aspirin under certain circumstances.

Twenty-six centers began a run-in phase in November 1995, although most did not begin recruiting until January 1996. Each center must have the study and its consent approved by their local Institutional Review Board. On May 1, 1996, the number of enrolling centers increased to 176 of the planned 200 with the goal of recruiting 5,300 patients over a 3-year period. As of January 1997, just under 1,000 patients had been randomized. Each patient will be followed to a common follow-up date 2 years after the last patient is recruited.

A number of other trials pertinent to AFFIRM are currrently at various stages. Pilot studies for similar trials in the Netherlands (Rate Control versus Electrical Cardioversion for Atrial Fibrillation (RACE)) and Germany (Prognosis in Atrial Fibrillation (PIAF)) are underway. A smaller U.S.A. Veterans Administsration study (DL-sotalol vs. amiodarone vs. placebo) and a proposed Canadian (amiodarone vs. DL-sotalol or propafenone) study are attempting to determine the best therapy for maintenance of sinus rhythm using the endpoint of time to first symptomatic recurrence. New drugs are also being tested in industry-sponsored trials. The results with bidisomide (GD Searle, Chicago, IL) were disappointing, showing virtually no efficacy.[5] Azimilide (Procter & Gamble Pharmaceutical, Cincinnati, OH) and dofetilide (Pfizer, Groton, CT) are currently being evaluated versus placebo.

References

1. Echt DA, Liebson PR, Mitchell LB, et al. Mortality and morbidity in patients receiving encainide, flecainide or placebo: The Cardiac Arrhythmia Suppression Trial. New Eng J Med 1991;324:781–788.
2. Andersen HR, Theisen L, Bagger JP, et al. Prospective randomised trial of atrial versus ventricular pacing in sick sinus syndrome. Lancet 1994;344:1523–1528.
3. Allessie MA, Konings K, Krichhof CJHJ, et al. Electrophysiologic mechanisms of perpetuation of atrial fibrillation. Am J Cardiol 1996;77:10A-23A.
4. NHLBI Working Group on Atrial Fibrillation. Atrial fibrillation: current understandings and research imperatives. J Am Coll Cardiol 1993;22:1830–1834.
5. Pritchett E, Anderson JL, Connolly SJ, et al. Treatment of symptomatic supraventricular arrhythmias with bidisomide. Circulation 1995;92:I-773. Abstract.

PART IV

The Electrophysiological Substrate of Atrial Fibrillation

CHAPTER 12

Animal Models of Atrial Fibrillation

Albert L. Waldo

The Early Models

The theme of this brief review is that models of cardiac arrhythmias, in this case atrial fibrillation (AF), are invaluable for gaining insights into the nature, mechanism, and treatment of their clinical counterpart. Although intuitively obvious, perhaps the simplest evidence in support of that statement is that, as emphasized by Cranefield,[1] on the basis of studies in the subumbrella of the jellyfish (Fig. 1), ray and dogfish auricles, and the turtle heart by Mayer[2,3] and Mines,[4,5] the basic principles of reentry were understood by 1914. Thus, the need for a tissue substrate with a central obstacle around which a reentrant wave front could rotate, the critical need for unidirectional block of an activation wave front in that substrate, and the need to have the wavelength of excitation shorter than the path length were already understood from some simple experiments in simple animal models.

The major points of this early work on reentry were particularly appreciated by Sir Thomas Lewis and his group. In fact, Lewis published simple diagrams illustrating the principles of reentry using a ring model (Fig. 2).[6] Importantly, this appreciation also produced an unspoken assumption that the center of the reentrant circuit was an anatomic obstacle. This apparently influenced Lewis and others for a long time. In fact, it does not seem that any investigators considered that the central area of block in the reentrant circuit could, in whole or in part, be functional, although the work on reentry due to reflection by Schmitt and Erlanger[7] could be interpreted otherwise. For instance,

Supported in part by grant RO1-HL38408 from the National Institutes of Health, National Heart, Lung, and Blood Institute, Bethesda, MD, and a grant from the Wuliger Foundation, Cleveland, OH.

From *Nonpharmacological Management of Atrial Fibrillation*, edited by F.D. Murgatroyd and A.J. Camm. © 1997, Futura Publishing Co., Inc., Armonk, NY.

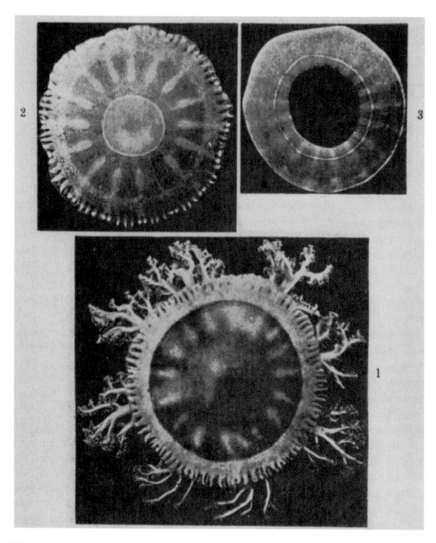

Figure 1. Three views of Cassiopea xamachana as published by A.G. Mayer. 1: An aboral view; 2: an oral view of the subumbrella with stomach- and mouth-arms removed; and 3: a ring of subumbrella tissue made by cutting off the marginal sense organs and removing the center of the disk. (Reproduced with permission from: Rytand DA. The circus movement (entrapped circuit wave) hypothesis of atrial flutter. Arch Intern Med 1966;65:125–159.)

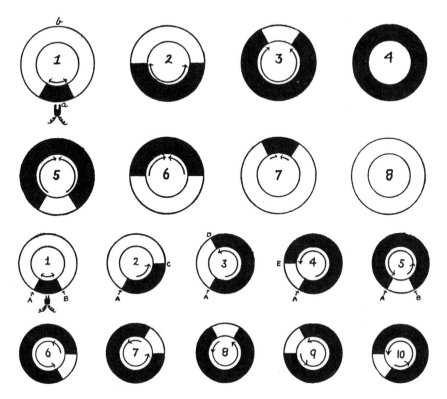

Figure 2. The **top two rows** illustrate the progress of a single wave passing through a ring of muscle as a result of stimulation at site a. The black portion of the ring represents the refractory state, and the figure shows its progress through the ring until in involves the whole (4); later, the figure shows its subsidence. The **bottom two rows** illustrate the establishment of a circus movement in a ring of muscle. The ring is stimulated in its lower quadrant, and the wave spreads to A and to B. At A it is blocked, but from B it continues around the ring. When it arrives at E (4), the refractory state at 4 is passing, and so the wave continues to travel around the circle (5 to 10). (Reproduced with permission from Lewis.[6])

in studies in the canine heart in which atrial flutter was initiated by Faradic stimulation of the atria and sequential site activation mapping from remarkably few atrial sites (usually 7 to 15) was performed, Lewis and colleagues concluded that atrial flutter was due to reentrant excitation around the superior and inferior venae cavae, two naturally occurring obstacles (Fig. 3).[8] However, implicit in this conclusion was the fact that there must be an area of functional block between the superior and inferior venae cavae. However, the latter was not discussed.

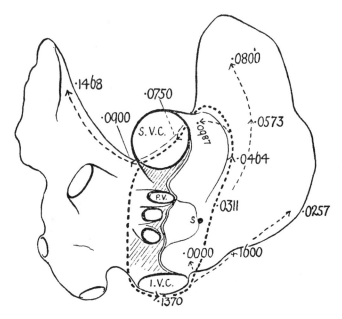

Figure 3. An accurate and natural-size outline of the auricle of dog KQ showing the readings obtained during the period of flutter. These have been reduced to a new common zero. The broken arrows represent the path pursued by the excitation wave, as ascertained from the direction of the deflections in direct leads and from the surface recordings; the former and latter evidences were entirely confirmatory of each other. An area is shaded to display the pericardial reflection more prominently. S.V.C. = superior and I.V.C = inferior vena cava; P.V. = right pulmonary veins. S marks the point stimulated. (Reproduced with permission from Lewis et al.[8])

Nevertheless, it should be emphasized that it was really quite difficult for these early investigators to develop animal models of atrial arrhythmias. It is noteworthy to quote a paragraph from the work of Lewis et al.[8]

"A chief difficulty is in obtaining flutter, or fibrillation when it is desired, of sufficient duration. The observations are to be made during the after-effect when stimulation has been withdrawn. In mapping out the auricle, during the progress of the flutter after-effect, an after-effect of considerable duration is essential. An after-effect lasting 20, 30, or more minutes is usually necessary. We know of no sure method by which these long after-effects are to be obtained, and this lack of knowledge adds much

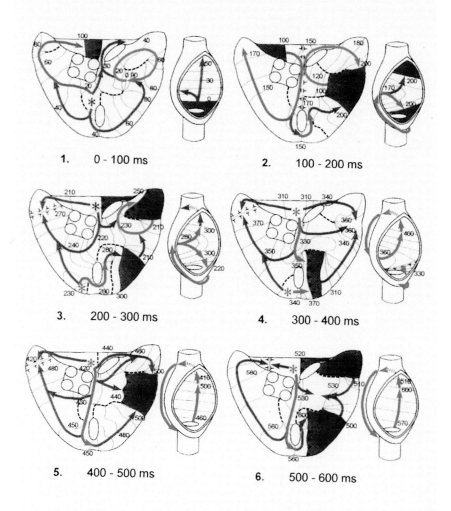

Figure 7. Representative example of the sequence of activation maps during 12 consecutive 100 msec windows (total of 1.2 sec of analysis) from an episode of sustained AF. The colored lines with arrows indicate the location of unstable reentrant circuits. The gray lines with arrows indicate the activation wave fronts which are not part of a reeentrant circuit. Thin lines represent isochrones at 10 msec intervals. The thick dashed lines represent lines of functional block. The closed asterisk indicates the epicardial break-through point of the wave front coming from the septum. The dark gray regions indicate atrial areas which were not activated during a 100 msec window. In the 1.2 sec episode, 18 reentrant circuits in total (mean: 1.5 reentrant circuits

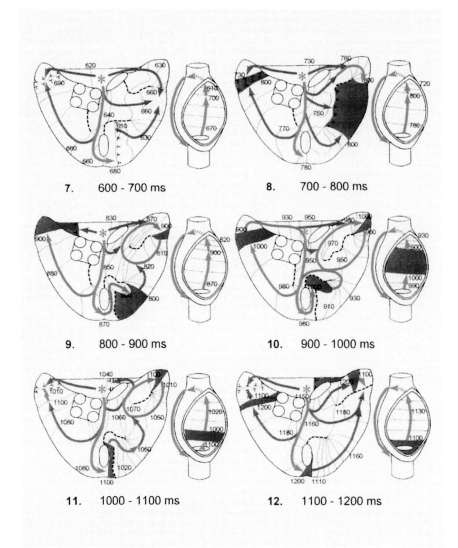

7. 600 - 700 ms

8. 700 - 800 ms

9. 800 - 900 ms

10. 900 - 1000 ms

11. 1000 - 1100 ms

12. 1100 - 1200 ms

Figure 7. *(continued).*
per 100 msec window) were observed (10 involving the septum and the atrial epicardium, 4 in the right atrial free wall, 2 around the pulmonary veins, 1 around the superior vena cava, and 1 around the inferior vena cava). Moreover, they had very short cycle lengths (mean: 104 msec), and 1 to 7.5 (mean: 2.6) consecutive rotations of the reentrant circuits, that is, these circuits disappeared and reformed. BB = Bachmann's bundle; IVC = inferior vena cava; LAA = left atrial appendage; PV = pulmonary veins; RAA = right atrial appendage; SVC = superior vena cava. (Reproduced with permission from Kumagai et al.[33])

to the difficulty of the work. It is impossible to say at the moment stimulation is withdrawn how long the after-effect will last. It is even impossible to say with certainty that an after-effect will be obtained. On many occasions, there will be no after-effect, on very many other occasions there will be a short after-effect, lasting a few seconds or perhaps a minute; on rare occasions an after-effect of many minutes' duration, very rarely of 30 or 60 minutes' duration, will be seen. It is upon these long after-effects that our observations have been undertaken. It will be apparent that there are many disappointments; some auricles will be stimulated repeatedly and only fleeting after-effects will be obtained; in others longer after-effects will be obtained, but these will cease spontaneously before the mapping out is complete; in yet others the after-effect will be of sufficient duration, but more often than not it will consist of fibrillation or impure flutter, to which the method of mapping out is unsuited."

Clearly, both the value of and the need for animal models of stable atrial arrhythmias was understood by Lewis and his group. However, it has taken many decades to make the last statement inappropriate, as multiplexing techniques and other contemporary technological advances make mapping during AF possible and informative.

At this point, the work of Walter E. Garrey should be mentioned. In a single study published in 1914,[9] and remarkable for the fact that it presented only descriptions of what the author had observed in dying hearts rather than any electrophysiological or even mechanical records, Garrey established a fundamental concept: a critical mass of tissue is necessary to sustain fibrillation of any sort (atrial or ventricular). He induced AF by Faradic stimulation from the top of one of the atrial appendages. When he separated the tip from the fibrillating atria, he found that "as a result of this procedure the appendage came to rest, but the auricles invariably continued their delirium unaltered." Simple but fundamental studies such as these permitted Garrey to conclude that "any small auricular piece will cease fibrillating even though the excised pieces retained their normal properties." Also, based on his studies, Garrey proposed[10] that fibrillation was due to " . . . a series of ring-like circuits of shifting location and multiple complexity." As we shall see, this has now been demonstrated. Interestingly enough, Lewis[11] proposed something similar, namely that, "In fibrillation. . . , according to my hypothesis a single circus movement does exist, but the path changes more grossly; but in general the same broad path is used over and over again. *A priori* it is possible to conceive of circus movements of many types. We might even assume several circuits, completely or transiently independent of each other, and each controlling for a time material sections of the muscle . . . " However, Lewis felt "that [in atrial fibrillation] the most mass of muscle is animated by a single circus movement . . varying with limits. . . .."

Development of Models of Atrial Fibrillation: Reentry Versus a Single Focus Firing Rapidly

The early assumption that anatomic obstacles served as the center of reentrant circuits is again seen in the important theoretical work of Wiener and Rosenblueth[12] in Mexico City in the mid-1940s. They calculated on the basis of estimates of the velocity of the potential circulating reentrant wave front that some anatomic orifices were too small to sustain reentrant excitation. However, their calculations indicated that the orifice of the inferior vena cava might be large enough for reentrant atrial flutter. They also inferred that the smaller orifice of the superior vena cava would serve for AF. Additionally, they mentioned "the possibility that the pulmonary veins, singly or jointly, may provide effective obstacles for flutter or fibrillation," but indicated that further investigation was necessary. Two important principles were implicit in this work. The first, similar to that of Garrey[10] and Lewis,[11] was that AF could be due to a single reentrant circuit generating a rhythm at such short cycle length that the remainder of the atria cannot follow 1:1. The second was the apparent assumption of constant conduction velocity in the reentrant circuit, something we now know is unusual. In fact, functional or anatomic areas of slow conduction in reentrant circuits probably is the rule.

Next came the important work from Scherf and colleagues,[13–15] also repeated by Kimura et al.[16] By placing aconitine on the heart, they demonstrated that both atrial flutter and AF could be generated from a single focus firing rapidly. When the site of aconitine application was excluded, the tachycardia was terminated. Additionally, it seemed that it was the degree of rapidity of firing at the aconitine site that determined whether the rhythm generated was atrial flutter or AF. Why aconitine would do this was not understood for years. As summarized recently,[17] studies done in rabbit atrial fibers ". . . found an increase in rate, flutter, and even fibrillation in the absence of early afterdepolarizations. In such preparations, it may be that the increase in background inward current caused by aconitine was sufficient to cause a marked increase in the rate of phase 4 depolarization." While there clearly is no clinical counterpart to aconitine-induced AF in patients, these findings do indicate that a single focus firing rapidly (whatever the cause) is capable of producing AF. As suggested above, it is assumed that the impulses generated from the aconitine site are so rapid that the atria cannot follow in a 1:1 fashion. The result is atrial fibrillation. As we begin to understand some of the more contemporary models of AF, this old concept is again quite relevant. That this is possible in patients is clearly demonstrated by the continuous rapid atrial pacing studies to precipitate and sustain AF deliberately as a therapeutic maneuver.[18,19]

In 1959, largely based on studies of a vagally mediated model of AF and the aconitine-induced model of AF in the canine heart, Moe and Abildskov proposed the multiple wavelet hypothesis and random reentry as the cause of AF.[20] This hypothesis has become generally accepted as the mechanism of AF. However, Moe and Abildskov still considered that AF could result from " . . . a single rapidly discharging ectopic focus, . . . multiple rapidly discharging foci, or . . . a rapidly circulating circus movement. . . ."

A Functional Model of Reentry

The need for an anatomic obstacle to develop and maintain reentrant excitation was either explicit or implicit until Allessie and colleagues[21-23] in the 1970s demonstrated in the isolated left atrium of the rabbit heart that reentrant excitation could occur in which the reentrant circuit was totally functionally determined. The requisite unidirectional block in response to a premature beat results from inhomogeneities of refractoriness. The center of the reentrant circuit is functionally determined, and is created by centripetal wavelets coming from the reentrant mother wave. By continuously bombarding the center of the reentrant circuit, these centripetal wavelets maintain a central area of functional block. This leading circle reentry (Fig. 4)[23] showed for the first time that the center of a reentrant circuit could be functionally determined. This was an important advance in our understanding of reentry, and of the excitable gap. In this form of reentry, the excitable gap is small and not fully excitable as the head of excitability always interacts with the tail of refractoriness. Thus, the excitable gap of a leading circle reentrant circuit consists of tissue in the relative

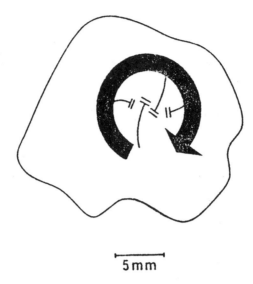

5 mm

Figure 4. Diagram of leading circle-type reentry showing a circuit consisting of a reentrant wave front (black arrow) circulating around a functionally refractory center produced by converging wavelets that block in the center. Block is indicated by double bars. (Reproduced with permission from Allessie et al.[23])

refractory period. Still, the presence of functional areas of slow conduction in the reentrant circuit was not greatly appreciated.

Stable Models of Atrial Fibrillation: The Era of Simultaneous Multisite Mapping Techniques

The next advance in the study of AF in animal models was largely because of the use of simultaneous multisite mapping techniques to analyze activation of the atria. Allessie and colleagues[24,25] developed a Langendorff-perfused canine atrial model of AF. In this model, sustained AF was initiated by rapid atrial pacing during infusion of acetylcholine. After cessation of rapid atrial pacing, AF persisted as long as acetylcholine was infused. By recording simultaneously from 192 electrodes of the 960 electrodes present in specially designed electrode arrays inserted through the tricuspid and mitral valve orifices, activation was recorded endocardially from either or both atria. Mapping during AF clearly demonstrated the presence of multiple, simultane-

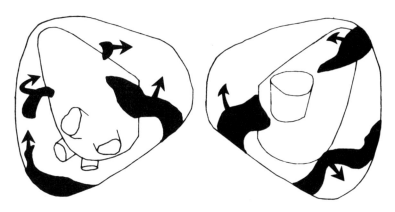

Figure 5. Multiple propagating wavelets in canine atria encountered at an arbitrary moment during self-sustained AF. A total of 7 wavelets were present, 3 in the right and 4 in the left atrium. The crest of the depolarization waves is indicated by arrows, which point to the general direction in which the wavelets propagate. (Reproduced with permission from Allessie et al.[25])

ously circulating reentrant wavelets of the random reentry type (Fig. 5). This was the first demonstration in an animal model that the multiple wavelet hypothesis as the mechanism of AF, proposed by Moe and Abildskov,[20] was, in fact, operative.

Simultaneous multisite (190 electrodes on the right atrial free wall) mapping studies of the sterile canine pericarditis atrial flutter model provided new insights into the evolution and maintenance of functionally determined reentrant circuits, and provided new insight into the interrelationship between AF and atrial flutter.[26] In particular, the onset of atrial flutter was shown to be preceded by a variable but usually relatively brief period of AF during which the requisites for the atrial flutter reentrant circuit form, namely, unidirectional block and a functional center around which a reentrant wave front can circulate (Figs. 6A and 6B).[26]

More recently, several new models of AF have been described. Most are still being characterized, are of considerable interest, and have already demonstrated usefulness. The first, an in vitro canine right atrial model described by Schuessler et al.[27] resulted from a figure of 8 reentrant circuit of very short cycle length induced by rapid pacing during acetylcholine infusion. The short cycle length of the reentrant circuit generated an AF rhythm in the remainder of the preparation. The second model produced in sheep simply by pacing the atria rapidly for a brief period[28,29] results in AF which persists for relatively long periods.

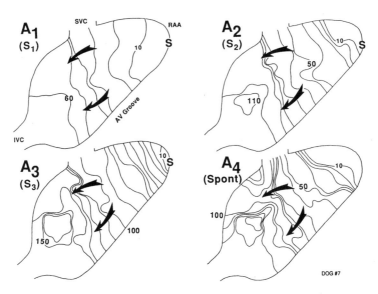

Figure 6A. Isochronous maps during the onset of atrial flutter in the canine pericarditis model induced by an eight-beat drive train (S_1) followed by two premature beats (S_2 and S_3, respectively) (300/130/80 msec) delivered from the right atrial appendage (RAA) at site S. Isochrones are displayed at 10-msec intervals. Arrows indicate the direction of the main activation wave front. Beats A_1, A_2, and A_3 represent isochronous maps corresponding to S_1, S_2, and S_3, respectively. Beat A_1 (S_1) was the last driven beat at a cycle length of 300 msec. Beat A_2 (S_2) was the first premature beat. Beat A_3 (S_3) was the second premature beat. In beats A_2 and A_3, radial activation preceded from the pacing site, and crowding of 10-msec isochrones developed in some areas. In beat A_4, the first spontaneous (Spont) beat, the earliest activated area was close to the pacing site. SVC = superior vena cava; IVC = inferior vena cava; AV = atrioventricular.

This model remains to be more fully characterized, but has already been used to study low energy atrial defibrillation.[28,29]

The third model of AF was developed by Cox and colleagues[30] by creating mitral regurgitation in the canine heart. This model appears to have been difficult to produce, as the consequence of producing acute mitral regurgitation was an associated high mortality rate. Initial simultaneous multisite mapping, which did not include the atrial septum, ". . . exhibited a spectrum of abnormal patterns ranging from the simplest pattern, in which a single reentrant circuit was present that activated the remainder of the atria, to the most complex cases, in which no consistent pattern of activation could be identified."

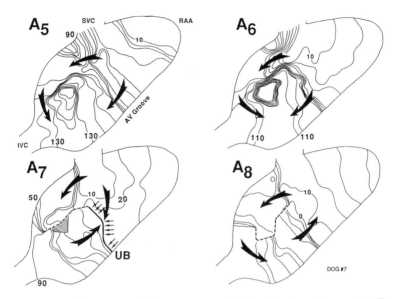

Figure 6B. Continuation of the sequence of activation from Figure 6A. Beats A_5 to A_8 represent subsequent spontaneous beats. Beats A_5 and A_6 showed development of the areas of slow conduction along the sulcus terminalis and in the pectinate muscle region. With beat A_7, unidirectional block (UB) (solid thick black line) of the inferior wave front occurred at the pectinate muscle region in the area of slow conduction. Then, the nonblocked superior activation wave front conducted around a line of functional block (dashed lines) and through an area of slow conduction close to the inferior vena cava to conduct through the areas of unidirectional block from the opposite direction. The shaded area represents an area of localized block. Beat A_8 was the first spontaneous atrial flutter beat, which traveled counterclockwise around an area of functional block (dashed line) at a cycle length of 152 msec. (Reproduced with permission from Shimizu et al.[26])

The fourth model of AF is the canine sterile pericarditis model.[31] It is produced the same way as the canine sterile pericarditis model of atrial flutter. The difference is that AF rather than atrial flutter is induced when the pacing induction protocol is initiated during days 1 and 2 after surgically creating the pericarditis. On postoperative days 3 and 4, the inducibility of AF decreases. Furthermore, the sterile pericarditis AF model appears to be a model of paroxysmal AF, since the duration of induced AF rarely exceeds 60 minutes. This model already has been used to study atrial defibrillation.[32] Most recently, simultaneous multisite mapping studies have shown that in this model, AF is produced by unstable reentrant circuits of very short cycle length which drive the atria at rates which cannot be followed in a 1:1 fashion (Fig. 7; see color insert after p. 144). These reentrant circuits are short lived (mean 3–4 rotations), but subsequently are reformed so that 1–4 such reentrant circuits are always present.[33] Continued study of this new model holds promise for providing better understanding of how antiarrhythmic drugs work to interrupt or prevent AF, and for providing better approaches for ablative cure of AF.[34]

The fifth model of AF is also in the canine heart. It is the same continuous vagal stimulation model used by Moe and Abildskov,[20] in which AF is initially induced by a burst of rapid atrial pacing.[35,36] Although not fully characterized, it is thought to resemble the model described by Allessie et al.[23,24] in the isolated Langendorff preparation and has been used to study antiarrhythmic drug action. The sixth model is that of AF produced by intermittent or sustained rapid atrial pacing in a goat heart or canine heart, respectively.[37,38] Although both models are still being characterized, the demonstration of pathophysiological changes (shortening of the atrial effective refractory period, histological changes consistent with hibernation) resulting from the persistent rapid atrial rate already have led to the appreciation that "atrial fibrillation begets atrial fibrillation," an important concept with enormous implications.

In sum, all these models provide new and important opportunities to understand better the nature and treatment of AF. Thus, it is clear that animal models already have provided significant insights into the nature and mechanism of AF. Surely, further studies and development of additional models will continue to provide valuable new insights which should continue to have important implications for patient care. Of course, the ultimate animal model to study is the human. Such studies have already begun during open heart surgery[30,39] and hold promise that with techniques of simultaneous multisite mapping and other new technologies, we will indeed continue to gain the requisite insights and understanding of AF to advance patient care.

References

1. Cranefield PF. The Conduction of the Cardiac Impulse. Mt. Kisco, NY: Futura Publishing Co, Inc; 1975:153–197.
2. Mayer AG. Rhythmical pulsation in scyphomedusae. Washington, DC: Carnegie Institution of Washington. Publication 47;1906:1–62.
3. Mayer AG. Rhythmical pulsation in scyphomedusae. II. In: Papers from the Tortugas Laboratory of the Carnegie Institution of Washington. 1908; 1:113–131.

4. Mines GR. On dynamic equilibrium in the heart. J Physiol (Lond). 1913; 46:349–383.

5. Mines GR. On circulating excitation in heart muscles and their possible relations to tachycardia and fibrillation. Trans R Soc Can 1914;43:8–52.

6. Lewis T. Observations upon flutter and fibrillation. IV: Impure flutter; theory of circus movement. Heart 1920;7:293–345.

7. Schmitt FO, Erlanger J. Directional differences in the conduction of the impulse through heart muscle and their possible relation to extrasystolic and fibrillary contractions. Am J Physiol 1928–29;87:326–347.

8. Lewis T, Feil HS, Stroud WD. Observations upon flutter and fibrillation. II: The nature of auricular flutter. Heart 1920;7:191–245.

9. Garrey W. The nature of fibrillary contraction of the heart: its relation to tissue mass and form. Am J Physiol 1914;33:397–414.

10. Garrey WE. Auricular fibrillation. Physiol Rev 1924;4:215–250.

11. Lewis T. The Mechanism and Graphic Registration of the Heart Beat. 3rd ed. London: Shaw & Sons; 1925:340–342.

12. Wiener N, Rosenblueth A. The mathematical formulation of the problem of conduction of impulses in a network of connected excitable elements, specifically in cardiac muscle. Arch Inst Cardiol Mex 1946;16:205–265.

13. Scherf D. Studies on auricular tachycardia caused by aconitine administration. Proc Exp Biol Med 1947;64:233–239.

14. Scherf D, Romano FJ, Terranova R. Experimental studies on auricular flutter and auricular fibrillation. Am Heart J 1958;36:241–251.

15. Scherf D. Terranova R. Mechanism of auricular flutter and fibrillation. Am J Physiol 1949;159:137–142.

16. Kimura E, Kato K, Murao S, et al. Experimental studies on the mechanism of auricular flutter. Tohoku J Exp Med 1954;60:197–207.

17. Cranefield PF, Aronson RS. Cardiac Arrhythmias: The Role of Triggered Activity and Other Mechanisms. Mt. Kisco, NY: Futura Publishing Co, Inc; 1988;426–465.

18. Waldo AL, MacLean WAH, Karp RB, Kouchoukos NT, James TN. Continuous rapid atrial pacing to control recurrent or sustained supraventricular tachycardias following open heart surgery. Circulation 1976;54:245–250.

19. Moreira DAR, Shepard RB, Waldo AL. Chronic rapid atrial pacing to maintain atrial fibrillation: use to permit control of ventricular rate in order to treat tachycardia induced cardiomyopathy. PACE 1989;12:761–775.

20. Moe GK, Abildskov JA. Atrial fibrillation as a self-sustaining mechanism independent of focal discharge. Am Heart J 1959;58:59–70.

21. Allessie MA, Bonke FIM, Schopman FJG. Circus movement in rabbit atrial muscle as a mechanism of tachycardia. Circ Res 1973;33:54–62.

22. Allessie MA, Bonke FIM, Schopman FJG. Circus movement in rabbit atrial muscle as a mechanism of tachycardia. II: The role of nonuniform recovery of excitability in the occurrence of unidirectional block as studied with multiple microelectrodes. Circ Res 1976;39:168–177.

23. Allessie MA, Bonke FIM, Schopman FJG. Circus movement in rabbit atrial

muscle as a mechanism of tachycardia. III: The "leading circle" concept: a new model of circus movement in cardiac tissue without the involvement of an anatomic obstacle. Circ Res 1977;41:9–18.

24. Allessie MA, Lammers W, Smeets J, et al. Total mapping of atrial excitation during acetylcholine-induced atrial flutter and fibrillation in the isolated canine heart. In: Kulbertus HE, Olsson SB, Schlepper M. eds. Atrial Fibrillation. Molndal, Sweden: AB Hassle; 1982:44–59.

25. Allessie M, Lammers WJEP, Bonke FI, Hollen J. Experimental evaluation of Moe's multiple wavelet hypothesis of atrial fibrillation. In: Zipes DP, Jalife J, eds. Cardiac Electrophysiology and Arrhythmias. New York: Grune & Stratton; 1985;265–275.

26. Shimizu A, Nozaki A, Rudy Y, Waldo AL. Onset of induced atrial flutter in the canine pericarditis model. J Am Coll Cardiol 1991;17:1223–1234.

27. Schuessler RB, Grayson TM, Bromberg BI, et al. Cholinergically mediated tachyarrhythmias induced by a single extrastimulus in the isolated canine right atrium. Circ Res 1992;71:1254–1275.

28. Powell AC, Garan H, McGovern BA, et al. Low energy conversion of atrial fibrillation in sheep. J Am Coll Cardiol 1992;20:707–711.

29. Ayers GM, Alferness CA, Ilina MI, et al. Ventricular proarrhythmic effects of ventricular cycle length and shock strength in a sheep model of transvenous atrial defibrillation. Circulation 1994;89:413–422.

30. Cox JL, Canavan TE, Schuessler RB, et al. The surgical treatment of atrial fibrillation. II: Intraoperative electrophysiologic mapping and description of the electrophysiologic basis of atrial flutter and atrial fibrillation. J Thorac Cardiovasc Surg 1991;101:406–426.

31. Ortiz J, Igarashi M, Gonzalez X, et al. A new, reliable atrial fibrillation model with a clinical counterpart. J Am Coll Cardiol 1993;21:183A. Abstract.

32. Ortiz J, Sokoloski MC, Geha AS, Waldo AL. Atrial defibrillation using temporary epicardial defibrillation stainless steel wire electrodes: studies in the canine sterile pericarditis model. Am Coll Cardiol 1995;26:1356–1364.

33. Kumagai K, Khrestian C, Waldo AL. Simultaneous multisite mapping during induced atrial fibrillation in the sterile pericarditis model: insights into the mechanism of its maintenance. Circulation. In press.

34. Kumagai K, Uno K, Khrestian C, Waldo AL. Single site radiofrequency catheter ablation of atrial fibrillation. J Am Coll Cardiol 1996;27:4A. Abstract.

35. Wang Z, Pagé P, Nattel S. Mechanism of flecainide's antiarrhythmic action in experimental atrial fibrillation. Circ Res 1992;71:271–287.

36. Wang J, Bourne GW, Wang Z, et al. Comparative mechanisms of antiarrhythmic drug action in experimental atrial fibrillation: importance of use-dependent effects on refractoriness. Circulation 1993;88:1030–1044.

37. Wijffels MCEG, Kirchhof CJHJ, Durland R, Allessie MA. Atrial fibrillation begets atrial fibrillation: a study in awake chronically instrumented goats. Circulation 1995;92:1954–1968.

38. Morillo CA, Klein GJ, Jones DL, Guiraudon CM. Chronic rapid atrial

pacing: structural, functional and electrophysiologic characteristics of a new model of sustained atrial fibrillation. Circulation 1995;91:1588–1595.

39. Konings KTS, Kirchhof CJHJ, Smeets JRLM, et al. High-density mapping of electrically induced atrial fibrillation in humans. Circulation 1994;89: 1665–1680.

CHAPTER 13

Determinants of Susceptibility to Atrial Fibrillation

Michiel J. Janse

Abnormalities in Transmembrane Potentials

Early studies in which transmembrane potentials were recorded from isolated preparations obtained from fibrillating human atria, either from atria of normal size or from dilated atria, showed that resting potentials were significantly reduced compared to resting potentials from cells in nonfibrillating atria.[1,2] In later studies, however, hypopolarized cells were found infrequently (15% of cells from fibrillating atria vs. 5% in normal atria).[3] The functional significance of the presence of partially depolarized cells is twofold: first, conduction velocity will be decreased because of the reduction of action potential upstroke velocity and amplitude as a consequence of the low resting membrane potential; second, since in partially depolarized cells the recovery kinetics of both the fast and the slow inward current are markedly delayed, the refractory period is prolonged, and lags behind completion of repolarization. This so-called post-repolarization-refractoriness results in a spatial dispersion of refractory periods. Both a reduced conduction velocity and an increase in dispersion of refractoriness predispose to reentry.

Attuel and colleagues[4] were the first to report on an intriguing abnormality observed in patients vulnerable to atrial arrhythmias, including fibrillation. In these patients there was no, or hardly any, adaptation of the atrial refractory period to changes in heart rate. At the most rapid rates investigated (cycle lengths in the order of 350–400 msec), the range of refractory period durations was similar to that of normal patients (approximately 160–250 msec). However, upon slowing of heart rate no prolongation of the refractory period was observed so that at cycle lengths between 800 msec to 1,000 msec, the refractory

From *Nonpharmacological Management of Atrial Fibrillation*, edited by F.D. Murgatroyd and A.J. Camm. © 1997, Futura Publishing Co., Inc., Armonk, NY.

periods of the atria of arrhythmic patients were much shorter than those of normals. These findings were largely supported by later studies, in which action potentials from isolated atria were recorded at different pacing rates.[3] Again, a poor adaptation of both action potential duration and refractory period to heart rate was found. Moreover, the effective refractory period was usually shorter in atrial tissue obtained from patients with AF than from normal atrial preparations, except at short cycle lengths where, because of post-repolarization-refractoriness, refractory periods were longer. In addition, it was found that in the AF group, the proportion of triangular action potentials was much greater than in the control group (97% vs. 23%). Finally, dispersion of action potential duration was much greater in the AF group than in the control group. Increased dispersion in refractoriness was also found by direct measurements during cardiac surgery in patients with chronic AF.[5] In that study, the average interval between local activations during AF, the so-called AF interval, was used as an index of local refractoriness (Fig. 1). As shown in Figure 2, there was a good correlation between the refractory period duration determined with the extrastimulus technique during regular pacing of the atria at a cycle length of 400 msec and the AF interval measured during AF at the same right atrial epicardial sites. The advantage of using the AF interval is that simultaneous recordings during brief episodes of AF could be made at 40 atrial sites, whereas classical determination of refractory periods at 40 sites with the extrastimulus technique would take an inordinate amount of time, and would in fact be impossible during an operation.

We employed this technique in 10 patients with idiopathic paroxysmal AF and in a control group of six patients. Reasons for operation were the "Corridor" operation for drug-refractory AF (eight patients), surgical ablation of accessory pathways in patients with AF (two patients) and surgical treatment of postinfarction ventricular tachycardia refractory to medical therapy (the six control patients). After a routine median sternotomy, a multielectrode grid with up to 40 electrode terminals was placed over the right atrium, and AF was induced by premature stimulation. The average AF interval in patients with paroxysmal AF, recorded at a total of 247 sites, was 152 ± 3 msec, compared to a value of 176 ± 8.1 msec recorded at 118 sites in the control group ($P < 0.05$). Dispersion in AF intervals, defined as the variance of the fibrillation intervals at all recording sites, was three times larger in the AF group than in the control group (Fig. 3). The question arises whether the short refractory period is the cause or the result of AF. Recent studies suggest that the latter is the case.

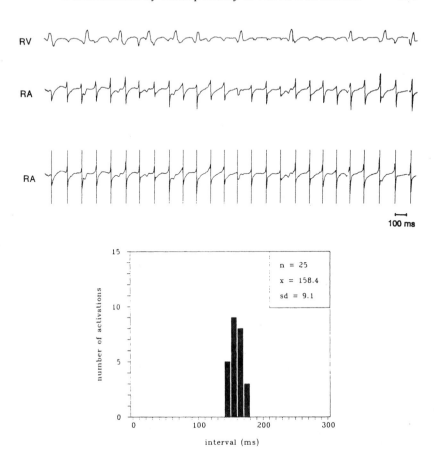

Figure 1. Upper two tracings: Electrograms during a 4-second period of AF recorded from an epicardial site on the right ventricle (RV) and a site on the right atrium (RA) in a patient during open-heart surgery. **Lower tracing**: Same tracing as the right atrium recording above, in which the vertical lines are the activation moments as determined by an interactive computer program. **Lower panel**: Twenty-five intervals between activation moments are expressed in a histogram. The mean AF interval at this particular site, that is, the index of local refractoriness, was 158.4 msec. (Reproduced with permission from Ramdat Misier et al.[5])

Electrical Remodeling

In an experimental model, the hypothesis was tested that AF itself causes the electrophysiological changes in the atrium that favor both induction and maintenance of AF.[6] In chronically instrumented con-

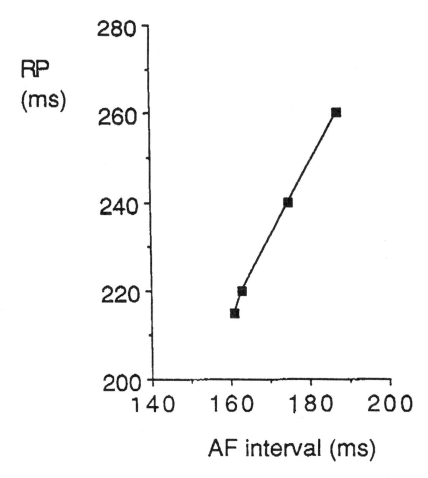

Figure 2. Relation between atrial fibrillation (AF) intervals and the refractory period, determined with the extrastimulus technique during regular pacing of the atria at a basic cycle length of 400 msec, at four epicardial sites. (Reproduced with permission from Ramdat Misier et al.[5])

scious goats, in which 27 electrodes were sutured onto the epicardium of both atria, a special device was implanted that could detect the presence or absence of AF and could also induce AF by delivering a 1-second burst of biphasic stimuli (strength four times diastolic threshold, interval 20 msec). Initially, electrically induced AF lasted only a few seconds before it terminated spontaneously. However, when the arrhythmia was repetitively reinduced, the episodes of AF became gradually longer, until chronic fibrillation (i.e., lasting longer than 24 hours) occurred

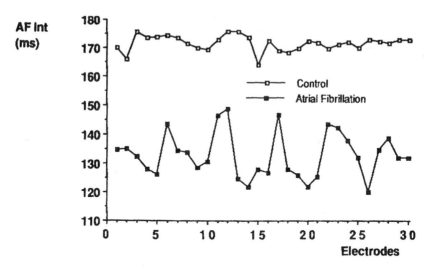

Figure 3. Atrial fibrillation intervals (AF Int) recorded simultaneously at 37 sites (Electrodes) in a control patient and at 32 sites in a patient with paroxysmal AF. (Reproduced with permission from Ramdat Misier et al.[5])

within periods varying among individual animals from several days to 2 weeks (Fig. 4). Repetitive induction of AF did not alter conduction velocity, but gave rise to a marked shortening of the refractory period from control values of 151 ± 12 msec to 93 ± 20 msec after 24 hours. In addition, the normal rate adaptation of the refractory period was abolished, or even reversed, resulting in a shortening of the refractory period at slower heart rates.

These changes could also be obtained by regular pacing at a rapid rate. When the atria were paced at a cycle length of 180 msec, the ventricles responded in a 2:1 fashion. After 24 hours, the atrial refractory period had shortened from 140 msec to 105 msec. When the atrial pacing cycle was lengthened to 360 msec, with the ventricles now being activated in a 1:1 manner so that ventricular rate and hemodynamic conditions remained constant, it took 24 hours before the atrial refractory period returned to its original value. These results indicate that following cardioversion of AF after 1 or 2 days, conditions remain favorable for reinduction of AF for at least 12 hours. This electrical remodeling may be responsible for the well-known fact that cardioversion has a much higher success rate when AF is of recent onset.[7]

On the ventricular level, persisting T-wave changes following a single paroxysm of ventricular tachycardia were already described in

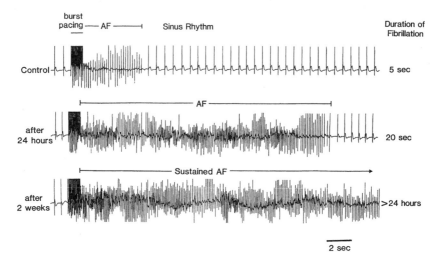

Figure 4. Prolongation of the duration of episodes of electrically induced atrial fibrillation (AF) after maintaining AF for 24 hours and 2 weeks respectively. The three tracings show a single atrial electrogram recorded from the same goat during induction of AF by a 1-second burst of stimuli (50 Hz, 4x threshold). In the upper tracing, the goat has been in sinus rhythm all the time and AF self-terminated within 5 seconds. The second tracing was recorded after the goat had been connected to the fibrillation pacemaker for 24 hours showing a clear prolongation of the duration of AF to 20 seconds. The third tracing was recorded after 2 weeks of electrically maintained AF. After induction of AF this episode became sustained and did not terminate. (From Wijffels et al.[6])

1935.[8] Rosenbaum and colleagues[9] used the term cardiac "memory" to describe the T-wave inversion that developed after about 24 hours of pacing and which could persist for several weeks after pacing was stopped. Katz[10] has suggested that such long-lasting T-wave abnormalities could be initiated by stretch, which would induce changes in gene expression that in turn would lead to the formation of abnormal potassium channels. It is possible that such a process might also occur on an atrial level. Future research concerning the changes in gene expression resulting in alterations of the ion channels involved in atrial repolarization, such as the transient outward current or the delayed rectifier, might unravel the mechanisms of the AF-induced and persisting shortening of the action potential and the refractory period. Once the mechanism is known, ways may be found to counteract the changes in gene expression.

The Wavelength and Inducibility of Atrial Fibrillation

It has been recognized for a long time that during reentrant rhythms, the conduction time of the reentrant impulse traveling around an area of block must be long enough to allow fibers proximal to the zone of block to recover their excitability. The wavelength for circus movement reentry has been defined as the distance traveled by the depolarization wave during the refractory period: wavelength = conduction velocity x refractory period. When the wavelength is short, because of depressed conduction, shortening of the refractory period, or both, small areas of conduction block may already be sufficient for the establishment of reentrant circuits. Since conduction block is more likely to occur in small areas than in a large segment of atrial myocardium, it is to be expected that inducibility of AF depends on wavelength. If wavelength during fibrillation is long, fewer wavelets can circulate through the atria and fibrillation may be self-terminating. If wavelength is short, a greater number of wavelets will be present, and fibrillation will tend to be stable and long-lasting. Wavelength is therefore also important for maintenance of fibrillation.

In conscious dogs in which multiple electrodes for recording and stimulation had been attached to both atria, refractory periods and conduction velocity were measured. To change wavelength, a variety of drugs (acetylcholine, propafenone, lidocaine, ouabain, quinidine, sotalol) were administered, and refractory period, conduction velocity, and their product were correlated with the induction of atrial arrhythmias during premature stimulation.[11] In all dogs (n = 19), atrial arrhythmias (n = 549) could be induced by a single premature stimulus including AF (n = 208). Although at shorter refractory periods a relatively high incidence of AF was observed, prolongation of the refractory period did not always prevent AF. In fact, the predictive power of refractory period duration alone or conduction velocity alone for induction of arrhythmias was poor. In contrast, wavelength correlated very well with inducibility of atrial arrhythmias. In Figure 5, the correlation between induction of AF and refractory period, conduction velocity and wavelength of the provoking impulse is plotted. The critical wavelength where atrial arrhythmias (repetitive responses or flutter) started to occur was 12 cm; the critical wavelength for AF was 8 cm. The values of premature beats that did not induce an arrhythmia are plotted with open symbols, those that induced AF with filled symbols. Because of

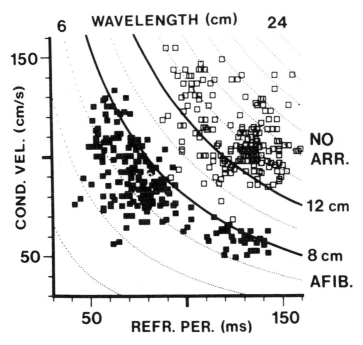

Figure 5. Relation between induction of atrial arrhythmias and refractory period, and conduction velocity and wavelength of the initiating premature beat. The refractory period is plotted on the abscissa and the conduction velocity on the ordinate. Because the wavelength is the product of refractory period and conduction velocity, "isowavelength" curves at 12 cm and 8 cm are drawn. Because of the natural dispersion in electrophysiological properties and the different effects of a wide variety of administered drugs, a wide range of refractory periods and conduction velocities was achieved. Different responses, i.e., either no arrhythmias or AF, were obtained over a wide range of conduction velocities and refractory periods. However, wavelength discriminated well between the two types of response. (Modified from Rensma et al.[11])

the use of a variety of drugs, values for refractory period and conduction velocity varied widely. It can be seen that AF could be induced over a wide range of refractory periods (between 50 and 150 msec) and over a wide range of conduction velocities (50–140 cm/sec). For each of these parameters there is a wide overlap between the population of "no arrhythmias" and "fibrillation". When, however, wavelength was used as a criterion, there was a clear separation between both populations. These findings were obtained in healthy dogs in which electrophysiological properties of the atria were acutely altered by the administration of drugs. Thus, extrapolation to spontaneous fibrillation in diseased atria must be made with caution.

Still, it is reasonable to assume that drugs that would increase wavelength, by prolonging the refractory period, increasing conduction velocity, or both, would be antifibrillatory. Indeed, mapping experiments in dogs with AF in which the arrhythmia was terminated by flecainide or propafenone[12,13] showed that, because of the use-dependent increase in refractoriness, the size of the reentrant circuits increased and the number of reentrant wavelets decreased, until block in the remaining circuit(s) occurred and sinus rhythm was restored.

Dispersion of Refractoriness

Although one factor predisposing to reentry, the shortening of the refractory period, may be the result of prolonged episodes of rapid atrial activity, another factor, dispersion of refractory periods, is unlikely to be due to rapid atrial excitation. Different factors may be involved in this dispersion. Vagal stimulation shortens the atrial refractory period in a nonuniform way,[14,15] possibly because "fibers immediately adjacent to vagal postganglionic endings are exposed to relatively high concentrations of the cholinergic mediator and are profoundly affected, while fibers more remote from sites of acetylcholine liberation are influenced to a much lesser degree".[14] Both the shortening of the refractory period and the increase in dispersion are arrhythmogenic because "an early ectopic impulse generated during a period of vagal stimulation is bound to be propagated along an irregular wave front as the impulse encounters areas in varying states of excitability. The likelihood of fibrillation must be enhanced by such irregularity".[14] These mechanisms may operate in the syndrome of vagally mediated paroxysmal AF occurring in relatively young patients without structural heart disease described by Coumel et al.[16] It is difficult to find an explanation for the much rarer adrenergically mediated paroxysmal AF,[17] since stellate ganglion stimulation was found to have no effects on atrial refractoriness.[15] Whereas vagal stimulation may result in functional inhomogeneities in normal hearts and cause AF, it has been suggested that fibrosis provides the pathological basis for electrophysiological inhomogeneities in AF in rheumatic heart disease. Extracellular electrograms from atrial strips from patients with rheumatic mitral stenosis were found to be fragmented ("toothbrush appearance") and this was attributed to fibrosis.[18] Similar fragmented electrograms have been found in patients with AF; the fragmentation increased during premature stimulation, and the conduction delay was greater in patients with AF than in control patients.[19]

Atrial fibrillation is more common with increasing age. Spach and Dolber[20] showed that with advancing age, extensive collagenous septa develop in the atria, leading to progressive electrical uncoupling of the side-to-side connections of parallel-oriented atrial fibers. This led to "zigzag" conduction in the transverse direction and to fragmented extracellular electrograms. Fibrosis may result not only in slow, zigzag conduction, but also in an increase in dispersion of refractoriness since, in well-coupled cells, the current flow during repolarization will tend to decrease dispersion by prolonging action potentials with a short duration and shortening action potentials with a long duration. Dispersion of atrial refractoriness does increase with age and is increased in patients with AF.[3,5] Another factor that could contribute to shortening of the atrial refractory period is the presence of partially depolarized cells,[1,2] because in these cells the recovery of excitability lags behind completion of repolarization (post-repolarization-refractoriness).

Multiple or Single Wave Reentry?

Although it is widely accepted that AF is a reentrant arrhythmia, various mechanisms may lead to the electrocardiographic manifestations of AF, as schematically depicted in Figure 6. Local application of aconitine results in AF which is dependent on a rapid focus at the site of application. When, after application of aconitine to the atrial appendage, the appendage was clamped off, sinus rhythm was restored promptly in the rest of the atria, whereas the clamped-off appendage showed a fast, regular tachycardia.[21] Thus, in this case, the arrhythmia was due to a focus that fired so rapidly that uniform excitation of the atria was no longer possible. This kind of fibrillation may best be described as "fibrillatory conduction". When AF is induced by rapid stimulation or by faradic shocks applied to an atrial appendage, it is usually short-lived, unless the atrial refractory period is shortened by vagal stimulation or administration of acetylcholine.[21] When during this type of fibrillation the appendage was clamped-off, fibrillation ceased in the appendage and continued in the rest of the atria[21].

To explain the characteristics of this type of fibrillation, Moe developed the multiple wavelet hypothesis,[22] which later was tested experimentally by Allessie and co-workers.[23] In the experiments of Allessie et al., the presence of multiple independent wavelets was demonstrated. The width of the wavelets could be as small as a few millime-

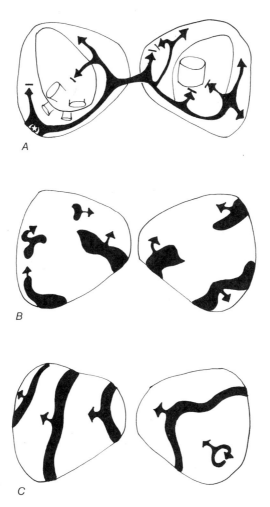

Figure 6. Schematic representation of different mechanisms that can give rise to AF. The left and right atria are depicted as in the study of Allessie and co-workers.[23] In (**a**), a rapid focus in the left atrium, indicated by an asterisk, gives rise to "fibrillatory conduction" in which, because of spatial dispersion in refractoriness, the propagating wave is blocked in several areas. In (**b**), the multiple wavelet reentrant pattern described by Allessie et al.[23] is shown. In (**c**), the mechanism described by Schuessler et al.[24] is depicted, where a single microreentrant circuit is responsible for the arrhythmia and where in a small time window, wavelets generated by four previous circuits are present. (Reproduced with permission from: M.J. Janse. Eur Heart J 1995;16(suppl G):2–6.)

ters, but broad wave fronts propagating uniformly over large segments of the atria were observed as well. Each wavelet existed for a short time, not longer than several hundred milliseconds. Extinction of a wavelet could be caused by fusion of collision with another wavelet, by reaching the border of the atria, or by meeting refractory tissue. New wavelets could be formed by division of a wave at a local area of conduction block or by an offspring of a wave, traveling to the other atrium. The critical number of wavelets in both atria necessary to maintain fibrillation was estimated to be between three and six. The presence of multiple reentrant wavelets during AF induced by single premature beats in the canine, isolated right atrium in the presence of acetylcholine was confirmed by Schuessler et al.[24] However, when, by increasing the dose of acetylcholine, the atrial refractory period became shorter than 95 msec, and AF became sustained, reentry tended to stabilize in a single, small circuit. Single reentrant circuits were also found during intraoperative mapping in humans during AF.[25,26] To quote Cox et al.: ". . . . it would be an oversimplification to categorize atrial flutter as an arrhythmia that is caused by a single reentrant circuit and AF as one caused by multiple reentrant circuits, as was thought in the past. Whereas atrial flutter appears always to occur on the basis of a single reentrant circuit, some forms of AF may also be caused by a single reentrant circuit and more complex forms result from multiple reentrant circuits".[25]

Konings et al.[26] classified AF into three categories on the basis of patterns of activation. In type I, single broad wave fronts propagated at normal speed, and only small areas of slow conduction or conduction block were found, which did not disturb the main course of activation. In type II, either single waves were seen with longer or multiple lines of conduction block and/or slow conduction, or two wavelets were present. In type III, there were three or more wavelets with multiple arcs of conduction block and areas of slow conduction. The average interval between depolarization was longest in type I (174 ms) and became shorter in type II (150 ms) and type III (136 ms). These different types are not separate entities, but rather a continuous spectrum of increasing complexity. Two types of reentrant excitation were seen: (1) leading circle reentry, in which tissue was reexcited by the same wave front that activated it before—this reentry was usually not stationary, but drifted through the tissue; and (2) random reentry, in which a propagating wavelet reexcited an area that had been excited by another wavelet shortly before. In type II and type III AF both forms of reentry were seen, but in type I leading circle reentry was occasionally observed while random reentry was not. Type I might be caused by a single macroreentrant circuit giving rise to irregular activation of other parts of the atria. It "might be regarded as a case of atrial flutter with such a high rate that it cannot be followed in a 1:1 fashion by all parts of the atria. If this were true, type I AF might be a good candidate for termination by rapid pacing".[26] In leading circle reentry, where the head of the circulating wave front bites into its own relative refractory tail, no excitable gap should be present and external stimuli are not expected to influence the arrhythmia. With random reentry, the tissue may not always be immediately re-excited by one of the wandering wavelets. Indeed, in the dog, overdrive pacing during AF did capture part of the atria over a distance of 3–4 cm from the pacing site, the window of entrainment being 12–16 ms.[27] The area of capture was limited because the paced wave front collided with fibrillatory waves and because of conduction block. The fibrillation in these experiments was classified as type II. Rapid pacing might be one of the options for termination of type I AF, catheter ablation might be another, and this has in fact been shown to be feasible.[28]

Summary

In summary, refractory periods of atria that have been fibrillating are shortened and the rate-adaptation of the refractory period is lost. This seems to be the result rather than the cause of AF. Dispersion of refractoriness may be caused by different factors, such as vagal stimulation, the presence of hypopolarized cells, and fibrosis. Fibrosis, whether caused by advancing age or by rheumatic heart disease, results in fragmented electrograms and slow-zigzag conduction. All these electrophysiological abnormalities favor reentry. Dispersion of refractoriness may provide the setting for unidirectional block when a premature impulse arising in a zone with short refractory periods fails to excite an area with long refractory periods. For the induction of reentry, the conduction time of the impulse propagating around the area of block must be long enough to allow fibers proximal to the line of block to recover their excitability. When the wavelength of the impulse is short because of a shortened refractory period, depressed conduction, or both, relatively small areas of conduction block may suffice to allow reentry.

Mapping studies of AF in normal dog hearts, usually in the presence of acetylcholine or vagal stimulation, have largely confirmed the multiple wavelet hypothesis of Moe and Abildskov. Both random reentry and leading circle reentry may occur. In random reentry, there is a short and variable excitable gap. Mapping studies in humans have shown a continuous spectrum of complexity of activations patterns. In type I, a single macroreentrant circuit may be present, with offsprings that excite the rest of the atria in an irregular fashion. In theory, this type of AF might be terminated by pacing or ablation. In types II and II, both random and leading circle reentry may be present.

References

1. Hordof AJ, Edie R, Malm JR, et al. Electrophysiologic properties and response to pharmacologic aspects of fibers of diseased human atria. Circulation 1976;54:774–779.
2. Ten Eick RA, Singer DH. Electrophysiological properties of diseased human atrium. I. Low diastolic potential and altered cellular response to potassium. Circ Res 1979;44:545–557.
3. Le Heuzey JY, Boutjdir M, Lavergne T, et al. Cellular aspects of atrial vulnerability. In: Attuel P, Coumel P, Janse MJ, eds. The Atrium in Health and Disease. Mt Kisco, NY: Futura Publishing Co; 1989:81–94.
4. Attuel P, Childers R, Cauchemez B, et al. Failure in rate adaptation of the atrial refractory period: its relationship to vulnerability. Int J Cardiol 1982; 2:179–197.
5. Ramdat Misier AR, Opthof T, van Hemel NM, et al. Increased dispersion of "refractoriness" in patients with idiopathic paroxysmal AF. J Am Coll Cardiol 1992;19:1531–1535.
6. Wijffels MCEF, Kirchhof CJHJ, Dorland R, et al. Atrial fibrillation begets atrial fibrillation: a study in awake chronically instrumented goats. Circulation 1995;92:1954–1968.
7. Crijns HJGM, van Wijk LM, van Gilst WH, et al. Acute conversion of atrial fibrillation to sinus rhythm: clinical efficacy of flecainide acetate. Comparison of two regimens. Eur Heart J 1988;9:634–638.
8. Graybiel A, White PD. Inversion of the T wave in lead I or II of the electrocardiogram in young individuals with neurocirculatory asthenia, with thyrotoxicosis, in relation to certain infections, and following paroxysmal ventricular tachycardia. Am Heart J 1935;10:345–354.
9. Rosenbaum MB, Blanco HH, Elizari WV, et al. Electrotonic modulation of the T wave and cardiac memory. Am J Cardiol 1982;50:213–222.
10. Katz AM. T wave "memory": possible causal relationship to stretch-induced changes in cardiac ion channels? J Cardiovasc Electrophysiol 1992;3: 150–159.
11. Rensma PL, Allessie MA, Lammers WJEP, et al. Length of excitation wave and susceptibility to re-entrant atrial arrhythmias in normal conscious dogs. Circ Res 1988;62:394–410.
12. Wang Z, Pagé P, Nattel S. Mechanism of flecainide's antiarrhythmic action in experimental atrial fibrillation. Circ Res 1992;71:271–287.
13. Villemaire C, Talajic M, Nattel S. Comparative mechanism of antiarrhythmic drug action in experimental atrial fibrillation: importance of use dependent effects on refractoriness. Circulation 1993;88:1030–1044.
14. Alessi R, Nusynowitz M, Abildskov JA, et al. Nonuniform distribution of

vagal effects on the atrial refractory period. Am J Physiol 1958;194: 406–410.

15. Zipes DP, Mihalick MJ, Robbins GT. Effects of selective vagal and stellate ganglion stimulation on atrial refractoriness. Cardiovasc Res 1974;8: 647–655.

16. Coumel P, Attuel P, Lavellée JP, et al. Syndrome d'arythmie auriculaire d'origine vagale. Arch Mal Coeur 1978;71:645–651.

17. Coumel P, Attuel P, Leclercq JF, et al. Arythmies auriculaires d'origine vagale ou catécholergique: effects comparés du traitement bêta bloqueur et phénomène d'échappement. Arch Mal Coeur 1982;75:373–388.

18. Van Dam RT, Durrer D. Excitability and electrical activity of human myocardial strips from the left atrial appendage in cases of mitral stenosis. Circ Res 1961;9:509–514.

19. Cosio FG, Pacacias J, Vidal JM, et al. Electrophysiological studies in atrial fibrillation: slow conduction of premature impulses. A possible manifestation of the background for reentry. Am J Cardiol 1983;51:122–130.

20. Spach MS, Dolber PC. Relating extracellular potentials and their derivatives to anisotropic propagation at a microscopic level in human cardiac muscle: evidence for electrical uncoupling of side-to-side connections with increasing age. Circ Res 1986;58:356–371.

21. Moe GK, Abildskov JA. Atrial fibrillation as a self-sustaining arrhythmia independent of focal discharge. Am Heart J 1959;58:59–70.

22. Moe GK. On the multiple wavelet hypothesis of atrial fibrillation. Arch Int Pharmacodyn Ther 1962;140:183–188.

23. Allessie MA, Lammers WJEP, Bonke FIM, et al. Experimental evaluation of Moe's multiple wavelet hypothesis of atrial fibrillation. In: Zipes DP, Jalife J, eds. Cardiac Arrhythmias. New York: Grune & Stratton; 1985: 265–276.

24. Schuessler RB, Grayson TM, Bromberg BI, et al. Cholinergically mediated tachyarrhythmias induced by a single extrastimulus in the isolated canine right atrium. Circ Res 1992;71:1254–1267.

25. Cox JL, Canavan TE, Schuessler RB, et al. The surgical treatment of atrial fibrillation. II. Intraoperative electrophysiologic mapping and description of the electrophysiologic basis of atrial flutter and atrial fibrillation. J Thorac Cardiovasc Surg 1991;101:406–426.

26. Konings KTS, Kirchhof CJHJ, Smeets JRLM, et al. High-density mapping of electrically induced atrial fibrillation in humans. Circulation 1994;89: 1665–1680.

27. Kirchhof C, Chorro F, Scheffer GJ, et al. Regional entrainment of atrial fibrillation studied by high-resolution mapping in open-chest dogs. Circulation 1993;88:736–749.

28. Haissaguerre M, Gencel L, Fischer B, et al. Successful catheter ablation of atrial fibrillation. J Cardiovasc Electrophysiol 1994;5:1045–1052.

CHAPTER 14

Electrophysiology of Atrial Fibrillation

Lessons from Patients in Sinus Rhythm

Panos Papageorgiou, Peter Zimetbaum, Kevin Monahan,
Charles Kirchhof, Mark E. Josephson

Introduction

Atrial fibrillation (AF) is not only the most common arrhythmia, it is also one of the earliest arrhythmias ever described.[1] Its impact on extended morbidities and high health care costs is unquestionable. The latter aspect of the disease is becoming even more important in today's era of health care reform and cost containment. Based on the most complete epidemiological data compiled by the Framingham Heart Study,[2] the incidence of AF reaches 4% in patients older than 60 years, and up to 15% in those older than 70 years. The changing demographics in the industrialized world due to an increasing proportion of the population older than 60 years indicate that the prevalence of the disease will increase dramatically in the future. Currently, in our hospital, AF is an admitting diagnosis in 3.4% of admitted patients. It becomes, therefore, exceedingly important to establish criteria of the arrhythmogenic substrate for AF, and to be able to identify individuals who will develop the arrhythmia. Such an understanding of the organization and substrate of human AF may eventually help us to devise ways to prevent the arrhythmia.

With the technical assistance of Philippa Beswick and Nanette Hallett
From *Nonpharmacological Management of Atrial Fibrillation*, edited by F.D. Murgatroyd and A.J. Camm. © 1997, Futura Publishing Co., Inc., Armonk, NY.

Arrhythmogenic Substrate in AF

There remains little doubt that most AF is a reentrant rhythm. Despite the apparent chaotic pattern of atrial activation during AF, experimental work done especially by Moe[3,4] and Allessie et al.[5] has consistently shown that AF consists of microreentrant wavelets that propagate, become extinct, or fractionate within the atrial tissue. The electrophysiological substrate for the development of reentry involves the presence of an area of unidirectional conduction delay or block and the ability to recover tissue excitability proximal to the area of the block. As mentioned above, epidemiological data indicate that the prevalence of AF rises dramatically with increasing age. Although there might be an association between the aging process and alterations in certain physiological parameters, such as autonomic tone, aging is basically accompanied by anatomic changes of the atria that involve the development of large collagen strands, which can create an electrophysiological substrate permissive to reentry. In addition to the anatomic separation of cells by connective tissue fibers, functional changes may also take place at the cellular level that need not be secondary to the aging process. Unidirectional delay or block may occur due to altered electrical connections between myocardial cells, perhaps due to a particular spatial expression of ion transport mechanisms, connexins, or other regulatory membrane proteins.[6,7]

Lessons from Surface Electrical Recordings

In accordance with the notion of reentry being the major mechanism of AF, the electrocardiographic hallmark in patients with a history of AF is the manifestation of intra-atrial conduction defects. In general, patients with a history of AF or atrial flutter display on the surface ECG intra-atrial conduction delays, as manifested by notched P waves and P wave durations of more than 110 ms. Several investigators[8-11] have found that the P wave duration was prolonged in patients with a history of AF compared with normal control individuals. Furthermore, it has been suggested that the P wave duration may have a positive predictive value for the development of postoperative AF. Buxton and Josephson[12] have demonstrated that 83% of patients who developed AF after coronary artery bypass surgery had an abnormally prolonged P wave more than 110 ms in duration. Patients who developed AF had a mean total P wave duration of 126 ms, whereas the mean P wave duration was 116 ms in patients who did not develop postoperative AF.

More specifcally, total P wave duration of more than 120 ms with an isoelectric interval of more than 10 ms in simultaneously recorded leads 1, 2, and 3, identifed a postoperative risk of AF of approximately 40%. Figure 1 shows the total P wave and isoelectric interval measurements by using the surface ECG leads 1,2, and 3.

A more sophisticated analysis of P wave by means of signal-averaged ECG has confirmed the significance of P wave durations on surface 12-lead ECGs. Fukunami and co-workers[13] have performed signal-

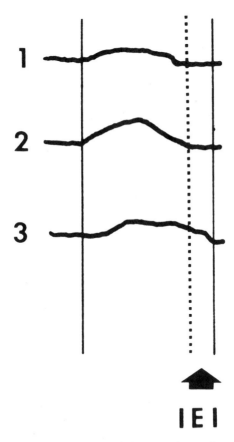

Figure 1. Simultaneous recordings of P waves in surface leads 1, 2, and 3. The two solid vertical bars define total P wave duration. The interval between the left solid bar and the dotted vertical bar is P wave duration of lead 2 (longest standard P wave in this example). The difference between these two intervals is the isoelectric interval (lEl). (Reproduced with permission from Buxton et al.[12])

averaged ECGs on patients with a history of paroxysmal AF and on normal individuals. They found that the presence of a P wave of more than 120 ms and a root mean square voltage for the last 20 ms of less than 3.5 mV offers a positive predictive value for the development of AF at the order of 90%. The problem, however with the noninvasive evaluation of intra-atrial conduction defects is that the measurement relies on the precise identifcation of the beginning and the end of the P wave on surface recordings. This task can be hampered by technical limitations, such as the absence of discrete P wave onset or the merging of the P wave offset with the QRS onset.

Lessons from Intracardiac Electrical Recordings

During long-term ECG monitoring, it has been demonstrated that the initiation of AF is invariably preceded by atrial premature depolarizations (APD). Given the reentrant nature of AF, the study of intracardiac electrograms during atrial extrastimulus testing in patients with a previous history of AF or with inducible AF can provide valuable information regarding the electrophysiological substrate, and it may identify intra-atrial regions critical for the initiation of AF. In 1968, Haft and co-workers[14] first demonstrated that closely coupled APDs, at coupling intervals ranging from 180 ms to 280 ms, were able to produce bursts of nonsustained AF. In patients with a history of paroxysmal AF or atrial flutter, atrial extrastimulus testing has been shown to be associated with intra-atrial delays of the impulse conduction toward the atrioventricular (AV) junction and coronary sinus ostium.[10,11] In addition, a close association between AF inducibility and fragmented atrial electrograms has been demonstrated. During sinus mapping of the right atrium and coronary sinus, Tanigawa et al.[15] have shown the presence of prolonged and fractionated electrograms in individuals with a history of paroxysmal AF. Furthermore, the fragmentation of atrial electrograms was even more pronounced during atrial extrastimulus testing in patients with a history of paroxysmal AF.[16]

It has been observed repeatedly that AF is readily induced by right atrial extrastimulus testing, whereas it is rarely induced by single extrastimuli delivered from the left atrium (i.e., the distal coronary sinus). We and others have demonstrated that right atrial stimulation is associated with longer intra-atrial conduction delays compared with coronary sinus stimulation. As a result, critical intra-atrial delays may allow the formation of reentry circuits and facilitate AF induction. We[17] recently tested the hypothesis that both greater overall intra-atrial conduction delays and, more specifcally, delays at critical sites are more often achieved from the high right atrium than the coronary sinus and result in site-dependent initiation of AF. We studied 17 individuals who were referred to our center for evaluation of symptomatic palpitations or history of supraventricular tachycardias. None of these individuals had a documented history of AF or flutter, or any identifable structural heart disease. We performed atrial extrastimulus testing with single APDs during basic pace drives from the high right atrium and the distal coronary sinus. We recorded bipolar electrograms from the high right atrium, along the tendon of Todaro, along the coronary sinus, and from the posterior triangle of Koch. We calculated the local delay at each intra-atrial site as the difference between the local atrial response (A1A2) minus the stimulus coupling interval (S1S2).

In 8 out of 17 patients, AF was induced only with high right atrial extrastimulus testing. Extrastimulus testing from the distal coronary sinus did not produce AF, atrial flutter, or any kind of reproducible atrial repetitive responses. In all patients, high right atrial stimulation was associated with marked intra-atrial conduction delays. Figure 2 (top panel) represents a three-dimensional isochronal landscape of intra-atrial anisotropic conduction from a single patient during high right atrial stimulation. The intra-atrial conduction delay at each intra-atrial site is plotted as a function of the coupling interval of the premature stimulus. It can be seen that significant conduction delays are encountered even with late-coupled APDs, with coupling intervals starting at approximately 60 ms before the atrial refractoriness. In contrast, coronary sinus stimulation only produced minimal amounts of intra-atrial conduction delays. This is clearly seen in Figure 2 (bottom panel), where coronary sinus extrastimulus testing in the same patient was associated with much smaller delays at comparable APD coupling intervals with high right atrial stimulation. It is unclear which fixed or functional areas of slow conduction can explain the observed conduction delays during high right atrial stimulation. It is possible that the crista terminalis can play such a role by intersecting the propagation of high right atrial stimuli, as recently suggested.[18]

The individuals in whom AF was induced had similar ages to the no-AF group and, during extrastimulus testing, they exhibited the same degree of local latency at the stimulus sites compared with the no-AF group. However, a critical area of delay that was associated with the development of AF was recorded in the posterior triangle of Koch. Figure 3 shows the maximal conduction times to all intra-atrial sites, normalized for local latency at the stimulus sites, during high right atrial and coronary sinus stimulation in patients with or without

HRA extrastimulus testing

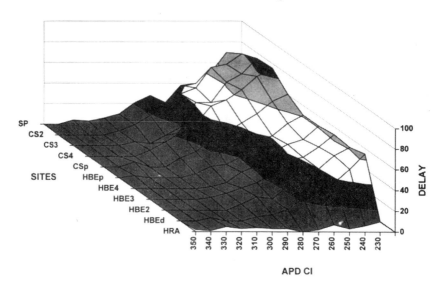

CS extrastimulus testing

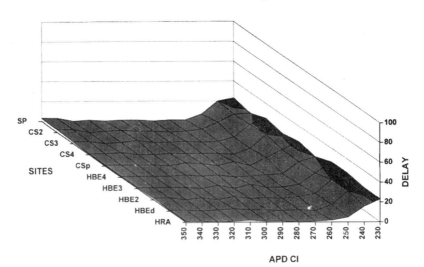

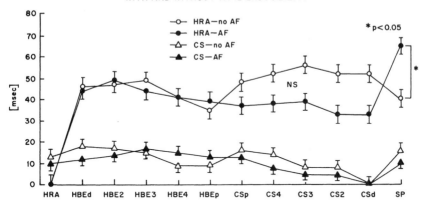

Figure 3. Mean normalized intra-atrial conduction times grouped according to the presence (n = 8, filled symbols) or absence (n = 9, open symbols) of AF inducibility, and displayed during HRA stimulation (circles) vs. CS stimulation (triangles). AF inducibility was associated with a statistically significant increase in conduction time to the posterior triangle of Koch (SP) during HRA stimulation. (Reproduced with permission from Papageorgiou et al.[17])

AF. It was noted that conduction times to all sites were remarkably prolonged during high right atrial stimulation. More importantly, in patients with AF inducibility there was a further increase in the conduction time toward the posterior triangle of Koch, which reached statistical significance when compared with the no-AF group. In addition, the local electrogram duration at the posterior triangle of Koch was longer in patients who developed AF during high right atrial extrastimulus testing. Figure 4 shows that the local electrogram width at the earliest achievable APD-coupling interval was significantly greater

---

Figure 2. Intra-atrial conduction times in a single patient, recorded in response to extrastimulus testing from the high right atrium (HRA) (**top panel**) and coronary sinus (CS) (**bottom panel**). Intra-atrial delay (y axis, in msec) is plotted in three dimensions, as a function of the intra-atrial recording sites (z axis) and the APD-coupling intervals (x axis, in msec). Note the presence of marked intra-atrial conduction delay when the extrastimuli are delivered at the HRA, as opposed to CS extrastimuli. The atrial effective refractory period was 220 msec during HRA stimulation and 220 msec during CS stimulation. HBE = His bundle electrogram; SP = posterior triangle of Koch (slow pathway region).

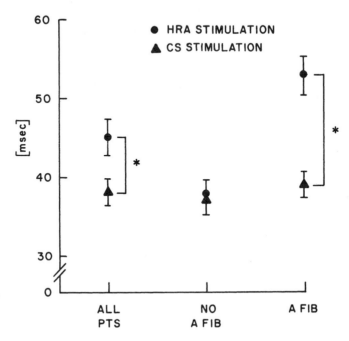

LOCAL ELECTROGRAM WIDTH AT
POSTERIOR TRIANGLE OF KOCH

Figure 4. The width of the local electrogram at the posterior triangle of Koch was measured during the most premature APDs achieved with HRA and the CS extrastimulus testing. In all 17 patients, the mean width of the local electrogram was significantly prolonged during HRA stimulation than during CS stimulation. This difference was further pronounced in patients with AF inducibility (n = 8), whereas it was abolished in patients without AF inducibility (n = 9). (Reproduced with permission from Papageorgiou et al.[17])

during high right atrial stimulation in patients with AF. Patients without AF inducibility, had comparable local electrogram widths during high right atrial and coronary sinus stimulation.

Our data suggest that prolonged conduction times during high right atrial extrastimulation appears to be a common property of atrial tissue regardless of AF inducibility. However, nonuniform anisotropy in the area of the posterior triangle of Koch, and perhaps elsewhere around the tricuspid annulus, seems to be critical for the initiation of AF. The fact that initiation of AF by left atrial extrastimuli is exceedingly rare, may be related to the lack of intra-atrial conduction delays, especially in the posterior triangle of Koch. These observations simply provide an association between AF and the described phenomena. More elaborate studies with extensive high-density mapping of the posterior triangle of Koch will be needed to prove a causal relationship between local reentry and AF initiation.

In addition to the abnormalities associated with intra-atrial conduction, patients with a history of atypical atrial flutter/AF have been shown to exhibit altered characteristics of atrial refractoriness. Josephson and colleagues[11,19,20] have described shorter atrial effective refractory periods (ERPs) measured from the high right atrium than measured from the coronary sinus in patients with atrial flutter/AF but not in patients without atrial arrhythmias. That relationship remained unchanged when tested with two basic pace drive cycle lengths of 600 ms and 450 ms (Fig. 5). Of note, although the atrial ERP shortened during the basic drive of 450 ms, the degree of ERP shortening differed between patients with and without atrial arrhythmias. Figure 6 shows that during high right atrial stimulation, the degree of ERP shortening in patients with atrial flutter/AF was by far less compared with normal

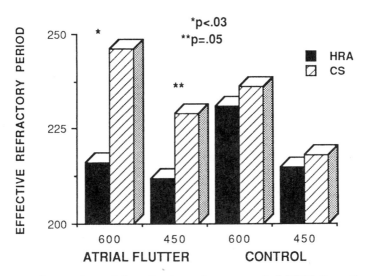

Figure 5. Comparison of the effective refractory period (ERP) from the high right atrium and coronary sinus in patients with and without AF/atypical flutter. The ERP is plotted on the y axis in msec. ERPs were determined from both the HRA (dark bars) and distal CS (hatched bars) at paced cycle lengths of 600 ms and 450 ms in patients with AF/flutter and in controls. (Reproduced with permission from Josephson.[20])

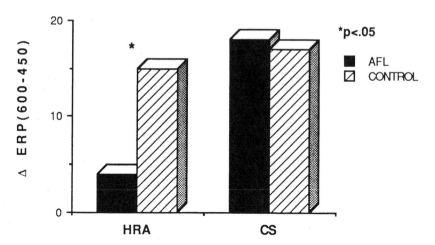

Figure 6. The effect of cycle length on atrial refractoriness. The difference in ERP (ERP) at cycle lengths of 600 ms and 450 ms is shown during HRA and distal CS extrastimulus testing in patients with AF/flutter (dark bars) and in controls (hatched bars). It is apparent that the HRA ERP fails to shorten in response to a decreased paced cycle length in patients with AF. (Reproduced with permission from Josephson.[20])

individuals, whereas during coronary sinus stimulation there was a comparable degree of ERP shortening in both groups of patients. Therefore, patients with atrial flutter/AF seem to fail to adjust their high right atrial ERPs in response to a shorter basic drive cycle length, or conversely fail to prolong them at longer drive cycle lengths.

Conclusions

Consistent with the notion of reentry in AF, initially set forth by the experimental work of Moe and Allessie,[3–5] surface recordings of electrical potentials, endocardial atrial mapping, and programmed electrical stimulation have all established that intra-atrial conduction delays and inhomogeneity of atrial refractoriness constitute the necessary substrates for AF development. It is conceivable that programmed atrial stimulation may have a role as a provocative test for patients with undocumented symptoms compatible with AF, or to select patients at high risk for AF development. Along these lines, preliminary work[21] has shown that intra-atrial delays during atrial extrastimulus testing via epicardial wires in post-CABG (coronary artery bypass grafting) patients can predict AF development. Our recent work[17] has proposed that the sufficient factor for AF initiation may be the presence of nonuniform anisotropic conduction in the low right atrium. New evidence from our laboratory[22] has suggested that prevention of local reentry at the posterior triangle of Koch via distal coronary sinus pacing can prevent AF induction by high right atrial extrastimuli. As our collective knowledge of the AF pathophysioloy expands, it is certain that more precise therapeutic modalities, such as highly specialized pacing algorithms or highly targeted RF ablations, will develop and greatly improve the treatment of the arrhythmia.

References

1. Lewis T. Auricular fibrillation: a common clinical condition. Br Med J 1909; 2:1528.
2. Kannel WB, Abbott RD, Savage DD, McNamara PM. Epidemiologic features of chronic atrial fibrillation: the Framingham study. N Engl J Med 1982;306:1018–1022.
3. Moe GK. On the multiple wavelet hypothesis of atrial fibrillation. Arch Int Pharmacodyn Ther 1962;140:183–188.
4. Moe GK, Rheinbolt WC, Abildskov JA. A computer model of atrial fibrillation. Am Heart J 1964;67:200–220.
5. Allessie MA, Lammers WJEP, Bonke FIM, Hollen J. Experimental evaluation of Moe's multiple wavelet hypothesis of atrial fibrillation. In: Zipes DP, Jalife J, eds. Cardiac Arrhythmias. New York: Grune & Stratton; 1985: 265–276.
6. Spach MS, Miller WT III, Geselowitz DB, et al. The discontinuous nature of propagation in normal canine cardiac muscle: evidence for recurrent discontinuities of intracellular resistance that affect the membrane currents. Circ Res 1981;48:39–54.
7. Saffitz JE, Kanter HL, Green KG, et al. Tissue-specific determinants of anisotropic conduction velocity in canine atrial and ventricular myocardium. Circ Res 1994;74:1065–1070.
8. Simpson RJ Jr, Foster JR, Gettes LS. Atrial excitability and conduction in patients with interatrial conduction defects. Am J Cardiol 1982;50: 1331–1337.
9. Simpson RJ Jr, Foster JR, Mulrow JP, Gettes LS. The electrophysiological substrate of atrial fibrillation. PACE 1983;6: 1166–1170.
10. Cosio FG, Palacios J, Vidal JM, et al. Electrophysiologic studies in atrial fbrillation: slow conduction of premature impulses. A possible manifestation of the background for reentry. Am J Cardiol 1983;51:122–130.
11. Buxton AE, Waxman HL, Marchlinski FE, Josephson ME. Atrial conduction: effects of extrastimuli with and without atrial dysrhythmias. Am J Cardiol 1984;54:755–761.
12. Buxton AE, Josephson ME. The role of P wave duration as a predictor of postoperative atrial arrhythmias. Chest 1981;80:68–73.

13. Fukunami M, Yamada T, Ohmori M, et al. Detection of patients at risk for paroxysmal atrial fibrillation during sinus rhythm by P wave-triggered signal-average electrocardiogram. Circulation 1991;83:162–169.

14. Haft JI, Lau SH, Stein E, et al. Atrial fibrillation produced by atrial stimulation. Circulation 1968;37:70–74.

15. Tanigawa M, Fukatani M, Konoe A, et al. Prolonged and fractionated right atrial electrograms during sinus rhythm in patients with paroxysmal atrial fibrillation and sick sinus syndrome. J Am Coll Cardiol 1991;17:403–408.

16. Ohe T, Matsuhisa M, Kamakura S, et al. Relation between the widening of the fragmented atrial activity zone and atrial fibrillation. Am J Cardiol 1983;53:1219–1222.

17. Papageorgiou P, Monahan K, Boyle NG, et al. Site-dependent intra-atrial conduction delay: relationship to initiation of atrial fibrillation. Circulation 1996;94:384–389.

18. Olgin JE, Kalman JM, Fitzpatrick AP, Lesh MD. Role of atrial endocardial structures as barriers to conduction during human type I atrial flutter: activation and entrainment mapping guided by intracardiac echocardiography. Circulation 1995;92:1839–1848.

19. Watson RM, Josephson ME. Atrial flutter. 1. Electrophysiologic substrates and modes of initiation and termination. Am J Cardiol 1980; 45:732–741.

20. Josephson ME. Clinical Cardiac Electrophysiology: Techniques and Interpretations. Philadelphia, PA: Lea & Febiger; 1993:275–310.

21. Chung MK, Pool DP, Leo HL, et al. Atrial conduction latency predicts occurrence of postoperative atrial fibrillation in patients undergoing coronary bypass surgery. J Am Coll Cardiol 1995;special issue:65A. Abstract.

22. Papageorgiou P, Anselme F, Monahan KM, et al. Coronary sinus pacing prevents induction of atrial fibrillation. J Am Coll Cardiol 1996;27(Suppl A):313A. Abstract.

CHAPTER 15

Lessons from Mapping Atrial Fibrillation in Humans:

Implications for Ablation

Gregory W. Botteron, Michael E. Cain

Introduction

Atrial fibrillation (AF) is the most common cardiac arrhythmia, responsible for over one-third of all arrhythmia hospitalizations. Although the prevalence of AF is less than 1% in the general population, up to 10% of individuals over the age of 75 years are affected.[1] While definitive pharmacological and nonpharmacological therapies for several ventricular and supraventricular arrhythmias have experienced unparalleled advances in the last several years, curative treatment of AF has been, until recently, only a concept.

The precedent of linking data acquired from intraoperative mapping of spontaneous or induced arrhythmias in humans to the development of surgical and then catheter-based therapies was established nearly 30 years ago. In 1968, Sealy and associates reported the first successful surgical division of an accessory pathway in a patient with Wolff-Parkinson-White syndrome.[2] Over the next 20 years large surgical series were reported with success rates at experienced centers exceeding 98%.[3] Novel approaches for the surgical treatment of atrioventricular nodal reentrant tachycardia soon followed.[4,5] The data acquired from analysis of intraoperative maps of cardiac activation and the success of surgery-based interventions provided new insight into the electrophysiology of these rhythm disorders, established that anatomically directed therapies could cure cardiac arrhythmias, and catalyzed the development of catheter-based systems for arrhythmia ablation. The

From *Nonpharmacological Management of Atrial Fibrillation*, edited by F.D. Murgatroyd and A.J. Camm. © 1997, Futura Publishing Co., Inc., Armonk, NY.

overwhelming success of catheter-based procedures, coupled with extremely low morbidity and mortality, has made catheter ablation of many cardiac arrhythmias commonplace,[6] and obviated the need for arrhythmia surgery in most instances.

Attention has focused recently on whether catheter-based procedures will one day supplant surgery for the treatment of patients with AF. If history is to repeat itself, the feasibility and time course of development of catheter-based procedures for curing AF will be dependent, at least in part, on the data obtained during intraoperative mapping of AF in humans. This chapter focuses on the intraoperative mapping studies of human AF and examines the impact of the data acquired so far on: (1) the pathogenesis of AF; (2) the development of surgery-based treatments that cure AF; and (3) the likelihood that effective and less technically demanding catheter-based therapies will be developed and implemented for the treatment of AF.

Methods for Mapping of AF in Humans

Intraoperative mapping of AF in humans has been performed at only a few centers[7,8] due, at least in part, to the tremendous investment in equipment and expertise required. Although the computer-assisted mapping systems used in these studies are detailed elsewhere,[7-9] a few principles of electrode design and signal processing merit review before discussing the mapping data acquired.

The Nyquist criteria specifies that for accurate resolution a bioelectrical signal must be sampled at at least twice the density at which it occurs. This criterion dictates the necessary temporal (digitization rate at least twice the highest frequency of interest in the signal) as well as spatial (distance between recording sites must be half the lengthscale to be resolved) sampling of bioelectrical signals. Accordingly, the total number of electrograms recorded simultaneously and the area they subserve define the minimal spatial resolution of any activation map.

Cardiac electrograms are a differential voltage recording between two electrodes. Electrodes are either unipolar or bipolar. A unipolar recording is between an electrode positioned in the field of interest and a far-removed reference electrode. A unipolar electrogram is a measure of the electrical state between the site of interest and the distant reference. Unipolar electrograms permit measurements of the true voltage throughout the cardiac cycle, and higher density spatial mapping since only one pole is in the mapping field. A disadvantage of unipolar recordings is that signal deflections indicating local tissue activation can be superimposed on far-field electrical activity hindering accurate assignment of the moment of local depolarization.

Bipolar electrodes measure the electrical gradients between two relatively closely spaced electrodes. With narrow-spaced bipoles, activation is discrete, permitting more accurate assignment of the timing of local tissue activation. Moreover, electrical noise in the local recording environment is represented similarly on each electrode of the bipole. Amplifiers with high common-mode rejection features effectively suppress noise, particularly 60 Hz powerline noise, obviating the need for notch filters, which can alter signals through filter ringing and phase shifts. However, because the amount of tissue between the electrode poles dictates the amount of electrical energy in their field, absolute information about local voltage cannot be obtained.

Advances in digital technology are continually improving the available tools for electrogram amplification, signal preprocessing, and data storage; therefore, only the basic components/concepts of computer-assisted mapping systems will be discussed. The signal recorded from unipolar or bipolar electrodes first passes through an isolation amplifier, both to provide for patient safety and to protect the system from power surges, such as those caused by defibrillation. It is then bandpass-filtered to limit the effect of nonphysiological noise and high frequency aliasing (i.e., direct current and signals typically greater than 500 Hz). Differential amplification with high signal-to-noise characteristics is necessary prior to digitization to ensure that the noise floor of the signal of interest is less than the least significant bit of the analog-to-digital converter. For example, with a 12-bit analog to digital converter that provides 72 dB of dynamic range, a $\pm$ 50 mV signal must have a noise level less than 25 μV. Ideally, digitization should be simultaneous in all channels, which can be achieved with either separate analog to digital converters for each channel that are each synchronized to a common clock trigger, or use of more recently developed multichannel converters that are capable of digitizing many channels without significant phase degradation. Finally, the data must be written to a storage device. To permit acquisition of long, continuous data streams, the digitized data must be written in the time interval prior to the next sampling of the data. Although these hardware and software tasks are not the problem they were a decade ago, the speed of data transfer becomes an issue as more channels are used. For example, 2,000 channels acquiring data at 2,000 Hz require that samples be transferred and written in an average of 4 μsec each.

The two studies of intraoperative mapping of AF in humans dis-

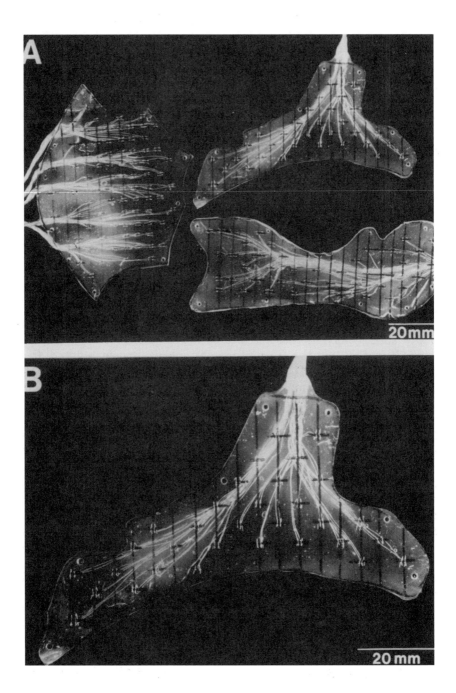

cussed in the section that follows differ in their approach. Our group[7,10] utilized large epicardial plaques with narrow-spaced bipolar electrodes to map 156 epicardial sites simultaneously from as much of the right and left atria as possible (Fig. 1). We optimized overall spatial sampling but sacrificed spatial resolution. The spatial resolution generally varied from 0.5 to 1.0 cm. The electrode density was greatest in the right atrium near the crista terminalis, and least in the posterior left atrium. Konings and colleagues utilized a single "spoon" electrode with 244 unipolar electrodes with a fixed interelectrode distance of 2.25 mm.[8] The electrode had an overall dimension of 3.6 cm and was placed at a single location on the lateral right atrium, thus optimizing spatial resolution at the expense of overall spatial sampling.

Results

In 1991, our group was the first to publish activation maps of AF in humans generated from data recorded with the use of high-density, computer-assisted intraoperative mapping systems.[7,10] The data were acquired from 13 patients with inducible AF who underwent arrhythmia surgery for Wolff-Parkinson-White syndrome. The left and right

---

Figure 1. Atrial epicardial electrode templates containing 156 bipolar electrodes. These templates, fashioned of silicone rubber (0.02-inch thickness, Dow Corning Corp., Midland, MI) were designed to conform to the epicardial surfaces of the atria. Fine silver wires (Quad Teflon-coated silver wire, 0.005 inch diameter. Medwire, Inc., Mt. Vernon, NY) were embedded in these silicone rubber templates at an interelectrode distance of 6 mm and an intraelectrode distance of 1 mm. The largest template, containing 80 electrodes, was placed over the posterolateral right atrium and extended from the interatrial groove posteriorly to the right atrial appendage and atrioventricular groove anteriorly. A second template with 64 electrodes covered the anterior aspects of both the right and left atria immediately behind the ascending aorta in the region of the transverse sinus. The third template, also containing 64 electrodes, covered the posterior left atrium inferior to the pulmonary veins and the posterior left atrial appendage. These templates were fixed in position on the epicardial surfaces of the atria with 4–0 silk sutures. The template on the left side of **A** covers the lateral right atrium. The upper right template in A covers the anterior right and left atria and the medial portion of the left atrial appendage. The lower right template covers the posterior left atrium. **B** shows an enlarged view of the anterior left and right atrial template. The holes on the edges of each template are for suture fixation to the atrium. (Reproduced with permission from Cox et al.[7])

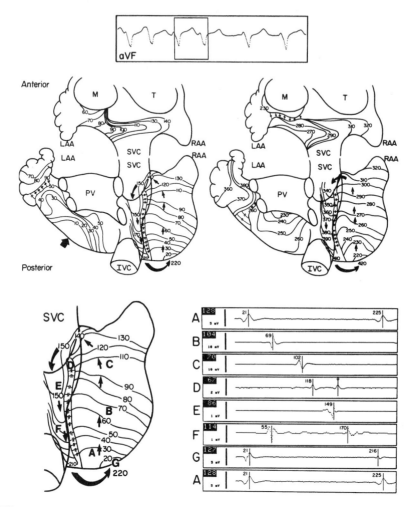

Figure 2. Right atrial reentrant activation during human AF. The activation sequence for the window marked by the *boxed area* on the ECG lead aVF is shown in the lower maps. A right atrial reentrant loop is seen rotating counterclockwise around a line of bidirectional block associated with the sulcus terminalis. In the *upper left panel*, the *dark arrow* marks the site of a left free-wall accessory pathway and shows retrograde activation from the ventricle entering the posterior left atrium. The total length of the window is 420 msec. The labels on each electrogram **A to G** (*lower right panel*) correspond to the letters on the lower left enlarged map denoting the location of seven selected electrodes of the 80 electrodes covering the posterior right atrium. LAA = left atrial appendage; RAA = right atrial appendage; SVC = superior vena cava; IVC = inferior vena cava; PV = pulmonary veins; M = mitral valve; T = tricuspid valve; mV = millivolts. (Reproduced with permission from Cox et al.[7])

atria were mapped simultaneously using epicardial plaques containing 156 bipolar electrodes. In nearly one-half of the subjects reentrant circuits could be demonstrated in the right atrium (Figs. 2 and 3). The conduction time around these reentrant circuits ranged from 180 msec to 210 msec. In the other patients, patterns of activation most consistent with large wave fronts were observed in the right atrium. Reentry was rarely seen in the left atrium, which largely exhibited fibrillatory conduction from right atrial wave fronts. However, mapping of the left atrium was less complete due to the pulmonary veins and its posterior location. Analysis of the data from the right and left atrial electrodes also, and importantly, showed marked intra- and interpatient spatial and temporal variability in the activation patterns with little reproducibility in the pathways of conduction.

Konings and co-workers analyzed high-density maps of induced AF from 25 patients undergoing surgical division of accessory pathways.[8] The spoon electrode containing 244 unipolar electrodes was manually held against the lateral wall of the right atrium. Three types

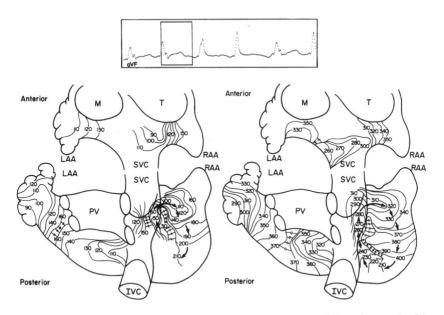

Figure 3. A right atrial reentrant circuit during human AF is shown. In this example, the rotation of the reentrant wave front is clockwise. The length of the window is 400 msec with the activation from the first 210 msec shown in the left map and 210 msec to 400 msec shown in the right map. Same abbreviations as Fig. 2. (Reproduced with permission from Cox et al.[7])

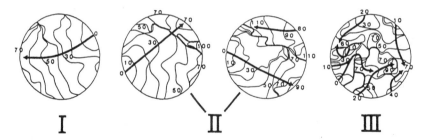

Figure 4. Illustration of the three types of activation during AF. The mapping electrode had a diameter of 3.6 cm and was positioned on the free wall of the right atrium. Type I is characterized by single uniformly propagating waves. During type II, single nonuniform conduction waves or two wavelets are present. In contrast, during type III AF a high degree of dissociation was present with three or more wavelets detected that were associated with multiple areas of slow conduction and arcs of conduction block. (Reproduced with permission from Konings et al.[8])

of AF were identified based on the spatial complexity of the isochronal atrial activation maps analyzed (Fig. 4). In type I AF (ten patients), the mapping area was activated by a single uniform wave front with minimal conduction delay. Type II AF, found in eight patients, was characterized by either one major wave front that conducted with significant conduction delay or by the presence of two separate wave fronts with a line of conduction block. In type III AF (seven patients), three or more wave fronts were identified along with multiple lines of conduction block and zones of slowed (<10 m/sec) conduction. Although more than one type of AF was observed in some patients, individual patients were classified according to the dominant pattern. While the demographics of the patients in these three groups were similar, there were statistically significant differences in the measured values of the fibrillation intervals and conduction times. During AF, the mean fibrillation interval was 174 ± 28 msec, 150 ± 14 msec, and 136 ± 16 msec in types I, II, and III, respectively. In addition, as the fibrillation interval shortened, the variability in the intervals increased significantly. Intraatrial conduction time was also observed to decrease progressively with type I having a velocity of 61 ± 6 cm/sec, type II was 54 ± 4 cm/sec, and type III, the slowest, with a mean velocity of 38 ± 10 cm/sec. In eight of the 25 patients, the left atrium was also mapped. The spatial complexity of activation in the left atrium compared to the right atrium was similar in five patients, more complex or spatially disorganized in two, and more organized in one patient. Fibrillation intervals measured in the right and left atria were not statistically different.

Analysis of the intraoperative mapping acquired in humans so far has confirmed Moe's prediction over 30 years ago that the mechanism of AF involves reentry with areas of fixed and functional conduction block.[11] The types of reentry observed in both studies can be broadly grouped as random and leading circle reentry. Random reentry describes a new wave front depolarizing tissue in what is now the recovered wake of another wave front. In leading circle or closed loop reentry, the same wave front depolarizes the same tissue a second (or more) time. Each relies on the availability of excitable tissue to sustain reentry. These findings provide the foundation needed for developing therapies that limit the amount of contiguous tissue available for activation, thus preventing reentry. Moreover, the measured mean conduction velocities of 40 cm/sec to 60 cm/sec, and estimated refractory periods of 140 msec to 200 msec, establish the relative length-scale over which this reentrant process occurs. But just as importantly, both studies have shown that the activation patterns in any individual are not fixed in either time or space, and that even within a homogeneous group of patients with structurally normal hearts, the spatial activation characteristics vary greatly.

Impact of Surgery for AF

The initial surgical procedure to interrupt AF was conceived without the benefit of mapping data during AF from humans. The first operation was based on the hypothesis that AF was the breakdown of variants of reentrant atrial flutter, and was designed to interrupt large, anatomically fixed pathways for reentry in the right and left atria. This relation between a stable tachycardia and fibrillation was based on evidence that ventricular fibrillation was often the result of degradation of ventricular tachycardia. A procedure based on this concept was performed in one patient, and while initially successful, AF recurred.

Subsequent analysis of the intraoperative mapping data acquired from patients with inducible AF undergoing arrhythmia surgery had a major impact on the evolution of surgical procedures for AF. The mapping studies proved that AF was due to reentry and demonstrated the relative length-scale over which reentry within the atria occurs. However, the findings in individual patients that the reentrant pathways were neither reproducible nor fixed, and that there was considerable temporal variability within patients were critical to the decision that a fixed, anatomically based, surgical procedure would be preferable to a map-guided or individual patient-tailored approach. Based on these data, Cox and co-workers at Washington University developed, implemented, and tested the Maze surgical procedure in an experimental animal model of AF. The pattern of surgical incisions was specifically designed to permit depolarization of all atrial tissue during sinus rhythm but restrict the amount of contiguous tissue so that reentry would not occur. The established success of the surgical Maze procedure in patients has definitively shown proof-of-concept that an anatomic-based approach that limits the amount of contiguous excitable atrial tissue prevents the sustained reentry responsible for AF.[12]

The success of the Maze operation, the analysis of activation maps of AF in humans, and the increasing experience with radiofrequency catheter ablation of supraventricular and ventricular arrhythmias have prompted investigators to focus on two new objectives: (1) To determine whether a catheter-based Maze procedure is feasible and effective; and (2) To determine with the use of a catheter-based procedure the extent to which less extensive tissue ablation that is tailored to an individual patient and not merely anatomically based would be beneficial.

Impact on Catheter Ablation

Conceptually, a catheter-based Maze procedure should be an effective alternative to surgery if a series of linear lesions could be produced that had an identical distribution to those of the Maze operation. Recently, Swartz, using specially designed vascular sheaths to better orient standard thermistor ablation catheters within the right atrium and left atrium (via transseptal puncture), produced a series of linear lesions with radiofrequency energy that approximated the incisions of the surgery-based MAZE operation. Results in the first seven patients, all of whom had chronic AF and structural heart disease, demonstrated proof-of-concept. Radiofrequency catheter ablation terminated AF and restored sinus rhythm acutely in six of the seven patients reported.[13] Recognized limitations such as exceedingly long procedure times, a high rate of atrial flutter following the procedure, and risk of cerebral embolic events are likely to improve as operators gain more experience with this procedure.

Although a catheter-based Maze procedure is technically feasible, the difficulties already encountered using present methods reduce the enthusiasm for performing this procedure on a large scale. We believe that research efforts focused on determining whether a less technically demanding catheter-based ablation procedure will be effective in selected patients demonstrating organized forms of AF will be more fruitful. One component that is essential to research aimed at testing the feasibility of developing a limited catheter-based Maze procedure is to determine the minimal mass of atrial tissue needed to support multiple, simultaneous, sustained reentrant wave fronts. Mapping data acquired intraoperatively from humans have provided the approximate length-scale necessary for reentry during AF. These data clearly demonstrate that this factor differs markedly among patients. For example, the iso-chronal maps constructed by Konings and co-workers[8] found that in some patients, the entire mapping electrode was repeatedly depolarized by a single wave front, suggesting that reentry was occurring over a distance that well exceeded the 3.6 cm covered by the plaque. In other patients, a complete reentrant wave front or multiple wave fronts were detected within the atrial tissue subserved by the plaque. Based on the data obtained with this high-density electrode plaque and assuming that the cycle lengths and conduction times measured adequately describe local tissue refractoriness and conduction velocity, the mean wavelengths calculated for type I, type II, and type III AF are 10.6 cm, 8.1 cm, and 5.1 cm, respectively. Thus, the length over which reentry during AF occurred in this group of highly selected patients varied by at least a factor of two.

The surgical Maze procedure has been successful across all patient populations, including those with paroxysmal or chronic AF as well as those with advanced structural heart disease.[12] Accordingly, the distribution of the surgical incisions must be sufficient to prevent AF regardless of wavelength size. Even AF due to reentry having very short wavelengths cannot recur because of insufficient contiguous excitable tissue to sustain reentry. Based on these findings one could hypothesize that in selected patients with AF characterized by a long wavelength, atrial partitions of much greater size would be equally efficacious and allow for a catheter-based procedure that was much less extensive and technically demanding. Several issues need to be addressed before this hypothesis can be adequately tested. First, we lack at present a reliable catheter-based method to measure the wavelength during AF and identify those who would likely benefit from a limited catheter-based procedure. Second, even the intraoperative data acquired so far are not temporally robust. It is not yet known whether individual patients will manifest all three types of AF given sufficient monitoring, or if other variables such as autonomic tone are altered. Therefore, determination of the complexity of activation patterns during AF based on analysis of a few seconds of data may be misleading. Nevertheless, the recent success by Haissaguerre and colleagues supports the concept that less extensive lesions produced with catheter-based procedures will be beneficial in some patients. This group used a specially designed, multipolar catheter to create three linear lesions in the right atrium of a patient with AF.[14] Analysis of electrograms recorded during AF prior to the procedure showed the fibrillation to be "organized" and confined to the right atrium. The procedure was successful although the reported follow-up was short.

Need for Additional Data

The number of patients studied in the two intraoperative mapping studies discussed is small (38 patients) and comprised predominantly of young adults with accessory pathway mediated tachycardias undergoing arrhythmia surgery. Only seven of the 38 patients in this highly selected group had a clinical history of AF and all were paroxysmal. Although there is little controversy that reentry is the mechanism of AF in other patient populations, specific data not yet available on conduction velocity, estimated refractoriness, and the spatial features of AF in the other populations, especially patients with structural heart disease in whom AF is persistent, are critical for determining the likelihood that less extensive procedures would be effective in curing AF. The spatial activation of AF in this group could be an order of magnitude different from that measured in the patient group with Wolff-Parkinson-White syndrome already studied. Additionally, analyzing longer intervals of data will better delineate the temporal characteristics of AF. The extent of variability detected in the spatial features of AF, particularly in those with highly organized AF, will be critical for determining whether a less extensive, patient-tailored approach is practical on a large scale.

Novel Catheter Techniques

Based on the concepts already discussed, it would be desirable to have a reliable catheter-based method to measure the wavelength during AF and identify those patients who would likely benefit from a limited catheter-based ablation procedure. Two groups have attempted to characterize the spatial features of activation during AF from data acquired using transvenous catheters. Swiryn and colleagues studied patients with AF using a catheter with orthogonal electrodes and discovered that the directions of the wave fronts of activation during AF followed preferential pathways of conduction in the right atrium and were not randomly distributed.[15] They also proposed that the magnitude squared coherence spectrum may provide a quantitative measure of the relative organization present in any wave front of activation.[16] This spectrum quantifies the phase relationship in activation between two recording sites in the right atrium. Although no reliable change in the magnitude squared coherence spectrum could be detected that presaged the spontaneous termination of AF,[17] it is possible that with increased spatial sampling a meaningful, quantitative measure of spatial organization of activation wave fronts will be achievable with this technique.

Recently, our group has used a decapolar electrode catheter and a novel signal-processing technique to quantify the correlation between activation sequences during AF at five sites in the right atrium.[18,19] The observed relationship between correlation and distance decreases monotonically with increasing electrode separation. Over very short distances, activation sequences between two sites correlate well because the likelihood that they are each activated by the same depolarization wave front is high. The correlation between activation sequences decreases exponentially as the distance between sites increases. This relationship decays slowly when the depolarization wave fronts are large and more quickly when the size of the wave fronts is relatively small. The relationship is reliably fit by a decaying exponential function. Solving for the exponential permits determination of the activation space constant, a single value that reflects the distance over which the correlation in activation decreases by $1/e$ and enables direct statistical comparisons between patient groups.

Results of the experiments performed in patients and in experimental animals support our hypothesis that the activation space constant quantifies the spatial organization of the activation process and is directly linked to wave front size. For example, activation space constants were significantly smaller in patients with chronic AF compared to the calculated values in patients with inducible but not clinical AF (Fig. 5). The range of values for the activation space constants calculated in patients having paroxysmal AF were wide and overlapped those in the other two groups.[19] It has been shown recently that among patients in AF, the activation space constant identifies those in whom intravenous procainamide is likely to terminate AF and restore sinus rhythm.[20] In work performed in experimental animals, a significant correlation was found between the spatial organization of AF and internal defibrillation thresholds and a significant increase in spatial orga-

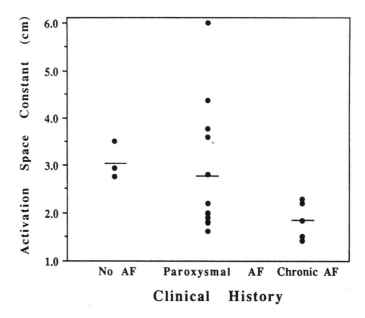

Figure 5. Plot of the activation space constants calculated from data acquired from patients with no clinical history of AF (n = 3), those with paroxysmal AF (n = 12), and those with chronic AF (n = 5). The group of patients with chronic AF had the lowest mean activation space constant (1.84 ± 0.36), the group with no clinical history of AF had the highest mean (3.06 ± 0.4), while the group with paroxysmal AF had a wide range of activation space constants, with a mean falling between the other two subgroups (2.8 ± 1.4). (Reproduced with permission from Botteron et al.[19])

nization was measured with antiarrhythmic drug loading preceding restoration of sinus rhythm.[21]

Although the overall experience with this technique is small and sampling has been limited to a single site in each patient (lateral right atrium), the data acquired to date using this minimally invasive, catheter-based procedure strongly suggest that the measurement of the spatial features of AF in patients will be useful to guide therapy.

Summary

Intraoperative mapping of AF in human hearts has provided conclusive evidence that AF is due to multiple, simultaneous, reentrant wave fronts in the atria. The trajectory of these wave fronts depends on the availability of excitable tissue for depolarization. It is no longer appropriate to view AF as a random or chaotic rhythm, but instead one with a measurable mean conduction velocity and refractory period and a measurable organization in the spatial activation pattern. The relative length-scale over which reentry occurs in AF in humans is highly variable but on the order of several centimeters. These data have greatly increased our fundamental understanding of AF, have refined our ability to design and implement further experimental studies into the mechanism of AF, and will ultimately result in improved therapies.

References

1. Halperin JL, Hart RG. Atrial fibrillation and stroke: new ideas, persisting dilemmas. (Review.) Stroke 1988;19:937–941.
2. Cobb FR, Blumenschwein SD, Sealy WC, et al. Successful surgical interruption of the bundle of Kent in a patient with Wolff-Parkinson-White syndrome. Circulation 1968;38:1018–1029.
3. Cox JL, Gallagher JJ, Cain ME. Experience with 118 consecutive patients undergoing operation for the Wolff-Parkinson-White syndrome. J Thorac Cardiovasc Surg 1985;90:490–498.
4. Ross DL, Johnson DC, Denniss AR, et al. Curative surgery for atrioventricular junctional ("A-V nodal") reentrant tachycardia. J Am Coll Cardiol 1985;6:1383–1392.
5. Cox JL, Holman WL, Cain ME. Cryosurgical treatment of atrioventricular node reentrant tachycardia. Circulation 1987;76:1329–1336.
6. Ganz LI, Friedman PL. Supraventricular tachycardia (see comments). (Review.) N Engl J Med 1995;332:162–173.
7. Cox JL, Canavan TE, Schuessler RB, et al. The surgical treatment of atrial fibrillation. II. Intraoperative electrophysiologic mapping and description of the electrophysiologic basis of atrial flutter and atrial fibrillation. J Thorac Cardiovasc Surg 1991;101:406–426.
8. Konings K, Kirchhof C, Smeets J, et al. High-density mapping of electrically induced atrial fibrillation in humans. Circulation 1994;89:1665–1680.
9. Witkowski FX, Corr PB. An automated simultaneous transmural cardiac mapping system. Am J Physiol 1984;247:H661-H668.
10. Cox JL, Boineau JP, Schuessler RB, et al. Surgical interruption of atrial reentry as a cure for atrial fibrillation. In: Olsson SB, Allessie MA, Campbell RWF, eds. Atrial Fibrillation: Mechanisms and Therapeutic Strategies. Armonk, New York: Futura Publishing Co; 1994:373–404.
11. Moe G. On the multiple wavelet hypothesis of atrial fibrillation. Arch Int Pharmacodyn Ther 1962;140:183–188.
12. Cox JL, Jaquiss RD, Schuessler RB, et al. Modification of the Maze procedure for atrial flutter and atrial fibrillation. II. Surgical technique of the Maze III procedure. J Thorac Cardiovasc Surg 1995;110:485–495.
13. Swartz JF, Pellersels G, Silvers J, et al. A catheter-based curative approach to atrial fibrillation in humans. Circulation. 1994;90(suppl):I-335. Abstract.

14. Haissaguerre M, Gencel L, Fischer B, et al. Successful catheter ablation of atrial fibrillation. J Cardiovasc Electrophysiol 1994;5:1045–1052.
15. Gerstenfeld E, Sahakian A, Swiryn S. Evidence for transient linking of atrial excitation during atrial fibrillation in humans. Circulation 1992;86: 375–382.
16. Ropella K, Sahakian A, Baerman J, et al. The coherence spectrum: a quantitative discriminator of fibrillatory and nonfibrillatory cardiac rhythms. Circulation 1989;80:112–119.
17. Sih HJ, Ropella KM, Swiryn S, et al. Observations from intraatrial recordings on the termination of electrically induced atrial fibrillation in humans. PACE 1994;17:1231–1242.
18. Botteron GW, Smith JM. A technique for measurement of the extent of spatial organization of atrial activation during atrial fibrillation in the intact human heart. IEEE Trans Biomed Eng 1995;42:579–586.
19. Botteron GW, Smith JM. Quantitative assessment of the spatial organization of atrial fibrillation in the intact human heart. Circulation 1996;93: 513–518.
20. Botteron G, Smith J. Spatial organization of electrical activation during atrial fibrillation in the intact human heart and its response to antiarrhythmic drug therapy. PACE 1994;17:750. Abstract.
21. Baker BM, Botteron GW, Ambos HD, et al. Vagal stimulation reduces spatial organization of atrial fibrillation and increases atrial defibrillation threshold. J Am Coll Cardiol 1996;27(suppl A):312A.

PART V

Intervention on the Atrial Fibrillation Substrate

CHAPTER 16

Atrial Fibrillation Surgery Now:

The Cardiologist's Perspective

Brett M. Baker, Joseph M. Smith

Atrial fibrillation (AF) affects up to 1% of the general population.[1-4] Those affected suffer a host of complications from the relatively benign (palpitations, fatigue, exercise intolerance, and breathlessness) to the malignant (stroke, systemic embolic complications, secondary cardiomyopathy, and increased cardiovascular mortality).[5] The relative risk for stroke associated with AF ranges from four- to sixfold for the average patient to as high as 17-fold for select subgroups.[6-8] Compared with age- and disease-matched controls, patients with AF suffer a twofold increase in cardiovascular mortality. Until recently, antiarrhythmic drug therapy was the only option available for the prevention of AF and maintenance of sinus rhythm. However, such therapy has been shown to be substantially less effective at maintaining sinus rhythm than first thought,[9-14] while exposing patients to potentially life-threatening side effects.[15-17]

The enormous societal costs of AF, the absence of a safe and effective pharmacological cure, and previous success of arrhythmia surgery in curing other supraventricular and ventricular arrhythmias have motivated the development of surgical procedures designed to cure AF. This review will cover the evolution of definitive surgical procedures for the treatment and cure of AF and will discuss the current role of cardiac surgery in the management of affected patients.

Electrophysiological Basis for Surgical Treatment of AF

AF is frequently but somewhat incorrectly described as the result of "chaotic and disorganized" atrial depolarization.[18] The inherent orga-

From *Nonpharmacological Management of Atrial Fibrillation*, edited by F.D. Murgatroyd and A.J. Camm. © 1997, Futura Publishing Co., Inc., Armonk, NY.

nization of atrial activation during AF has only recently been quantified,[19,20] but it was the appreciation that reentrant activation underlies AF and that reentry imparts physical and physiological constraints on atrial activation which suggested a role for surgical therapy in treating AF. The rationale underlying the development of surgical therapy for AF is likely traced back to Moe's presentation of the multiple wavelet hypothesis for AF. In a series of papers, Moe and colleagues clearly elucidated the concept that AF is the result of multiple wavelets of atrial activation which migrate over the surface of the atria in ever-changing patterns.[21] Moe's work illustrated that the maintenance of sustained AF was dependent upon (among other things) a critical mass of contiguous atrial tissue. In the absence of such a critical mass, the number of wavelets which could simultaneously coexist on the atrial surface was small enough to allow for coalescence, collision, and self-extinction. These concepts immediately gained acceptance as they were consistent with earlier observations that AF was infrequently seen in laboratory animals with small atria, and that dissection of a fibrillating heart into smaller segments could stop fibrillation.[22–24]

Early attempts at surgical treatment of AF had the goal of reducing the mass of contiguous atrial tissue available for participation in sustained reentry. The first of these techniques involved the surgical isolation of the left atrium,[25] which was accomplished by surgical separation and/or cryoablation of all connections between the left and right atria. This procedure resulted in restoration of sinus rhythm to the right atrium, with resultant physiological control of ventricular rate. A substantial portion of the left atrium remained electrically silent after the procedure, with subsequent return of fibrillation to the isolated left atrium in some cases. Although this procedure restored sinus control to the right atrium as well as the ventricles, loss of left atrial transport function made this approach suboptimal. Additionally, as the left atrium was either electrically quiescent or continued to fibrillate, it was unclear that this procedure offered any reduction in stroke risk.

The Corridor Procedure

The Corridor procedure involves partial isolation of the sinus node complex from the rest of the right atrium; a small "corridor" of right atrial tissue is left in place which extends from the sinus node to the atrioventricular (AV) node.[26–28] Incisions are made surrounding the sinus node, with extension in a parallel fashion across the interatrial septum to the AV node, maintaining a small bridge of atrial tissue between the two incisions. Cryocoagulation is utilized along each of the incisions to insure electrical isolation of the enclosed tissue. The Corridor procedure is designed to restore the propagation of atrial activation from the sinus node across the corridor to the isolated AV node, while atrial tissue outside the bounds of the corridor remains in fibrillation.

Guiraudon and his colleagues developed the Corridor procedure and have reported the largest operative experience with the procedure thus far.[28] Between 1987 and 1993, 36 of their patients underwent the procedure for the treatment of drug-refractory AF. Nine of the patients had recurrent AF resulting from incomplete isolation of the corridor region. Subsequent surgical exploration suggested residual electrical connections between left atrial tissue and corridor tissue adjacent to the coronary sinus. Despite additional dissection and cryoablation in this area, five of the nine patients experienced recurrent AF within the corridor region and were eventually treated with His bundle ablation and ventricular pacing. In 25 of the 36 patients (69%) sinus rhythm was restored and maintained over a 41 ± 14 months. Of the 31 patients who had successful isolation of the corridor region, three patients have had recurrent AF, while three patients experienced atrial flutter (two patients) or atrial tachycardia (one patient) within the corridor region. These arrhythmias were successfully controlled with antiarrhythmic drugs. Ten of the 36 patients eventually required permanent cardiac pacing.

As with left atrial isolation, the Corridor procedure restores sinus control of ventricular rate, but is not designed to extinguish fibrillation within the atria, leaving patients at continued risk for thromboembolic complications related to AF. Predictably, atrial transport function also appears impaired following the Corridor procedure; echocardiographic evaluation revealed an absence of left atrial contraction in all 31 of Guiraudon's patients in whom corridors were successfully isolated.[28]

The Maze Procedure

The Maze procedure was developed with the intention of permanently interrupting AF and restoring both sinus rhythm and biatrial transport function. As with left atrial isolation, surgically created lines of conduction block are employed to reduce the amount of contiguous atrial tissue available for reentrant activation, thus inhibiting sustained fibrillation. The Maze procedure, like the Corridor operation, directs atrial activation from the sinus node to the AV node by creating constraining lines of conduction block.[29-31] In the Maze procedure, however, the sinus impulse is directed not only to the AV junction, but also to the complete extent of the residual right and left atria via a series of insulating atrial incisions. Electrical activation which originates at the sinus node propagates between the suture lines inferiorly and anteriorly around the base of right atrium to the cranial portion of the interatrial septum. Activity then separates into two wave fronts, one activating the posteromedial walls of the right and left atria and the other to the left atrial wall, finally propagating to the AV node. This pattern of activation is designed to preserve physiological AV synchrony on both the left and right sides of the heart (Fig. 1). The only electrically isolated region is that of the left atrium immediately adjacent to the pulmonary veins. Additionally, both the right and left atrial appendages are amputated.

Since the development of the Maze procedure (Maze I) by Cox and his colleagues, the procedure has been modified twice (Maze II and Maze III) with substantial improvement in outcomes.[31-33] The Washington University experience with the Maze procedure spanning from 1987 to 1995 consists of 139 patients (95 men, 44 women) with an average age of 53 years (range 22 to 77 years). Nine patients in the series had a history of previous cardiothoracic surgery. Forty-three of these patients underwent concomitant cardiac surgical procedures at the time of their Maze operations. Eight of the patients had a history of atrial flutter, while the remainder of the patients had either paroxysmal or chronic atrial fibrillation that was refractory to medical management.

AF was extinguished acutely and AV synchrony was restored in all patients. Episodes of postoperative AF were seen in almost 50% of patients, but this was readily and routinely managed with a brief course of antiarrhythmic therapy. Late recurrence of AF has occurred in less than 7% of patients. Atrial transport function has been extensively evaluated in these patients. In those patients treated with Maze I or II, 70% had documented left atrial transport by at least one of the following: intraoperative visualization, transthoracic or transesophageal echocardiography, three-dimensional magnetic resonance scanning, and/or hemodynamic assessment *with and without AV synchrony*. At least one form of evidence of left atrial transport has been documented in 90% of those treated with Maze III. Perioperative mortality was 2.2%, and all patients in this group had significant underlying cardiac or pulmonary disease in addition to AF. The incidence of transient ischemic attacks was 3% of patients with Maze I or II and 1% in those with Maze III. The percentage of patients requiring permanent

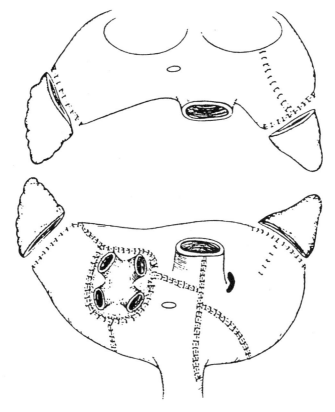

Figure 1. Maze III procedure: This is a schematic representation of the second modification of the Maze procedure. The atria are viewed anteriorly (above) and posteriorly (below). Both atrial appendages are removed and suture lines partition atrial tissue as shown. Note that the orifices of the pulmonary veins are isolated from the rest of the atrial tissue. (From: Cox JL. Evolving applicaions of the Maze procedure for atrial fibrillation (invited editorial). Reprinted with permission from The Society of Thoracic Surgeons, Annals of Thoracic Surgery 1993;55:578–580.)

pacemakers decreased from 54% with Maze I and II to 9% with Maze III. Blunting of the sinus node response to exercise, potentially a result of sinus node devascularization and/or denervation, dropped from 65% with Maze I and II to 8% in Maze III. In summary, the Maze III modifications have significantly reduced the incidence of the four most common complications of Maze I and II, namely: a blunted chronotropic response to exercise, the requirement for permanent pacemaker implantation, the recurrence of atrial fibrillation/flutter, and the absence of postoperative left-sided atrial transport function.

Similar success with the Maze III procedure for the treatment of AF refractory to medical management has been achieved at other centers. Between 1993 and 1995, 19 patients at the Mayo Clinic underwent the procedure for the treatment of nonvalvular AF.[33] These patients had been unsuccessfully treated with an average of five different antiarrhythmic agents each, including amiodarone in seven patients. Mean patient age was comparable to that of patients in the Washington University series (54 years) and concomitant cardiac procedures were performed in six of the 19 patients (repair of atrial septal defects in three patients, coronary artery bypass grafting in three patients).

Sinus rhythm was restored all 19 of these patients, with no operative deaths. Restoration of atrial transport function was confirmed with echocardiography in 18 of 19 patients. At a mean follow-up of 10 months, none of the patients had experienced recurrent AF or required pacemaker placement. Interestingly, four patients with tachycardia-related depression of left ventricular function had improvement of left ventricular ejection fraction into the normal range by three months after the procedure.

Kosakai and his colleague have integrated the Maze procedure into combined surgery for the concomitant treatment of AF and mitral valve disease.[34] Sixty-two patients underwent the Maze procedure combined with mitral valve repair (n = 26) or replacement (n = 36). In addition, aortic valve replacement (n = 22), tricuspid annuloplasty (n = 28), and atrial plication were performed in selected patients. Forty-one of the patients underwent a modified version of Maze III which involved the use of cryoablation in place of some of the suture lines typically used in an effort to reduce procedure duration. The Maze III atriotomies were also altered to better preserve the sinus node artery.

Sinus rhythm was restored in 52 of the 62 patients (84%), despite a mean duration of AF of 8.3 years. Mean cardiac arrest times averaged 142 minutes (range 92 to 212 minutes), with cardiopulmonary bypass times averaging 226 minutes (range 148 to 295 minutes). There was no perioperative or postoperative mortality. Two patients (3.2%) required pacemaker placement postoperatively for sinus node dysfunction and one patient experienced a transient ischemic attack four months after the procedure. Echocardiography was used to document atrial A waves indicating transmitral flow in 71% of the patients in whom sinus rhythm was restored. The investigators observed that the 10 patients in whom sinus rhythm was not restored had significantly larger left atrial dimensions and longer durations of AF prior to surgery. They concluded that combining the Maze procedure with mitral valve surgery is a safe and effective option for patients with chronic AF and mitral valve disease.

Considerations in Selecting Patients for the Surgical Treatment of AF

Surgical treatment of AF in patients whose arrhythmias are refractory to medical therapy has been shown to be feasible, although the data currently available do not clearly demonstrate which subgroups of patients will benefit most from this type of intervention. A series of questions arise when considering the recommendation for a patient to undergo surgery for AF :

1. Will surgery cure the arrhythmia?

Experience with the Maze procedure has demonstrated it to be an effective technique for the restoration of sinus rhythm in patients with AF refractory to medical management. With the most recent version of this procedure (Maze III), restoration of physiological (sinus) control of heart rate with restoration of atrial transport function and mechanical synchrony can be accomplished in over 90% of patients with a risk profile consistent with that associated with open heart surgery.[30–33]

2. Will surgery eliminate the risk of thromboembolism associated with AF?

This is a critically important question, and the data currently available are not conclusive. Since stroke risk is to some degree dependent on altered atrial hemodynamics and absence of active atrial transport attributable to AF, there is a rationale for the Maze procedure decreasing stroke risk. In patients with multiple thromboembolic events or thromboembolism despite optimum medical therapy with warfarin anticoagulation, the risk of subsequent thromboembolic events may exceed 30% in 12 months. The Maze procedure with surgical evacuation of the left atria, amputation of the left atrial appendage, restoration of sinus rhythm, and restoration of atrial transport would appear to offer the best strategy for avoiding the extremely high risk of recurrent stroke in these patients.

3. Will surgery eliminate symptoms?

The symptoms associated with AF are many and varied, and the proximate causes of these symptoms appear multifactorial. The extremes of ventricular rate response (tachycardia and/or bradycardia), the loss of AV synchrony and/or its attendant hemodynamic sequela, the irregularity of the pulse rate, the absence of a physiological rate response to exercise, the absence of physiological neurohumoral control of heart rate, and combinations of these have all been implicated as causal determinants of the adverse symptom profile of AF. To the extent to which a patient's symptoms can be directly linked to any or all of these attributes of the fibrillating atria, symptomatic relief may be expected with the surgical cure of AF. It is important to note, however that complaints such as fatigue, diminished exercise tolerance, or dyspnea may have many potential etiologies, particularly in patients predisposed to having AF.

4. What are the alternatives?

In those patients refractory to pharmacological therapy, alternatives to the Maze procedure include radiofrequency catheter modification of the AV node,[35,36] radiofrequency ablation of the AV node[37] with permanent pacemaker placement, implantation of an implantable atrial defibrillator,[38] or catheter-based atrial ablation emulating the concepts embodied in the Maze procedure.[39] Modification of the AV node is acutely successful at controlling the rate of ventricular response in more than 90% of patients, although up to 20% of patients may require permanent pacemaker placement for high-degree AV block. While these techniques effectively control ventricular response to AF, they do not restore physiological (sinus) control of heart rate nor do they restore atrial transport function or AV mechanical synchrony. As a result, these procedures are unlikely to completely eliminate all symptoms associated with AF. Additionally, there is concern regarding an increased postprocedure sudden death rate in patients treated with AV junction ablation and permanent pacemaker implantation, with speculation that these procedures unveil susceptibility to bradycardia-dependent tachyarrhythmias by exposing patients to relative bradycardia. More importantly, as both atria continue to fibrillate, it is unlikely that these procedures attenuate the risk of thromboembolism.

The implantable atrial defibrillator is a device and concept in evolution. It will likely play a role in patients with drug-refractory paroxysmal AF, or in patients with relativly rare episodes of AF in whom chronic antiarrhythmic drug therapy for a rare event would be unacceptable. Catheter-based atrial ablation procedures for the cure of AF have been recently demonstrated to be feasible and effective. Although technological developments hold the promise of making such procedures even more safe and less technically demanding, ultimately increasing the availability of this therapeutic modality, the role of these procedures in managing patients with AF cannot be reliably assessed at present.

5. Who should be considered for a surgical curative procedure for AF?

The available data would suggest that several patient groups be considered for surgical cure of AF. It is reasonable to describe the risks and benefits of this procedure to patients with symptomatic AF refractory to medical management in whom other therapeutic modalities have failed to relieve symptoms. A minority of such patients will be so limited by their symptoms that the >90% likelihood of alleviating symptoms will outweigh the 2–3% risk of important complications.

In patients with thromboembolic events attributable to AF in whom anticoagulation is constraindicated, or in patients who suffer such events despite therapeutic anticoagulation, a surgical procedure that evacuates the left atrium, amputates the left atrial appendage, and restores atrial transport function seems a rational therapeutic strategy. While we await conclusive data, the grave prognosis of these patients when treated with optimal medical management together with our current understanding of the pathophysiological links between AF and stroke make the suggestion of a surgical procedure to cure AF reasonable.

Finally, in patients with medically refractory AF who are undergoing cardiac surgery for other reasons, surgical cure of AF should be considered. Total bypass times are extended with combined procedures, but this can be minimized by an experienced surgeon.

Summary

The substantial societal costs of AF have motivated the development of surgical techniques for the treatment of this arrhythmia. Based on Moe's multiple wavelet hypothesis of the development of AF, surgical techniques have been created which utilize suture lines as barriers to reentrant conduction and effectively reduce the amount of contiguous atrial tissue available for maintenance of sustained AF. Among these surgical options, the Maze procedure best treats AF, with restoration of sinus control to both the atria and the ventricles, as well as return of atrial transport function.

Catheter-based alternatives to the Maze procedure effectively control ventricular response to fibrillation, but likely do not reduce patients' risk of future thromboembolic events. Patients with AF and cardiogenic thromboembolic events despite warfarin anticoagulation, or patients with AF and stroke in whom antiacoagulation is contraindicated may benefit from restoration of sinus rhythm with the Maze procedure. Patients with AF who are undergoing cardiac surgery for other reasons may experience the benefits of this procedure with little additional risk.

References

1. Onundarson PT, Thorgeirsson G, Jonmundsson E, et al. Chronic atrial fibrillation: epidemiologic features and 14 year follow-up. A case control study. Eur Heart J 1987;8:521–527.
2. Cameron A, Schwartz MJ, Kronmal RA, et al. Prevalence and significance of atrial fibrillation in coronary artery disease (CASS Registry). Am J Cardiol 1988;61:714–717.
3. Diamantopoulos EJ, Anthopoulos I, Nanas S, et al. Detection of arrhythmias in a representative sample of the Athens population. Eur Heart J 1987;8(suppl D):17–19.
4. Hirosawa K, Sekiguchi M, Kasanuki H, et al. Natural history of atrial fibrillation. Heart Vessels 1987;2(suppl):14–23.
5. Kannel WB, Abbott RD, Savage DD, et al. Epidemiologic features of chronic atrial fibrillation: the Framingham study. N Engl J Med 1982;306: 1018–1022.
6. Wolf PA, Dawber TR, Thomas HE Jr, et al. Epidemiologic assessment of chronic atrial fibrillation and risk of stroke: the Framingham study. Neurology 1978;28:973–977.
7. Wolf PA, Abbott RD, Kannel WB. Atrial fibrillation: a major contributor to stroke in the elderly. The Framingham study. Arch Intern Med 1987; 147:1561–1564.
8. Halperin JL, Hart RG. Atrial fibrillation and stroke: new ideas, persisting dilemmas. Stroke 1988;19:937–941.
9. Reimold SC, Cantillon CO, Freidman PL, et al. Propafenone versus sotalol for suppression of recurrent symptomatic atrial fibrillation. Am J Cardiol 1993;71:558–563.
10. Middlekauff HR, Wiener I, Saxon LA, et al. Low-dose amiodarone for atrial fibrillation: time for a prospective study? Ann Intern Med 1992;116: 1017–1020.
11. Suttorp MJ, Kingma JH, Koomen EM, et al. Recurrence of paroxysmal atrial fibrillation or flutter after successful cardioversion in patients with normal left ventricular function. Am J Cardiol 1993;71:710–713.
12. Anderson JL, Gilbert EM, Alpert BL, et al. Prevention of symptomatic recurrences of paroxysmal atrial fibrillation in patients initially tolerating antiarrhythmic therapy: a multicenter, double-blind, crossover study of flecainide and placebo with transtelephonic monitoring. Circulation 1989; 80:1557–1570.
13. Pritchett EL, McCarthy EA, Wilkinson WE. Propafenone treatment of symptomatic paroxysmal supraventricular arrhythmias: a randomized, placebo-controlled, crossover trial in patients tolerating oral therapy. Ann Intern Med 1991;114:539–544.
14. Coplen SE, Antman EM, Berlin JA, et al. Efficacy and safety of quinidine therapy for maintenance of sinus rhythm after cardioversion: a meta-analysis of randomized controlled trials. Circulation 1990;82:1106–1116.

15. Flaker GC, Blackshear JL, McBride R, et al. Antiarrhythmic drug therapy and cardiac mortality in atrial fibrillation. J Am Coll Cardiol 1992;20: 527–532.
16. The Cardiac Arrhythmia Suppression Trial (CAST) Investigators. Preliminary report: effect of encainide and flecainide on mortality in a randomized trial of arrhythmia suppression after myocardial infarction. N Engl J Med 1989;321:406–412.
17. Falk RH. Proarrhythmia in patients treated for atrial fibrillation or flutter. Ann Intern Med 1992;117:141–150.
18. Zipes D. Genesis of cardiac arrhythmias: electrophysiological considerations. In: Braunwald E, ed. Heart Disease: A Textbook of Cardiovascular Medicine. Philadelphia, PA: WB Saunders Co; 1988:667.
19. Botteron GW, Smith JM. A technique for measurement of the extent of spatial organization of atrial activation during atrial fibrillation in the intact human heart. IEEE Trans Biomed Eng 1995;42:579–586.
20. Botteron GW, Smith JM. Quantitative assessment of the spatial organization of atrial fibrillation in the intact human heart. Circulation 1996;93: 513–518.
21. Moe GK. On the multiple wavelet hypothesis of atrial fibrillation. Arch Int Pharmacodyn Ther 1962;140:183–188.
22. Allessie MA, Rensma PL, Brugada J, et al. Pathophysiology of atrial fibrillation. In: Zipes DP, Jalife J, eds. Cardiac Electrophysiology. From Cell to Bedside. WB Saunders Co: Philadelphia; 1990:548.
23. Cox JL, Canavan TE, Schuessler RB, et al. The surgical treatment of atrial fibrillation. II. Intraoperative electrophysiologic mapping and description of the electrophysiologic basis of atrial flutter and atrial fibrillation. J Thorac Cardiovasc Surg 1991;101:406–426.
24. Allessie MA, Bonke FIM, Schopman FJG. Circus movement and rapid atrial muscle as a mechanism of tachycardia. III. The "leading circle" concept: a new model of circus movement in cardiac tissue without the involvement of an anatomic obstacle. Circ Res 1977;41:9–18.
25. Williams JM, Ungerleider RM, Lofland GK, et al. Left atrial isolation: a new technique for the treatment of supraventricular arrhythmias. J Thorac Cardiovasc Surg 1980;80:373–380.
26. Defauw JAMT, Guiraudon GM, van Hemel NM, et al. Surgical therapy of paroxysmal atrial fibrillation with the corridor operation. Ann Thorac Surg 1992;53:564–571.
27. van Hemel NM, Defauw JAMT, Kingma JH, et al. Long-term results of the corridor operation for atrial fibrillation. Br Heart J 1994;71:170–176.
28. Leitch JW, Klein G, Yee R, et al. Sinus node-atrioventricular node isolation: long term results with the corridor operation for atrial fibrillation. J Am Coll Cardiol 1991;17:970–975.
29. Cox JL, Schuessler RB, D'Agostino HJ, et al. The surgical treatment of atrial fibrillation. III. Development of a definitive surgical procedure. J Thorac Cardiovasc Surg 1991;101:569–583.
30. Cox JL, Boineau JP, Schuessler RB, et al. Successful surgical treatment of atrial fibrillation: review and clinical update. JAMA 1991;266:1976–1980.
31. Cox JL, Boineau JP, Schuessler RB, et al. Modification of the Maze procedure for atrial flutter and atrial fibrillation: I. Rationale and rationale and surgical results. J Thorac Cardiovasc Surg 1995;110:473–484.

32. Cox JL. Personal communication. February, 1996.
33. Morris J, Stanton M, Hammill S. The Maze procedure: a reproducibly safe and effective cure for refractory nonvalvular atrial fibrillation. Circulation 1995;92:I-264.
34. Kosakai Y, Kawaguchi AT, Isobe F, et al. Cox Maze procedure for chronic atrial fibrillation associated with mitral valve disease. J Thorac Cardiovasc Surg 1994;108:1049–1054.
35. Kunze KP, Schluter M, Geiger M, et al. Modulation of atrioventricular nodal conduction using radiofrequency current. Am J Cardiol 1988;61: 657–658.
36. Williamson BD, Man KC, Daoud E, et al. Radiofrequency catheter modification of atrioventricular conduction to control the ventricular rate during atrial fibrillation. N Engl J Med 1994;331:910–917.
37. Morady F, Calkins H, Langberg JJ, et al. A prospective randomized comparison of direct current and radiofrequency ablation of the atrioventricular junction. J Am Coll Cardiol 1993;21:102–109.
38. Griffin J. Personal communication. December, 1995.
39. Swartz JF, Perells G, Silvers J, et al. A catheter-based approach to atrial fibrillation in humans. Circulation 1994;90:I-335.

CHAPTER 17

Atrial Fibrillation in the Future: The Surgeon's Perspective

Gerard M. Guiraudon, Colette M. Guiraudon, George J. Klein, Raymond Yee

Atrial fibrillation (AF) has long been defined by its electrocardiographic pattern. It has been considered an elusive target for electrophysiological interventions until recently, when the first successful direct approach was developed.[1] Since then, during the last 10 years, new interventions were designed using surgical or catheter delivery. Rationales for intervention are based on reconciliation of multiple premises, namely: atrial anatomy and function, atrial pathology, and mechanism of AF. Rationales are also determined by the patient's condition and symptoms, as well as the pecking order of various therapeutic endpoints.

Premises Conducive to Rationale

Atrial Anatomy

The atria are two compliant pouches between the continuous venous flow return and the intermittent ventricular flow output. The anatomy of atria may appear simple at first, but is in fact very complex.[2] Atria are made of a grossly spherical wall which is especially irregular and rugged on the endocardial side. Its thickness varies from place to place, being paper thin between pectineal muscle, or very thick as for the pectineal muscle or other trabeculation (Fig. 1) The myocardial synthetium look in total disarray on histological sections. The myocardium is not a uniform piece of "fabric" but is perforated by many large orifices or interrupted by the absence of myocardial cells, and has a

From *Nonpharmacological Management of Atrial Fibrillation*, edited by F.D. Murgatroyd and A.J. Camm. © 1997, Futura Publishing Co., Inc., Armonk, NY.

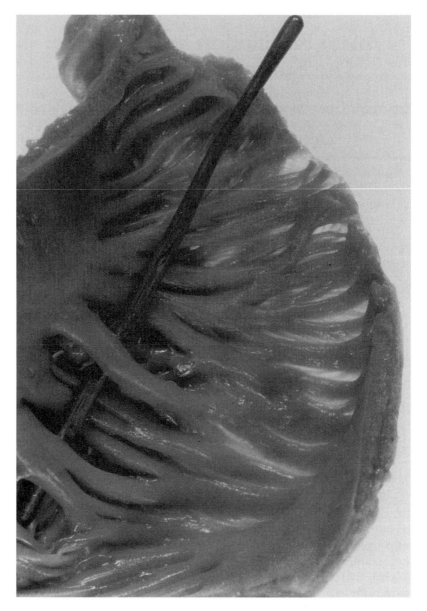

Figure 1. Photograph of the endocardial aspect of the right atrial wall in a human heart specimen. The pectineal segment is most complex with a lattice pattern: transerval "free" bundles and vertical bundles. The lattice pattern shows beyond any doubt that the right atrium is a three-dimensional structure with separate epicardial and endocardial bundles.

lattice pattern. Atria constitute a complex heterogenous tridimensional structure in the shape of a sphere.

Atrial Function

Atria harbor the heart chronotropic function which is located within the sinus node and the atrioventricular (AV) node areas. Cardiac chronotropic function is the main determinant of increased cardiac output during exercise, combined with increased contractility.[3] Atrial contraction is critical to maintain cardiac output of the failing heart by increasing the ventricular end-diastolic pressure and/or volume (Starling Law).[3] In the normal heart, atrial contraction does not seem to play a significant role in cardiac physiology, except as part of the compliance (recoil) of the atrial "pouch".[4] The respective role of chronotropic function and atrial contraction (normal sinus rhythm versus normal venticular chronotropic function without concomitant atrial contraction) has not been elucidated as yet.

Prevention of intra-atrial thrombus formation is a major function of atria. The normal atrial anatomy, especially the left atrial appendage is prone to intracavitary thrombus. The causes of thrombus formation include: alteration of atrial geometry (increased left atrial dimension), pathological alteration of atrial wall (endothelium), loss of contraction, and concomitant loss of the left atrial appendage washout. Left ventricular failure as well as mitral valve stenosis are independent causes of left atrial thrombus in the absence of AF. Mitral valve regurgitation seems to decrease the risk of intracavitary thrombus. But overall, whatever the mechanism involved, the left atrial appendage is the main site of left atrial intracavitary thrombus.[5,6]

To conclude, AF has a global impact on atrial function and anatomy: namely atrial size, contraction, chronotrophic function, and thrombus prevention.

Atrial Pathology

Atrial fibrillation is commonly associated with structural heart disease: rheumatic heart disease, mainly mitral valve disease; dilated cardiomyopathy; and chronic pericarditis. AF is uncommon in ischemic heart disease, unless complicated with cardiac failure (dilated cardiomyopathy) or acute myocardial infarction. Lone AF has occurred in patients without structural heart disease and other known causes of AF (AF without a cause).

Gross pathology shows enlarged and thickened atria, with accentuation of their rugged anatomy.[7] There is alteration of the endocardium. The incidence of the presence of intracavitary thrombus depends on associated heart disease (mitral valve disease, dilated cardiomyopathy) and history of AF. Thrombi are essentially found in the left atrial appendage, the left atrial posterior wall (mitral valve disease), free in the left atrium (mitral valve stenosis), and in the right atrium.

Histology of AF associated with structural heart disease has been well reported.[8,9] Recent work has focused on "lone atrial fibrillation", which seems to occur in the absence of structural heart disease.[10,11] We have reported atrial pathology in 12 patients with lone AF who had a corridor operation.[12,13]

Atrial pathology of lone AF documented the following striking features: (1) Some atria presented with evidence of primary atrial cardiomyopathy (Fig. 2); (2) Some atria showed only myocardial hypertrophy consistent with tachycardia-induced cardiomyopathy (remodeling) (Fig. 3); (3) Significant pathology of sinus node tissue, even in the absence of sinus node dysfunction; and (4) A dramatic decrease in nerve

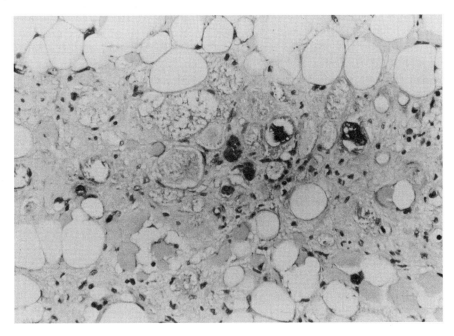

Figure 2. Atrial pathology in lone atrial fibrillation: severe cardiomyopathy with atrial adiposis and fibrosis.

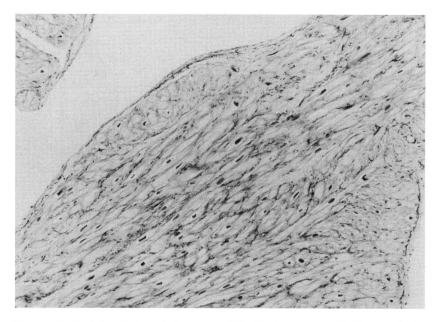

Figure 3. Atrial pathology in lone atrial fibrillation: myocardial hypertrophy.

endings, confirming the critical role of the autonomous nervous system, albeit these findings appeared paradoxical.

Mechanism of AF

Atrial fibrillation was long considered due to rapid, chaotic atrial activation associated with irregular fast ventricular contraction. Moe speculated, on a computer model, that atrial fibrillation was associated with concomitant multiple wavelets of activation.[14] Allessie et al. confirmed Moe's hypothesis on an animal model.[15] Currently, the accepted mechanism for "common" AF is random reentry:[16] four to six activation fronts are moving randomly (Fig. 4). Although activation fronts are short-lived, new fronts are generated by bifurcation of existing fronts. Atrial propensity to sustain AF (atrial vulnerability) is determined by atrial size, wall structure, and spatial distribution of electrophysiological characteristics (dispersion). These conditions vary over time depending on the underlying mechanism and history of AF. The more the atria fibrillate, the more sustained the fibrillation (atrial remodeling):

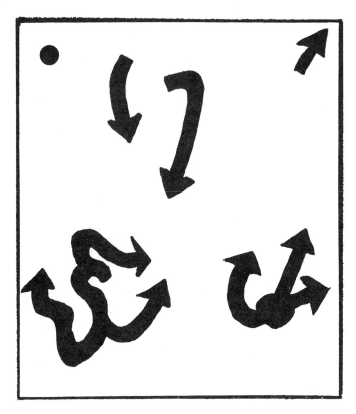

Figure 4. Schematic depiction of random reentry in the atria. The atria are depicted as a quadrangular structure with the sinus node in one corner (●). This model implies a two-dimensional structure, in contradiction to Figure 1.

atrial fibrillation begets atrial fibrillation.[17] This currently accepted mechanism may not be the only one.

Mapping AF provides insights into initiation and perpetuation of AF.[18] Mapping the atria in experimental animals has confirmed the speculations of Moe. The atrial activation could be "organized" in one segment and chaotic in the rest of the atria, with variation over time. A rapid sustained stationary reentry circuit may be identified as the perpetuating mechanism.[19,20] Mapping of human AF, although less extensive, has documented both types: reentry circuit perpetuating the AF[21] or self-sustained multi-wavelet mechanism.[22]

Recently, Jalife and his group have studied the mechanism of initiation of AF.[23] A reentry circuit (rotor) may transform into a drifting spiral which may bifurcate and produce sustained AF. This research may change our view on AF and our approaches.

To conclude, AF can be focal in nature in terms of initiation and perpetuation. Consequently, its interventional therapy should be focal as well. The chaotic atrial activation could hide the working focal mechanism.

Clinical Presentation

Patients with atrial fibrillation have multiple protean presentations.[24] The presenting symptoms can be associated with the arrhythmia itself, the associated structural heart disease, or the left atrial thrombosis. AF is considered a significant aggravating factor in the natural history of the heart disease. This may be revisited with the progress in drug management.[25]

Interventional Rationales

Although current surgical rationales are based on the assumption that atrial random reentry is the perpetuating self-sustained self-aggravating mechanism, prevention of random reentry should prevent AF to develop, whatever the initiating mechanism may be. Current rationales are used based on that concept and are: exclusion/reduction, fragmentation and channeling (Fig. 5).

Exclusion/reduction is aimed at isolating the fibrillating atrium, while reducing the surface area in the rest of the atria and preventing AF.

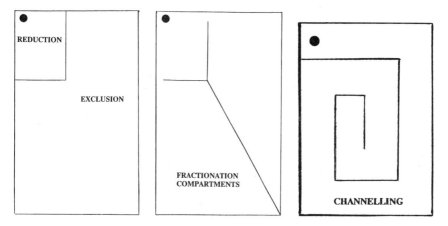

Figure 5. Surgical rationale based on random reentry (see text for discussion).

Fragmentation uses atriotomies to construct semi-excluded atrial segments where random rentry cannot sustain while they all can contract in harmony.

Channeling transforms the two-dimensional atria into a one-dimensional structure by construction of narrow strips of atrial tissue, where random reentry cannot occur.

Focal discrete interventions are not used as yet because intra-operative complete atrial mapping is not available at most institutions. The second concern is that vicarious perpetuating reentrant circuits can occur at other sites. "Random" linear ablation (atriotomies) have been performed using catheter techniques with positive results, although long-term follow-up is needed. It is ironic to remember that atriotomies have been documented as the cause of postoperative atrial tachycardias.[26] In another perspective, focal ablation of tachycardia associated with the Wolf-Parkinson-White syndrome, AV nodal reentrant tachycardia, or other focal atrial tachycardia may prevent atrial fibrillation to occur.

Cardiac denervation, or modification of the autonomous nervous system has not been developed. We failed in the mid-1970s to achieve adequate cardiac denervation in humans and failed to interrupt vagal-induced AF.[27] These difficulties were encountered with cardiac denervation aimed at controlling coronary artery vasospasm during the same period.

Cardiac autotransplantation, used by Batista et al.[28] to allow easier in vitro mitral valve repair, is associated with an unexpected restoration of sinus rhythm function. The role of cardiac denervation, albeit combined with subtotal exclusion of the left atrium, could be the main effective mechanism. There is more and more evidence that atriotomies and/or linear catheter ablation alter the atrial autonomic innervation.[29]

Other interventional rationales should be developed to make the intervention easier and simpler.

Interventional Endpoints

Three *primary endpoints* are paramount: stroke prevention, cardiac function, and symptom relief. In terms of stroke prevention, no study to date has documented that any surgical technique significantly decreases the risk of stroke more than long-term warfarin therapy. The magnitude of the sample size may preclude the design of a significant clinical trial. Improved cardiac function should be associated with increased exercise capacity and potentially prolonged life expectancy.

Studies showed improved cardiac index,[30] and/or improved left ventricular ejection fraction.[31] No study has specifically assessed exercise tolerance. Good symptom relief is provided by all surgical techniques. However, the least invasive intervention such as radiofrequency ablation combined with pacemaker implantation provides excellent control of symptoms.[32]

Secondary endpoints are essentially a way to assess the effect of the intervention rather than its efficacy: i.e., interruption of AF, restoration of sinus rhythm, restoration of adequate chronotropic function, and evidence of atrial contraction.

Other endpoints can be considered, such as cessation of antiarrhythmic drug therapy, absence of pacemaker implantation, etc.

The large number of endpoints suggest that the criteria for success, as far as electrophysiological interventions are concerned, are multiple and controversial. The same ambiguity exists for the medical therapy: heart rate control, maintenance of sinus rhythm, stroke prevention, symptom relief, etc.

Indications for surgical electrophysiological interventions are far from being defined. Patient selection is based on associated heart disease, duration of AF and its prevention, arrhythmia symptoms, cardiac function, left atrial dimension, drug efficacy, and associated structural heart disease. Currently, selected patients requiring mitral valve repair seem to be the best candidates for concomitant surgery for AF.

Current Surgical Techniques

The following surgical techniques have been reported: (1) The Corridor operation based on an excluded channel which houses the sinus node and the AV node; (2) The Maze operation which combines exclusion/reduction with the subtotal exclusion of the left atrium, and channeling and fragmentation; (3) The left atrial exclusion which isolates the fibrillating left atrium; (4) The compartment operation which fragments the atria into two or three segments; (5) The Spiral operation which "channels" the left and right atria; and (6) Cardiac autotransplantation which combines cardiac denervation with subtotal exclusion and remodeling of the left atrium.

The Case for the Left Atrial Appendectomy

Although all reported surgical approaches for AF do not include a left atrial appendectomy, we strongly believe that the *left atrial appendage* should be excluded in all patients operated on for or with AF, as well as all patients having cardiac surgery, for the following considerations. The left atrial appendage is the site of left atrial thrombi in 50% of patients with rheumatic AF[33] and in 90% of patients with nonrheumatic AF.[34] Suppression of the left atrial appendage should decrease the incidence of stroke dramatically, by more than 50%.[35] Suppression of the left atrial appendage itself has no known side effects and/or complications because, although its function is not known, its presence is a potential source of left atrial thrombus even in patients in sinus rhythm. Left atrial appendectomy is not associated with any specific complications, as it is well documented by the worldwide experience of left atrial ligation after closed mitral valve repair carried out via the left atrial appendage.[36]

Left atrial appendectomy should be a routine fixture of all cardiac surgery considering the life expectancy of the population and the increased prevalence of AF as the population gets older.

The Corridor Operation

A strip (channel) of atrial tissue (corridor) is isolated to restore sinus node function (Fig. 6).[1,37-39] The strip of atrial tissue has a small surface area and should not be able to sustain AF. The Corridor operation is performed under cardiopulmonary bypass and cold cardioplegic cardiac arrest. The surgical technique comprises exclusion of the left atrial free wall by using a horseshoe incision along the attachment of the left atrial wall onto the atrial septum. Construction of the corridor itself uses a horseshoe incision attaching onto the tricuspid anulus delineating the corridor, which includes a cuff of right atrium that harbors the sinus node region, the AV node region, and a strip of atrial septum bridging the two nodes.

We have reported our experience with nine patients.[37] Nine patients with drug-refractory AF underwent this operation; four patients had chronic AF and five had paroxysmal AF; the mean duration of symptoms was 12 ± 8 years. Patient ages ranged from 25 to 68 years (mean 48 ± 12). At preoperative electrophysiological study, no patient had evidence of an accessory AV pathway or AV node reentry. Sinus node recovery time could not be determined in five patients because of recurrent AF during or before programmed stimulation.

At operation, the corridor of atrial tissue harboring the sinus and AV nodes was successfully constructed in all patients. There were no perioperative complications. One patient required early reoperation to

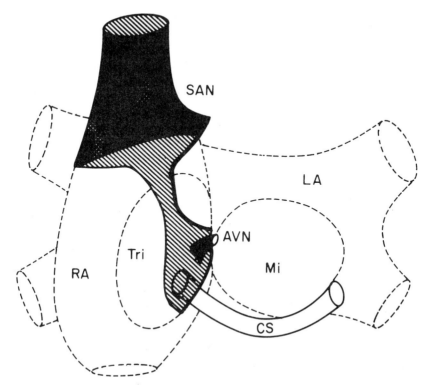

Figure 6. Corridor operation.

complete the corridor isolation. At the predischarge electrophysiological study, the corridor remained isolated in all patients except for one patient who had intermittent conduction between the corridor and excluded right atrium. One patient had nonsustained AF and one had atrial tachycardia within in the corridor. Atypical AV node reentry of uncertain significance was induced in one other patient. At exercise testing before discharge, the heart rate in the nine patients increased from a mean of 78 ± 20 beats per minute to 114 ± 17 beats per minute, the maximal heart rate achieved ranged from 41% to 84% (mean 68 ± 17%) of the predicted maximal heart rate based on age and gender criteria. The total follow-up time was 191 patient months (mean, 21 months; range, 3 to 52 months). Seven patients remain free of symptomatic supraventricular tachycardia. Two patients (cases 6 and 7) have had recurrences of AF during follow-up. The arrhythmia in one of these patients has been well controlled with propafenone (no recurrence in

36 months); the other patient has experienced paroxysmal episodes of AF (approximately weekly) while taking quinidine and verapamil. A permanent ventricular pacemaker was implanted in three patients after surgery. In two patients, a pacemaker was implanted after symptomatic sinus pauses and a pacemaker was implanted prophylactically when prolonged sinus pauses were demonstrated at the postoperative electrophysiological study. A patient who had undergone previous cardiac surgery and pacemaker implantation had an atrial pacemaker reimplanted postoperatively because of prolonged sinus pauses associated with bradycardia-dependent atrial arrhythmias.

These initial results demonstrate that the Corridor operation can maintain sinus rhythm in patients with AF.

Since then five additional patients have had a Corridor operation. Improved selection criteria allowed normal sinus node function after surgery in all.

Gursoy et al. reported five patients with the corridor operation for "lone atrtial fibrillation". Sinus node chronotropic function was normal postoperatively with good exercise tolerance.[40]

Vigano et al. recently reported 13 patients (nine males and four females) with the Corridor operation for paroxysmal lone AF (10 patients) and for atrial flutter (three patients).[41] The follow-up ranged from 9 months to 47 months. There were no surgical complications. All patients were in sinus rhythm with adequate exercise capacity. No patients were on antiarrhythmic drugs or had a pacemaker implanted.

Van Hemel et al. reported 36 patients with the Corridor operation for paroxysmal lone AF.[42] The follow-up was 41 ± 16 months. Thirty-one patients had successful construction of the corridor. Twenty-five patients were arrhythmia-free without medication (4-year actuarial freedom, 72 ± 9%). Twenty-six patients had normal sinus node function at rest and during exercise (4-year actuarial freedom of sinus node dysfunction, 81 ± 7%). Five patients had pacemaker implantation.

Overall, the Corridor operation gave good control of the arrhythmia and restored sinus rhythm, with a good functional capacity. One patient from Utrecht (the Netherlands) ran a marathon.

The Maze Operation

Since the first report,[22] the Maze operation has undergone many modifications and alterations by its designer and others. The master plan comprises a partial left atrial exclusion and multiple atriotomies combined with cryoblation. One left atriotomy divides the circular cuff of the left atrium around the mitral valve. Multiple right and septal atriotomies fragment and channel the right atrium and septum (Maze III) (Fig. 7).

Cox et al.[43-47] reported 87 patients with the Maze procedure for the treatment of atrial flutter and/or fibrillation. There were 64 males and 23 females with an average age of 54 years. The presenting arrhythmia was paroxysmal atrial flutter in six patients, paroxysmal AF in 37 patients, and chronic AF in 44 patients. All patients had failed extensive medical therapy with an average of five drugs per patient (36% had failed amiodarone).

Forty-three patients had paroxysmal atrial flutter or fibrillation (49%) and 44 patients had chronic AF (51%). The first 33 patients had the standard Maze procedure, whereas the remainder had variants that did not differ significantly from the original technique but were aimed at better preservation of the sinus node function. Twenty-four patients had concomitant cardiac repair, and seven had previous cardiac surgery.

Three patients died during surgery. Two patients had postoperative transient ischemic attacks. Early in the series, patients had postoperative fluid retention and pulmonary edema. This was caused by atrial natriuretic factor and was treated by spirolactone, which is now routinely prescribed. In the first 3 months after surgery, 47% of patients had recurrence of AF or atrial flutter. Of the 78 patients with more than 3 months of follow-up, 32 requried permanent pacing (AAI). Some patients had sinus node dysfunction before surgery. All patients were assessed in terms of exercise tolerance, arrhythmia (Holter), and cardiac function (atrial contraction). Overall, AF/flutter was controlled by surgery alone in 71 of 78 patients, whereas 32 patients (41%) required a pacemaker implantation. Since then, Cox has presented his continuing experience with 90 patients, confirming good results with the Maze III procedure.

Morris et al.[31] reported their experience with the Maze operation in 19 patients with nonvalvular AF. There was no mortality and all patients were in sinus rhythm 6 months after surgery with documented right and left atrial contraction.

Not all authors report such excellent results, with an average success of restoration of sinus rhythm in approximately 80% of patients.[48,49]

Left Atrial Isolation

Graffigna et al. have reported left atrial isolation in 184 patients with concomitant mitral valve surgery.[30] Seventy-one per cent of pa-

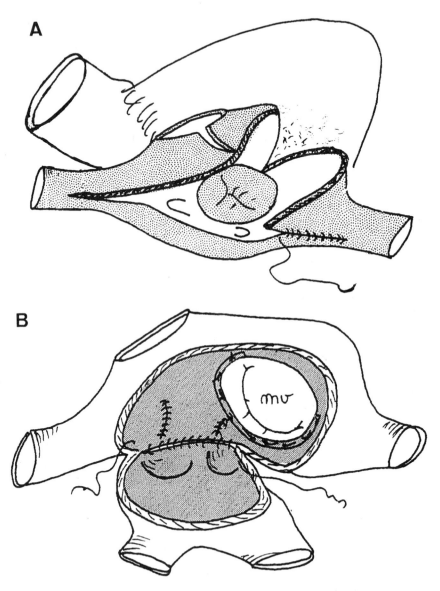

Figure 7. Maze operation. **A** = right atrial incisions; **B** = left atrial incisions.

tients returned to sinus rhythm after surgery, whereas 19% of patients with only mitral valve surgery returned to sinus rhythm (no controlled trial; $P < .001$). Patients with restored sinus rhythm had significantly greater cardiac index at discharge.

Boriani et al. recently reported a comparative study in patients with left atrial isolation combined with mitral valve surgery.[50] At 6 months, the mVO_2 was not significantly different than control, 23.3 ± 7.25 ml/min/m² versus 22 ± 5.6 ml/min/m².

Fragmentation or Compartment Operation (Open Corridor)

Shyu et al.[51] reported their experience with the Compartment operation in 22 patients. All patients had concomitant mitral valve surgery. The Compartment operation is best described as an open Corridor operation, the atriotomy which "normally" isolates the left atrium and the corridor itself is left incomplete and allows persistent connections between the three constructed segments of atria.

The Compartment operation was not associated with increased surgical morbidity. Fourteen patients (64%) were in sinus rhythm at 6 months of follow-up. Atrial mechanical function, as assessed by echo Doppler studies, was not always present after restoration of sinus rhythm.

The Spiral Operation

We have designed a new surgical technique to control AF, based on channeling of the right and left atria. The surgery is performed in three steps: modified extended vertical trans-septal approach, mitral valve surgery (if indicated), and spiraling of the left atrium combined with left atrial appendectomy (Fig. 8). A quasi-circumferential incision of the right atrium is performed (transplant incision). The right atrial free wall is incised along the right AV sulcus and is prolonged by a vertical septal incision through the fossa ovale. The incision of the superior wall (roof) of the left atrium extends from the septal incision and curves to reach the mitral valve anulus. The mitral valve is exposed using essentially stay sutures, and mitral valve surgery can be performed at that time. Spiraling of the left atrium is performed using a left atrial incision that is started at the mitral valve anulus in the left posterior septal region. The incision circumscribes the right pulmonary veins and proceeds transversely to circumscribe the left pulmonary

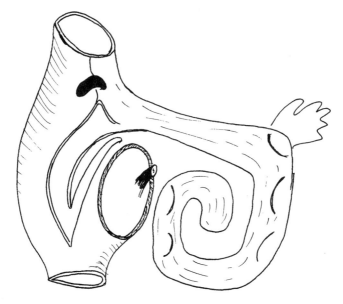

Figure 8. Spiral operation.

veins, traveling at the inferior pole of the left atrial appendage orifice. At that point, the incision involves the left atrial posterior wall. The extent of the spiraling incision depends on the posterior wall. The spiral incision can be done using conventional radiofrequency cauterization. The incision is not transmural with coagulation of the deeper layer by radiofrequency energy. The spiral incision is repaired by running sutures for safety, as well as other atriotomies.

Our initial experience comprised six patients (three with lone AF and three with mitral valve disease). Early good results need longer follow-up to be reliably assessed.

Cardiac Autotransplantation[28]

Recently Batista et al. (Brazil) advocated, at the 9th annual meeting of the European Association for Cardio-Thoracic Surgery (EACTS) in Paris, France, the use of cardiac autotransplantation for in vitro repair of complex cardiac lesions. Their experience comprised 84 patients. Sixty-two were female and 22 male (ages 18 to 75 years). Eighty-three patients were in chronic AF and one presented with the long QT syndrome. The left atrial diameter was greater than 6 cm, including

10 giant left atria in 68 patients. The left atrial diameter was between 6 cm and 4 cm in 16 patients. Cardiac pathology was as follows: mitral valve disease, 64 patients; aortic valve disease, 21; tricuspid valve disease, 4; and left atrial thrombosis, 13. Cardiac repair was performed, in vitro, on the warm cardioplegic heart. All patients were in sinus rhythm in the early postoperative period. Thirteen patients died postoperatively. At six months follow-up, 5 of 71 survivors were in AF (left atrial dimension >4.5 cm). All patients with a left atrial dimension smaller than 4 cm postoperatively were in sinus rhythm.

These remarkable results have been duplicated by other teams recently in Buffalo, NY and Bristol, England.[52] This reminds us that the role of the autonomic nervous system has been underestimated or neglected by electrophysiological interventionists.

Comments

Although surgical techniques are associated with good surgical results, surgical successes are not evidence that the surgical rationales are valid.

Surgical techniques may fail to meet the secondary end points: failure to interrupt AF, failure to reestablish sinus node function with adequate chronotropic response to exercise, and failure to restore atrial contraction.

Failure to Interrupt Atrial Fibrillation: The identical AF mechanism could be present postoperatively because: (1) The surgical rationale is inappropriate; (2) The working mechanism is a variant of the one currently accepted (focal mechanism?); or, (3) The surgery was not adequately executed. Failure to interrupt AF may be an illusion because new atrial tachycardia, such as multifocal atrial tachycardia, which can mimic the clinical presentation of AF are present after surgery. Current catheter electrophysiological studies have inherent limitations in distinguishing among these various mechanisms. These postoperative arrhythmias may be transitory, but are disturbing evidence that our understanding of AF is rudimentary and that there might be more than one working mechanism.

Failure to Restore Sinus Node Function: Sinus node dysfunction may be present before surgery and is part of AF pathophysiology. It can be induced surgically because of the site of atriotomies and/or associated ischemic changes. Although AAI pacemaker implantation can restore atrial contraction and chronotropic function, sinus dysfunction is a significant setback.

Atrial Contraction: Loss of atrial contraction can be part of surgical design (corridor or left atrial exclusion) or because of irreversible myocardial damage.

Underlying cardiac pathology has been overlooked in most studies. Surgery could fail to meet the primary end points. Unfortunately, reported studies did not or could not address these issues. This constitutes a serious flaw in our experience. Secondary end points document that the surgery has been achieved, as graft patency for coronary artery bypass surgery, but does not document that the surgery has a significant impact on patient outcome.

Surgical Indication: Surgical indications remain controversial, because the primary end points have not been validated. Other nonpharmacological electrophysiological interventions provide excellent control of arrhythmia with fewer side effects and/or risks. Patients with mitral valve disease, who require concomitant mitral valve surgery, seem to be an acceptable indication and this is currently used by some surgical teams.[53-56] Concomitant surgery for AF seems a benign adjunct to mitral valve surgery although it may increase surgical risk in various ways: atriotomies, prolongation of aortic cross-clamping and/or cardiopulmonary bypass time. Mitral valve disease associated with AF is a complex entity with multiple components: valvular anatomy, left ventricular function, left atrial dimension, duration of symptoms, age, sex, etc. Recent studies show that left ventricular function is the main independent prognostic marker. A recent review[57] of long-term follow-up of patients after mitral valve repair shows no difference between patients with or without AF in terms of survival and even morbidity at five years. Despite the large number of reported patients with combined surgery for AF, no comparative randomized series has been published in terms of outcome. AF might share the same fate as ventricular arrhythmia in patients with coronary artery disease: the premier prognostic marker is cardiac function, and it dwarfs all other markers or symptoms, even when those symptoms are the primary clinical presentation.

Further Directions

If electrophysiological assessment of AF becomes more precise, new rationales may develop guided by atrial mapping. AF may be associated with a focal perpetuating site which could be ablated.

However, it should be expected that surgery for AF shares the fate of other surgical approaches to supraventricular arrhythmias. Surgical techniques are associated with significant morbidity, and should be used to collect data and to assess new rationales and techniques which could be delivered by less invasive approaches.

Recently, catheter ablation techniques have been used to control AF. First, Haissaguerre et al. used catheter ablation techniques for unusual forms of AF.[58] These developments suggest that catheter ablation of AF may be common practice in the foreseeable future.[59,60]

Recent meetings of the American Heart Association (AHA) (1995) and the American College of Cardiology (ACC) (1996) have seen a flourish of presentations regarding catheter techniques and catheter ablation of AF. These studies have presented two new concepts: (1) Catheter techniques can safely produce linear transmural ablation (like incisions),[61–63] and (2) Segmental linear ablation can prevent either initiation[64] or perpetuation[65–67] of AF. Current surgical techniques may be "overkill" without added benefit.

The Case for Video Assisted Surgery for Atrial Fibrillation

Video assisted thoracic surgery (VATS) can provide an excellent approach to:[68] (1) the left lateral wall of the left atrium and the left atrial appendage; and (2) the wall of the right atrial free wall. VATS can also provide access to the posterior wall of the left atrium and the roof of the left atrium. Via this access, the atrial wall can be mapped using multielectrode plaques as well as "neutralized" using various tools and energies (RF, cryoablation, etc.). VATS can be associated with good control of the arrhythmia and with minimal side effects.

VATS allows the surgeon to carry out a left atrial appendectomy which may prove to be the most beneficial intervention for AF.

References

1. Guiraudon GM, Campbell CS, Jones DL, et al. Combined sino-atrial node atrio-ventricular isolation: A surgical alternative to His bundle ablation in patients with atrial fibrillation. Circulation 1985;72(suppl 2):III–220. Abstract.
2. Guiraudon GM, Guiraudon CM. Atrial functional anatomy. In: Kingma JH, van Hemel NM, Lie KI, eds. Atrial Fibrillation: A Treatable Disease? Boston, MA: Kluwer Academic; 1992:23.
3. Lamas GA. Physiological consequences of normal atrioventricular conduction: applicability to modern cardiac pacing. J Cardiac Surg 1989;4:89.
4. Robinson TF, Factor SM, Sonnenblick EH. The heart as a suction pump. Sci Amer 1986;254(6):84.

5. Aberg H. Atrial fibrillation. I. A study of atrial thrombosis and systemic embolism in a necropsy material. Acta Med Scand 1969;185:373–379.
6. Acar J, Cormier D, Grimberg G, et al. Diagnosis of left atrial thrombi in mitral stenosis: usefulness of ultrasound techniques compared with other methods. Eur J Cardiol 1991;12(suppl B):70–76.
7. Cormier B, Serafini D, Grimberg D, et al. Detection of thrombosis of the left atrium in mitral valve stenosis. Arch Maladies Coeur Vaisseaux 1991; 84:1321–1326.
8. James TN. Diversity of histopathologic correlates of atrial fibrillation. In: Kulbertus HE, Olson SB, Schlepper M, eds. Atrial Fibrillation. Modudal, Sweden: Astra; 1982:13.
9. Bharati S, Lev M. Histology of the normal and diseased atrium. In: Falk RH, Podrid PJ, eds. Atrial Fibrillation: Mechanisms and Management. New York: Raven Press; 1992:15.
10. Frustaci A, Caldarulo M, Buffon A, et al. Cardiac biopsy in patients with "primary" atrial fibrillation: histologic evidence of occult myocardial diseases. Chest 1991;2:303.
11. Sekiguchi M, Hiroe M, Kasanuki H, et al. Experience of 100 atrial endomyocardial biopsies and the concept of atrial cardiomyopathy. Circulation 1984; 70(suppl 2):118. Abstract.
12. Guiraudon CM, Ernst NM, Guiraudon GM, et al. The pathology of drug resistant lone atrial fibrillation in eleven surgically treated patients. In: Kingma JH, van Hemel NM, Lie KI, eds. Atrial Fibrillation: A Treatable Disease? Boston, MA: Kluwer Academic; 1992:41.
13. Guiraudon CM, Ernst NM, Klein GJ, et al. The pathology of intractable "primary" atrial fibrillation. Circulation 1992;86(suppl I),(4):I-662. Abstract.
14. Moe GK. On the multiple wavelet hypothesis of atrial fibrillation. Arch Int Pharmacodyn 1962;140:183.
15. Allessie MA, Lammers WJEP, Bonke FIM. Experimental evaluation of Moe's multiple wavelet hypothesis of atrial fibrillation. In: Zipes DP, Jalife J, eds. Cardiac Electrophysiology and Arrhythmias. New York: Grune & Stratton; 1985:265.
16. Allessie M, Kirchhof C. Termination of atrial fibrillatioin by class IC antiarrhythmic drugs: a paradox? In: Kingma JH, van Hemel NM, Lie KI, eds. Atrial Fibrillation: A Treatable Disease? Boston, MA: Kluwer Academic; 1992:265.
17. Wijffels M, Kirchhof C, Frederiks J, et al. Atrial fibrillation begets atrial fibrillation. Circulation 1993;86(suppl I):I–18. Abstract.
18. Allessie MA. Reentrant mechanisms underlying atrial fibrillation. In: Zipes DP, Jalife J, eds. Cardiac Electrophysiology: From Cell to Bedside. 2nd ed. Toronto: WB Saunders Co; 1995:562–566.
19. Schuessler RB, Grayson TM, Bromberg BI, et al. Cholinergically mediated tachyarrhythmias induced by a single extrastimulus in the isolated canine right atrium. Circulation Res 1992;71(5):1254–1267.
20. Morillo CA, Klein GJ, Jones DL, et al. Chronic rapid atrial pacing: structural, functional, and electrophysiological characteristics of a new model of sustained atrial fibrillation. Circulation 1995;91(5):1588–1595.
21. Harada A, Sasaki K, Fukushima T, et al. A atrial activation during chronic

atrial fibrillation in patients with isolated mitral valve disease. Ann Thorac Surg 1996;61:104–112.
22. Cox JL, Canavan TE, Schuessler RB. The surgical treatment of atrial fibrillation: II. Intra-operative electrophysiologic mapping and description of the electrophysiologic basis of atrial flutter and atrial fibrillation. J Thorac Cardiovasc Surg 1991;101:406–426.
23. Pertsov AM, Davidenko JM, Salomonsz R, et al. Spiral waves of excitation underlie reentrant activity in isolated cardiac muscle. Circulation Res 1993;631–650.
24. Stanton MS, Miles WM, Zipes DP. Atrial fibrillation and flutter. In: Zipes DP, Jalife J, eds. Cardiac Electrophysiology: From Cell to Bedside. Toronto: WB Saunders Co; 1990:735–742.
25. Stevenson WG, Stevenson LW, Middlekauff HR, et al. Atrial fibrillation no longer increases mortality in advanced heart failure: a longitudinal study of 750 patients. JACC 1996;27(2)(suppl A):89A. Abstract.
26. Waldo AL. Animal models of atrial arrhythmias. In: DiMarco JP, Prystowsky EN, ed. Atrial Arrhythmias: State of the Art. Armonk, NY: Futura Publishing Co; 1995:213–240.
27. Guiraudon GM, Coumel C. Personal communication. London, Ontario; Paris, France.
28. Batista RJV, Cunha MA, Takeshita N, et al. Cardiac autotransplantation: a new approach for the treatment of complex cardiac problems (Abstract). In: Programme Book, 9th Annual Meeting, The European Association for Cardio-Thoracic Surgery, Paris, France, September 24–27, 1995, p. 248.
29. Elvan A, Pride HP, Eble JN, Zipes DP. Radiofrequency catheter ablation of the atria reduces the inducibility and duration of atrial fibrillation in dogs. Circulation 1995;91:2235–2244.
30. Graffigna A, Ressia L, Pagnani F, et al. Left atrial isolation for the treatment of atrial fibrillation due to mitral valve disease: hemodynamic evaluation. N Trend Arrhyth IX 1993;4:1069.
31. Morris JJ, Stanton MS, Hammill SC. The Maze procedure: a reproducibly safe and effective cure for refractory nonvalvular atrial fibrillation. Circulation (suppl I) 1995;92(8):I–264. Abstract.
32. Haissaguerre M, Gaita F, Fischer B, et al. Elimination of atrioventricular nodal reentrant tachycardia using discrete slow potentials to guide application of radiofrequency energy. Circulation 1992;85:2162–2175.
33. Shrestha NK, Moreno FL, Narciso GV, et al. Two-dimensional echocardiographic diagnosis of left atrial thrombus in rheumatic heart disease: a clinicopathologic study. Circulation 1983;67:341–347.
34. Leung DYC, Black IW, Crannery GB, et al. Prognostic implications of left atrial spontaneous echo contrast in nonvalvular atrial fibrillation. J Am Coll Cardiol 1994;24:755–762.
35. Blackshear JL, Odell JA. Appendage obliteration to reduce stroke in cardiac surgical patients with atrial fibrillation. Ann Thorac Surg 1996;61: 755–759.
36. Christides C, Cabrol C, Cabrol A, et al. Reinterventions sur protheses valvulaires mitrales. A propos de 16 malades. Coeur 1974;Numero special: 515–523.
37. Leitch JW, Klein G, Yee R, et al. Sinus node-atrioventricular node isolation:

long term results with the Corridor operation for atrial fibrillation. J Am Coll Cardiol 1991;17(4):970.

38. Guiraudon GM, Klein GJ, Yee R. Supraventricular tachycardias: the role of surgery. PACE 1993;I,16,1:658–670.

39. Guiraudon GM, Klein GJ, Guiraudon CM, Yee R. Treatment of atrial fibrillation: preservation of sinoventricular impulse conduction: the Corridor operation. In: Olsson SB, Allessie MA, Campbell RWF, eds. Atrial Fibrillation: Mechanisms and Therapeutic Strategies. Armonk, NY: Futura Publishing Co; 1994:349–371.

40. Gursoy S, de Bruyne B, Atie J, et al. Interatrial dissociation following the corridor operation: role of atrial contraction in thrombogenesis. Eur Heart J 1991;12(suppl):337. Abstract.

41. Vigano M, Graffigna A, Pagnani F, et al. The surgical treatment for supraventricular arrhythmias. In: D'Alessandro LC. Heart Surgery. Rome, Italy: Casa Editrice Scientifica Internazionale, 1993:403.

42. van Hemel NM, Defaux JJAMT, Kingma JH, et al. Long-term results of the "Corridor" operation for atrial fibrillation. Br Heart J 1994;71:170.

43. Cox JL. Evolving applications of the Maze procedure for atrial fibrillation. Ann Thorac Surg 1993;55:578–580.

44. Cox JL, Boineau JP, Schuessler RB, et al. Successful surgical treatment of atrial fibrillation: review and clinical update. JAMA 1991;266:1976–1978.

45. Cox JL, Boineau JP, Schuessler RB, et al. Five-year experience with the Maze procedure for atrial fibrillation. Ann Thorac Surg 1993;56:814–824.

46. Cox JL, Boineau JP, Schuessler RB, et al. Surgical interruption of atrial reentry as a cure for atrial fibrillation. In: Olsson SB, Allessie MA, Campbell RWF, eds. Atrial Fibrillation: Mechanisms and Therapeutic Strategies. Armonk, NY: Futura Publishing Co; 1994:373–404.

47. Cox JL, Schuessler RB, Cain ME, et al. Surgery for atrial fibrillation. Sem Thorac Cardiovasc Surg 1989;1(1):67–73.

48. Kim Y-J, Sohn D-W, Park Y-B, et al. Restoration of atrial mechanical function after Maze operation: is it affected by the same factors as the restoration of sinus rhythm? JACC 1996;27(2)(suppl A):261A. Abstract.

49. Izumoto H, Kawazoe K, Mukaida M, et al. Is the Maze procedure safely combined with mitral valve repair? JACC 1996;27(2)(suppl A):261A. Abstract.

50. Boriani G, Capucci A, Marinelli G, et al. Left atrial isolation combined with mitral valve surgery: hemodynamic evaluation during cardiopulmonary exercise test. JACC 1996;27(2)(suppl A):260A. Abstract.

51. Shyu K-G, Cheng J-J, Chen J-J, et al. Recovery of atrial function after atrial compartment operation for chronic atrial fibrillation in mitral valve disease. J Am Coll Cardiol 1994;24(2):392–398.

52. Salerno TA, Bhazana S. Buffalo General Hospital, Buffalo, NY. Personal communication.

53. Brodman RF, Frame R, Fisher JD, et al. Combined treatment of mitral stenosis and atrial fibrillation with valvuloplasty and left atrial Maze procedure. J Thorac Cardiovasc Surg (letter) 1994;107:622.

54. Hioki M, Ikeshita M, Iedokoro Y, et al. Successful combined operation for mitral stenosis and atrial fibrillation. Ann Thorac Surg 1993;55:776–778.

55. McCarthy PM, Cosgrove DM, Castle LW, et al. Combined treatment of

mitral regurgitation and atrial fibrillation with valvuloplasty and the Maze procedure. Am J Cardiol 1993;71:483–486.

56. Kosakai Y, Kawaguchi AT, Isobe F, et al. Cox Maze procedure for chronic atrial fibrillation associated with mitral valve disease. J Thorac Cardiovasc Surg 1994;108:1049–1055.
57. Chua YL, Schaff HV, Orszulak TA, Morris JJ. Outcome of mitral valve repair in patients with preoperative atrial fibrillation. J Thorac Cardiovasc Surg 1994;107:408–415.
58. Haissaguerre M, Marcus FI, Fischer B, Clementy J. Radiofrequency catheter ablation in unusual mechanisms of atrial fibrillation: report of 3 cases. J Cardiovasc Electrophysiol 1994;5:743–751.
59. Haissaguerre M, Gencel L, Fischer B, et al. Successful catheter ablation of atrial fibrillation. J Cardiovasc Electrophysiol 1994;5:1045–1052.
60. Swarz J, Pellersels G, Silvers J, et al. A catheter-based approach to atrial fibrillation in humans. Circulation 1994;90(suppl 4):I–335. Abstract.
61. He DS, Mackey S, Marcus FI, et al. Radiofrequency energy for cardiac ablation using a multipolar catheter in sheep. Circulation (suppl I);92(8):I–265. Abstract.
62. Nakagawa H, Yamanashi WS, Pitha JV, et al. Creation of long linear transmural radiofrequency lesions in atrium using a novel spiral ribbon: saline irrigated electrode catheter. JACC 1996;27(2)(suppl A):188A. Abstract.
63. Avitall B, Helms RW, Chianng W, Periman BA. Nonlinear atrial radiofrequency lesions are arrhythmogenic: a study of skipped lesions in the normal atria. Circulation (suppl I)1995;92(8):I–265. Abstract.
64. Tondo C, Otomo K, Antz M, et al. Successful radiofrequency catheter ablation of atrial fibrillation by a single lesion to the inter-atrial septum. Circulation (suppl I);92(8):I–265. Abstract.
65. Haines DE, McRury IA. Primary atrial fibrillation ablation (PAFA) in a chronic atrial fibrillation model. Circulation (suppl I);92(8):I–265. Abstract.
66. Natale A, Tomassoni G, Kearney MM, et al. Catheter ablation approach on the right side only for paroxysmal atrial fibrillation therapy. Circulation 1995;92(8):I–266. Abstract.
67. Man KC, Daoud E, Knight B, et al. Right atrial radiofrequency catheter ablation of paroxysmal atrial fibrillation. JACC 1996;27(2)(suppl A):188A. Abstract.
68. Inderbitzi R. Surgical Thoracoscopy. Berlin, Germany: Springer-Verlag, 1994.

CHAPTER 18

Catheter Ablation as a Curative Approach to the Substrate of Atrial Fibrillation

Francis D. Murgatroyd, David E. Haines, John F. Swartz

Introduction

Atrial fibrillation is the most common sustained arrhythmia, affecting 0.4% of the general population and over 10% of the elderly.[1-3] Aside from its symptomatic effects (palpitation, dyspnea, dizziness, and sometimes, angina and syncope), it is associated with an adverse long-term prognosis due to an increased risk of systemic thromboembolism and impaired hemodynamic function. Conventional therapy is directed at one of two strategies. One is the restoration and maintenance of sinus rhythm using antiarrhythmic drugs and transthoracic cardioversion when necessary. The alternative approach is to improve symptoms by controlling the ventricular rate and giving anticoagulant therapy to decrease the risk of thromboembolism. Long-term antiarrhythmic therapy is neither uniformly effective nor uniformly safe, and anticoagulation is inconvenient and carries the risk of bleeding complications.

A variety of nonpharmacological strategies have been investigated in the management of atrial fibrillation (AF), including the attempt to use implanted devices to terminate and suppress arrhythmic episodes. Until recently, the only applications of catheter ablation in patients with AF were as nonpharmacological means of ventricular rate control—complete ablation[4] or attempted modification[5] of atrioventricular nodal conduction. However, the results of surgical division of the atria[6,7] indicate that sinus rhythm and atrial contractility can be restored, even in patients with long-standing AF associated with valvular heart disease. Recently, there have been indications that similar cura-

From *Nonpharmacological Management of Atrial Fibrillation*, edited by F.D. Murgatroyd and A.J. Camm. © 1997, Futura Publishing Co., Inc., Armonk, NY.

tive procedures can be successfully developed using transvenous catheter ablation. In this chapter, we will describe experimental studies and the early clinical experience in this field, and discuss some of the technical issues related to catheter design and procedure safety.

The Feasibility of Catheter Ablation to the Atrial Substrate

Atrial fibrillation has been shown to consist of multiple reentrant wavelets, circulating around both anatomical obstacles and lines of functional block using the "leading circle" mechanism described by Moe[8] and Allessie et al.[9] A critical mass of atrial myocardium is required for the sustenance of AF.[10,11] Several surgical procedures have been developed for the treatment of AF, based on the reduction of this critical mass of tissue. Atrial compartmentation[6,12,13] and the "Corridor" operation[14] provide, as a minimum, an alternative to atrioventricular nodal ablation, with the sinus node driving the ventricle via tissue that is excluded from the fibrillating mass. They may also have a genuine antiarrhythmic action by dividing this fibrillating mass and thus reducing the likelihood of AF.

More radically, the "Maze" operation was devised on the basis of mapping studies in animals and patients, and alters the anatomical substrate in such a way that reentry is impossible other than with very small wavelets.[15-18] However, this operation is a major undertaking with significant morbidity and cost implications: its broad application, other than as an adjunct to other open heart procedures (such as mitral valve surgery and possibly septal myectomy for hypertrophic cardiomyopathy), may be limited. As in the Wolff-Parkinson-White syndrome, however, the surgical operation has demonstrated the validity of the concept of a curative procedure. The ability to reproduce the success of the Maze operation by catheter ablation would be a very attractive prospect for electrophysiologists and their patients. The feasibility of such an approach has been demonstrated both in a number of animal models and recently in patients, and will be discussed later.

Technical Considerations for Catheter Ablation to the AF Substrate

In both the Maze[17] and Corridor[19] operations, it was found that the incision/suture lines must be complete and continuous to obtain procedural success. Conducting gaps in the lines of block may require repeat surgery or difficult mapping and ablation procedures to extinguish intra-atrial reentrant tachycardias. Similarly, successful ablation between the inferior vena cava and tricuspid annulus for common atrial flutter is correlated with the appearance of complete bidirectional conduction block in the isthmus.[20] The linear lesions required for catheter ablation to the AF substrate therefore need to be continuous and transmural. Achieving this result represents a considerable challenge even in the smooth, thin-walled areas of the atria. The difficulty is greater around the tricuspid and mitral annuli and at the crista terminalis, where greater tissue penetration of energy is required because of the tissue thickness, and around the atrial appendages and the right atrium anterior to the crista, where tissue contact is difficult because of trabeculation.

Currently available steerable ablation catheters can be used with a drag technique to produce a chain of conventional lesions, but this technique is painstaking and technically very difficult where the ablation line is perpendicular to the catheter shaft. Swartz et al.[21] addressed this problem using a series of long, shaped sheaths (Daig Corp., Minnetonka, MN, USA) to guide a 4 mm or 5 mm tip ablation catheter of relatively conventional design. For each line of ablation, a sheath was selected that would deliver the catheter to the distal end, in the direction of the line. After performing repeated dry runs to verify good atrial contact and a smooth pullback along the desired course, each line was then ablated using continuous energy delivery, moving the catheter by 2–3 mm every 30 seconds. Continuous temperature monitoring was used. This technique has proved very successful in restoring sinus rhythm in a group of patients with long-standing AF that is resistant to antiarrhythmic drug therapy. However, the procedure is lengthy (frequently more than 10 hours), and technically demanding, as an incomplete line of block requires mapping to identify the "gap," or repeat ablation of the whole line. In approximately half of the patients, atrial tachycardias occurred after a few days. These were found to be due to reentrant circuits, usually related to the mitral valve annulus or left superior pulmonary vein, and were abolished by local ablation.

The success achieved by Swartz et al. has demonstrated that catheter ablation of the substrate of AF is conceptually valid. However, the painstaking nature of the linear drag technique has prompted the development of catheters specifically designed to create lesions that are several centimeters long, without the need for frequent repositioning. A number of investigators have recently reported initial results with these catheters in animal preparations. The technology that is required differs in many respects from that of conventional radiofrequency catheters.

Electrode Design

First, the use of a single, long electrode would not be appropriate; this would result in nonuniform tissue heating, in part due to the "edge" effect (current density being naturally highest at the ends of a long electrode), and in part due to local variation in tissue contact. All linear ablation catheter designs have therefore used multiple poles, and the construction and spacing of the electrode segments affects the lesions produced. Fleischman et al. investigated the mechanical properties of catheters with 12.5 mm coil electrodes and 2 mm spacing.[22] The greatest flexibility (smooth curvature without sharp angles at the interelectrode spacing) and maneuverability were achieved by avoiding the tight winding of round wire, or by the use of flat wire for the coils. Demazumder et al. investigated the maximum interelectrode spacing compatible with continuous lesions of at least 3 mm depth, in an in vitro model,[23] and found the flow of the superfusing blood analogue to be an important determinant. Compared with static superfusate, a flow rate of 0.5 m/s increased thermal diffusion, causing the power requirement for a tissue interface temperature of 70°C to rise from 9 W to 25 W. This thermal diffusion increased the maximum interelectrode spacing compatible with continuous lesions from 5 mm to 9 mm. It was also noted that with flow, conventionally measured electrode temperature overestimated the tissue interface temperature by up to 20°C. These experimental results may not translate easily between species; Tomassoni et al. attempted linear ablation in the pectinate muscle of the right atrial appendage, and found that 1 mm interelectrode spacing created continuous lesions in dogs, but not in sheep.[24]

Temperature Control

The issue of temperature control is more complex in linear multielectrode catheters than in conventional radiofrequency ablation catheters. Whayne et al.[25] compared three multipolar linear ablation catheter systems in the canine atrium. In two systems—one with ring electrodes, the other with stiff coils—energy was delivered to each electrode in sequence. Each electrode had individual conventional temperature control (70°-80°C). The third system (MECA℠, EP Technologies,

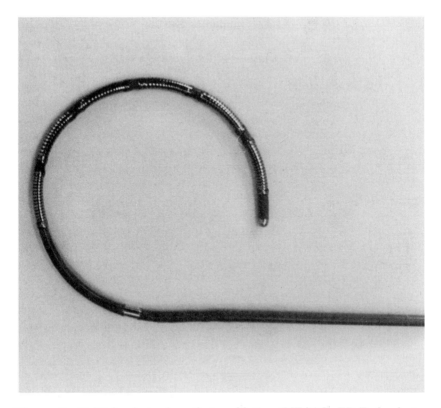

Figure 1. Multiple electrode catheter ablation (MECA℠, EP Technologies, Sunnyvale, CA, USA) catheter.[25]

Sunnyvale, CA, USA, Fig. 1), was able to deliver energy simultaneously to all the electrodes. In this system, each electrode segment was a flexible coil provided with a pair of thermistors, at either end and opposite sides of the coil, and the higher of the two measured temperatures was used by the system for feedback power control.[26] Due to the "edge" effect on current density, a conventional centrally located thermistor may not be ideal, and the dual thermistor system appears more likely to detect peak tissue rather than blood temperature.[27] Only 6% of the ablation lines delivered with the ring electrodes catheter were correctly targeted, continuous and transmural, compared with 36% of those delivered with sequential coil catheters and 76% of those using the MECA system. Probable reasons for these differences include the additive effect of heating adjacent electrodes simultaneously, improved flexibility yielding better tissue contact, and more accurate temperature monitoring. It is not clear, however, to what extent the latter advantage came from the presence of two thermistors as opposed to their location at the end rather than the centre of the electrode.

Temperature control is critical not only for the creation of continuous transmural lesions, but also for the avoidance of char and coagulum, and this is especially important in the left atrium because of the risk of systemic thromboembolism. Many studies have indicated that excessive temperatures are associated with the risk of char and coagulum. Strickberger et al. reported the use of linear ablation catheters in dogs, with energy delivered in sequence to each of four electrodes and a target temperature of 70°–85°C.[28] A total of 20 ablation lines (80 energy deliveries) was created, of which 14 were transmural throughout the length, and two through part of the length. Four (5%) of the lesions resulted in coagulum formation, in all cases associated with temperature rises >85°C. Kalman et al. used intracardiac echocardiography to guide catheter placement and ensure tissue contact in a model of AF in eight dogs.[29] Three ablation lines were created in the right atrium and two in the left: six lesions caused endocardial char formation—all associated with currents >0.9 A—and one sudden death (myocardial infarction, possibly related to coronary embolism) occurred during left atrial ablation. The same group used intracardiac echocardiography to guide the placement of three right atrial lesions in each of six pigs, and obtained complete linear block without any char or thrombus formation. In a comparative study of catheter systems with multiple electrodes of 12.5 mm length and a target temperature of 70°C, McRury et al.[27] found coagulum present after 51/99 energy deliveries by electrodes with single central thermistors, and 1/138 energy deliveries with the MECA dual thermistor system described above.

Local atrial electrogram amplitude may serve in addition to temperature control for evaluating the result of energy delivery on-line. Avitall et al. monitored this parameter continuously during energy delivery with a multipolar catheter system.[30] Power was titrated to each electrode until a 50% reduction in local electrogram amplitude was achieved, or a maximum 25 W of power had been delivered for 45 seconds. Postmortem examination indicated that contiguous transmural lesions were achieved when the electrogram amplitude was attenuated by more than 25% and a temperature >55°C was reached. Char was seen on two electrodes, both associated with >90% electrogram attenuation and temperature >100°C. It was concluded from this study that targets of 70°C for temperature and of 50%–80% for electrogram attenuation are appropriate.

A novel approach to the production of linear lesions without thrombus or char resulting from overheating is the use of saline perfused balloon catheters. Wharton et al.[31] used radiofrequency catheters with twelve 2 mm rings connected to form two six-ring electrodes. Each was surrounded by a 14 French angioplasty balloon with pores to allow saline outflow. Thus, the entire content and surface of the balloon was heated to the target temperature without the possibility of local "hot spots". Of 12 attempted linear ablations in sheep, optimal catheter seating was obtained on seven occasions, and five of these were found at subsequent histological examination to result in continuous transmural lesions. No ulceration, thrombus, or char was seen. This technique may offer an improved safety profile compared with direct electrode-tissue contact, but improved deployment systems are clearly needed.

Other Aspects of Catheter Design

As previously described, most animal and clinical investigations of linear ablation in the atria have used conventional catheters with deflectable tips or nonsteerable multipolar catheters.[32] The delivery of conventional catheters to the desired location and orientation may be assisted by the use of long single- or multielement preshaped sheaths.[21] Multipolar ablation allows the creation of a line of lesions from a single fixed position, but requires the catheter body to be positioned tangentially to the atrial wall. Positioning of these catheters can be difficult, especially when the desired line of ablation lies perpendicular to the direction from which the catheter is delivered, such as horizontal lines in the right atrium, or vertical lines in the left atrium via a transseptal approach. Steerability in two planes is a feature of some multipolar catheter designs and is likely to be highly advantageous. Even when the catheter is delivered to the correct location and orientation, ensuring adequate tissue contact may prove difficult. For this purpose, the San Francisco group strongly advocates the use of intracardiac echocardiography.[29] It is not known whether other imaging methods, such as transesophageal echocardiography, or electrical parameters, such as impedance or electrogram morphology, could also serve as adequate guides to tissue contact prior to energy delivery.

Another proposed means of optimizing tissue contact is the use of a multipolar catheter in the form of a loop deployed from a sheath. Haines et al. tested a design with a loop formed from two splines with ring or coil electrodes along their length.[33] Approximately 75% of 35 lesions created in canine left and right atria were in part transmural,

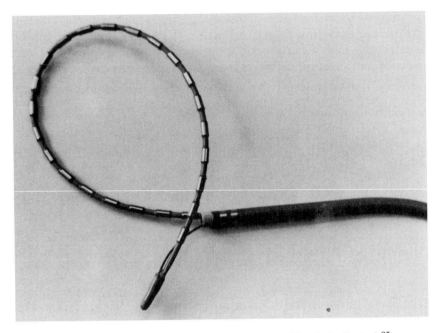

Figure 2. "Atrial ablater" catheter, devised by Avitall et al.[35]

but contiguity of lesions was never seen with ring electrodes, and was seen in only 25% when coils were used. Avitall et al. successfully used a similar system to create right lesions in the right atrium, and with various orientations via a transseptal approach in the left atrium.[34] A monorail guidewire was used both to position the catheter tip in a pulmonary vein or mitral valve orifice, and to deploy the loop (Fig. 2).[35] Continuous transmural lesions were created that extinguished sustained AF in four dogs.

Selection of Atrial Lesion Locations and Outcomes

The animal studies of atrial ablation described above have for the most part concentrated on the technical aspects of lesion delivery. In some, lines of block were created in locations selected on the basis of theoretical antiarrhythmic efficacy, while others have made no attempt to place "therapeutic" lesions. Some studies have been conducted in sinus rhythm, and a variety of models of AF have been utilized. In most cases where ablation has been performed in an AF model, the arrhythmia has either been extinguished or rendered noninducible. Clinical AF is a heterogeneous condition, and it is simplistic to assume that the disposition of lesions found to be effective in animal models can be translated directly to patients. As yet, only a few clinical studies exist of ablation to the AF substrate,[21,32,36] but a number of philosophies may be followed in the selection of lesion locations.

Catheter "Maze" Procedures

First, a procedure can be designed to eliminate the possibility of AF due to functional reentry. The prototype of this is the "Maze" procedure devised by Cox et al. on the basis of epicardial atrial mapping in dogs and man,[17,18] and subsequently revised on the basis of initial clinical findings (Fig. 3a).[37,38] In the catheter-based procedure described by Swartz et al., eight lines of block were created (three right atrial, four left atrial, one in the interatrial septum).[21] The lesion placement was broadly based on that of the Maze operation, the most important differences being in the treatment of the appendages and the posterior left atrium. In the Maze procedure, the appendages are amputated, and a large portion of the posterior left atrium, containing the four pulmonary venous orifices, is effectively isolated. In theory, this island would be noncontractile and might constitute a locus for thrombus formation. The catheter-based procedure spares both appendages and separates the pulmonary veins with intersecting horizontal and vertical lesion lines (Fig. 3b). The procedure has been performed in a number of patients with long-standing, drug-refractory AF, often in the setting of significant structural heart disease. In these patients, it was noted that the rhythm of each atrium became progressively organized with the completion of ablation lines on that side. Atrial fibrillation was, however, not usually extinguished without the completion of linear lesions in both atria. The procedure, though time-consuming, has proved to be highly effective in the treatment of patients with chronic AF. However, because of the extent of left atrial ablation, there is a significant potential for thromboembolism. If the procedure is to be more widely adopted, adequate precautions will be necessary to ensure the absence of char or coagulum formation.

In addition to providing anatomical obstacles to functional reentry, a catheter-based "Maze" procedure may have a second, indirect benefit, by altering the electrophysiological properties of the atria. Elvan et al. performed (epicardial) catheter ablation to the left and right atria (Fig.

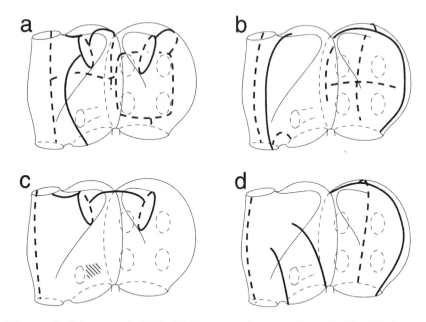

Figure 3. Schemas of atrial ablation procedures, as described by (a) Cox et al.,[37] (b) Swartz et al.,[21] (c) Elvan et al.,[39] (d) Kalman et al.[29]

3c) in a canine model using a combination of atrial pacing and vagal stimulation or methacholine infusion.[39] After ablation, there was marked attenuation of effective refractory period shortening by vagal stimulation but not by methacholine infusion, both in segments that were electrically isolated by lesions and in those that were not. Similar effects were seen on the inducibility of AF with vagal stimulation and methacholine. In the chronic state, the dose-response curve of the duration of AF inducible after methacholine infusion was shifted down and to the right. The procedure would therefore appear to have reduced AF inducibility both by causing lines of anatomical block, and by causing partial vagal denervation of the atrial myocardium.

Staged Ablation of the Atria

A second approach to ablation of the AF substrate is to reduce the occurrence of arrhythmia by performing more limited ablation, in a staged manner starting on one side alone. In a canine model of sustained AF (induced by rapid pacing over a period of weeks), Kalman et

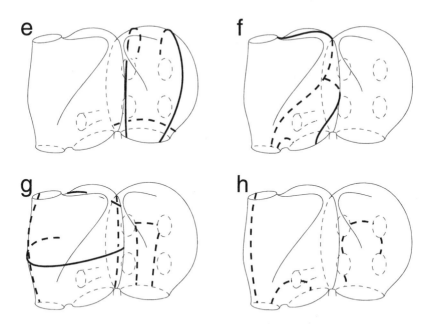

Figure 3. *(continued)* (e) Avitall et al.,[35] (f) Riccardi et al.,[36] (g) Haïssaguerre et al.,[32] and (h) Zarse et al.[47] Note that these figures are only approximate illustrations of the procedures described by each author. They are not intended to be anatomically accurate, but to give an indication of the variety in the extent and location of lesions.

al. found that fibrillation was abolished in 4/8 dogs by lesions on the right side alone, and in three dogs when left atrial lesions were also delivered (Fig. 3d).[29] An even more limited right atrial procedure has been suggested by Nakagawa et al.,[40] who found that a single large radiofrequency lesion interrupting Bachmann's bundle (created with a cool-tip electrode) was sufficient to terminate AF and prevent its reinduction in 8/9 cases of the canine sterile pericarditis model. Avitall et al. were able to extinguish sustained AF in four dogs using three lesions on the left side alone (Fig. 3e).[35]

The clinical experience of Haïssaguerre, which is described in the following chapter, is that paroxysmal AF can often be extinguished without the need for lesions in both atria, especially when the initial ablation lines result in an organized rhythm amenable to map-guided focal ablation. Riccardi et al. also reported some success with ablation limited to the right atrium in a group of 12 patients with paroxysmal AF of the vagal type, and structurally normal hearts (Fig. 3f).[36] No recurrences occurred in six patients (four of whom had previously taken ineffective antiarrhythmic drugs), three suffered recurrences of AF, and three, of atrial flutter. However, Haïssaguerre's group recently found that left atrial linear ablation significantly increases the success rate when added to right atrial lesions, and may on its own be more effective than purely right side ablation (Fig. 3g).[41]

The staged approach to ablation of the atrium is dependent on the type of AF, relying on the greater degree of organization in paroxysmal AF in structurally normal hearts compared with that in permanent arrhythmia. This difference was demonstrated by Kirchhof et al. who performed high-density mapping during cardiac surgery in patients with electrically induced AF and preexisting chronic AF.[42] In the latter group, atrial activation was more complex, and involved multiple simultaneous waves circulating around arcs of functional block. These arcs were usually perpendicular to the atrioventricular groove, suggesting an important role for tissue anisotropy. Thus, a staged or partial procedure has the advantage of causing less tissue destruction, and may avoid the left atrium altogether. However, it seems likely to be effective chiefly for paroxysmal or recent-onset AF in patients with relatively normal hearts. Furthermore, where it is associated with structural heart disease, AF might relapse months or years after an initially successful procedure due to progression of the underlying pathology.

Interruption of Anatomical Reentry

Zarse et al. from the Maastricht group have proposed a simple procedure based on the premise that macroreentry involving anatomical obstacles is more common than that purely around lines of functional block.[47] The successful elimination of all possible circuits based on anatomical reentry (Fig. 3h) was achieved in 14 Langendorff-perfused rabbit hearts with biatrial dilatation. The intra-atrial pressure required for sustained AF to be inducible rose from 9.2 ± 1.6 cm H_2O to over 14 cm H_2O in two, and over 20 cm H_2O in the remaining 12. This procedure has not been reported in other models or in humans.

Ablation of Underlying Repetitive Arrhythmias

Jaïs et al. have noted that in some cases the surface electrocardiographic appearance of AF may arise from a focal arrhythmia with fragmented interatrial conduction.[43] Intracardiac mapping can identify the source that is amenable to conventional catheter ablation. This arrhythmia characteristically occurs in young patients with frequent episodes, and conversion into a monomorhpic atrial tachycardia can often be seen. Similarly, the same group has sometimes found that after the creation of only one or two right atrial linear lesions, a highly organized repetitive form (reentrant flutter circuit or focal activity) is unmasked that is amenable to map-guided focal ablation.

Individualized Mapping and Ablation of the AF Substrate

In the future, the possibility of mapping AF in a patient, perhaps using an endocardial basket catheter, might allow the identification of favored locations for reentry and "streaming"[44] of depolarizing wave fronts, and also allow a tailor-made ablation procedure to be devised for that individual. Even with sufficient technological advancement to allow real-time high-density mapping of AF, the concept is based on two doubtful premises: (1) that such favored locations exist and are critical to the sustenance of AF, and (2) that the anatomical substrate in a given patient will not change with time. Truly individualized procedures are only likely to be applicable to patients with arrhythmias that are highly organized, or become so after a small number of standard lesions have been delivered. However, it is to be hoped that mapping of clinical AF in large numbers of patients will lead to the identification of the ideal sites for these initial, standard lesions. This will minimize procedure times and tissue destruction.

Summary

The conceptual validity of a curative treatment for AF based on the creation of lines of conduction block has been demonstrated in the operating room and by recent initial experience with transvenous catheter ablation. In patients with paroxysmal AF, a limited procedure in only one atrium may yield an organized atrial rhythm that is amenable to conventional mapping and focal ablation. Long-standing AF in the presence of structural heart disease has more electrophysiological complexity, and suppression of this type of arrhythmia appears to require a more extensive ablation procedure involving both atria. Clinical investigation of catheter ablation for AF is in its infancy, and the best pattern of ablation lines for each type of arrhythmia remains to be determined. However, any effective procedure requires the creation of lines of ablation lesions in the atrial myocardium that are continuous and transmural. Improvements in technique and technology are required to allow more rapid, precise, and reliable placement of these lines.

Excessive heating, causing char and thrombus, is a constant risk—in the left atrium, this can have grave embolic consequences. Good tissue contact and precise temperature control are necessary to avoid these complications. The likelihood of other potential adverse consequences from linear ablation in the atrium is unclear. Atrial proarrhythmia can occur due to the creation of inappropriate or incomplete lesions around which flutter circuits can turn.[45] Impairment of atrial contractile function due to tissue damage has been reported,[46] but is not seen uniformly[39]; conversely, patients in previously established AF may obtain hemodynamic improvement from the restoration of sinus rhythm.[21] Finally, these procedures involve the usual risks associated with transseptal puncture and long procedure and fluoroscopy times.

The benefit of a catheter-based procedure that provides long-term suppression of AF could be substantial, especially if the risks mentioned can be avoided, and the procedure duration significantly reduced. In addition to obtaining symptomatic improvement, patients may be able to avoid the inconvenience, risk, and cost of other antiarrhythmic therapies and anticoagulation. The economic benefits could significantly outweigh the initial outlay for the procedure itself.

References

1. Martin A, Benbow LJ, Butrous GS, et al. Five-year follow-up of 101 elderly subjects by means of long-term ambulatory cardiac monitoring. Eur Heart J 1984;5:592–596.
2. Petersen P, Godtfredsen J. Atrial fibrillation: a review of course and prognosis. Acta Med Scand 1984;216:5–9.
3. Ostrander LD Jr, Brandt RL, Kjelsberg MO, Epstein FH. Electrocardiographic findings among the adult population of a total natural community: Tecumseh, Michigan. Circulation 1965;31:888–898.
4. Scheinman MM, Morady F, Hess DS, Gonzalez R. Catheter induced ablation of the atrioventricular junction to control refractory supraventricular arrhythmias. JAMA 1982;248:851–855.
5. Williamson BD, Man KC, Daoud E, et al. Radiofrequency catheter modification of atrioventricular conduction to control the ventricular rate during atrial fibrillation. N Engl J Med 1994;331:910–917.
6. Shyu KG, Cheng JJ, Chen JJ, et al. Recovery of atrial function after atrial compartment operation for chronic atrial fibrillation in mitral valve disease. J Am Coll Cardiol 1994;24:392–398.

7. Cox JL, Boineau JP, Schuessler RB, et al. Five-year experience with the Maze procedure for atrial fibrillation. Ann Thorac Surg 1993;56:814–823.
8. Moe GK. On the multiple wavelet hypothesis of atrial fibrillation. Arch Int Pharmacodyn Ther 1962;140:183–188.
9. Allessie MA, Lammers WJEP, Bonke FIM, Hollen JM. Experimental evaluation of Moe's multiple wavelet hypothesis of atrial fibrillation. In: Zipes DP, Jalife J, eds. Cardiac Electrophysiology and Arrhythmias. Orlando, FL: Grune & Stratton; 1985:265–275.
10. Garrey WE. Auricular fibrillation. Physiol Rev 1924;4:215–250.
11. West TC, Landa JF. Minimal mass required for induction of a sustained arrhythmia in isolated atrial segments. Am J Physiol 1962;202:232–236.
12. Williams JM, Ungerleider RM, Lofland GK, Cox JL. Left atrial isolation: a new technique for the treatment of supraventricular arrhythmias. J Thorac Cardiovasc Surg 1980;80:373–380.
13. Harada A, D'Agostino HJJ, Schuessler RB, et al. Biatrial isolation with preservation of normal sinus node function and sino-ventricular conduction: a surgical treatment for supraventricular tachycardias. J Am Coll Cardiol 1987;9:100. Abstract.
14. Guiraudon GM, Campbell CS, Jones DL, et al. Combined sino-atrial node atrioventricular node isolation: a surgical alternative to His bundle ablation in patients with atrial fibrillation. Circulation 1985;72:III:220. Abstract.
15. Cox JL, Schuessler RB, Boineau JP. The surgical treatment of atrial fibrillation. I. Summary of the current concepts of the mechanisms of atrial flutter and atrial fibrillation. J Thorac Cardiovasc Surg 1991;101:402–405.
16. Cox JL, Canavan TE, Schuessler RB, et al. The surgical treatment of atrial fibrillation. II. Intraoperative electrophysiologic mapping and description of the electrophysiologic basis of atrial flutter and atrial fibrillation. J Thorac Cardiovasc Surg 1991;101:406–426.
17. Cox JL, Schuessler RB, D'Agostino HJJ, et al. The surgical treatment of atrial fibrillation. III. Development of a definitive surgical procedure. J Thorac Cardiovasc Surg 1991;101:569–583.
18. Cox JL. The surgical treatment of atrial fibrillation. IV. Surgical technique. J Thorac Cardiovasc Surg 1991;101:584–592.
19. Leitch JW, Klein GJ, Yee R, Guiraudon GM. Sinus node-atrioventricular node isolation: long-term results with the "Corridor" operation for atrial fibrillation. J Am Coll Cardiol 1991;17:970–975.
20. Cosio FG, Lopez Gil M, Goicolea A, et al. Radiofrequency ablation of the inferior vena cava-tricuspid valve isthmus in common atrial flutter. Am J Cardiol 1993;71:705–709.
21. Swartz JF, Pellersels G, Silvers J, et al. A catheter-based curative approach to atrial fibrillation in humans. Circulation 1994;90:I-335. Abstract.
22. Fleischman SD, Thompson R, Panescu D, et al. Flexible electrodes for long atrial lesions. Circulation 1996;94:I-676. Abstract.
23. Demazumder D, Dillon SM, Gottlieb CD, et al. Maximal interelectrode spacing requirements for creating continuous myocardial lesions using multielectrode catheters. PACE 1996;19:714. Abstract.
24. Tomassoni G, Dixon-Tulloch E, Newby KH, et al. Linear lesions in the right atrium with multipolar catheters: effects of the interelectrode distance and different animal models. Circulation 1996;94:I-558. Abstract.

25. Whayne JG, Haines DE, Panescu D, et al. Catheter system designs to facilitate RF ablation of atrial fibrillation. PACE 1996;19:650. Abstract.
26. Panescu D, Haines DE, Fleischman SD, et al. Atrial lesions by temperature-controlled radiofrequency ablation. Circulation 1996;94:I-493. Abstract.
27. McRury ID, Mitchell MA, Whayne JG, et al. Prevention of coagulum formation during radiofrequency ablation with long electrodes: the importance of the edge effect. Circulation 1996;94:I-6. Abstract.
28. Strickberger SA, Davis J, Maguire MA. Radiofrequency ablation of the atrium using sequential coil electrodes. J Am Coll Cardiol 1996;27:400A. Abstract.
29. Kalman JM, Olgin JE, Karch MR, et al. Are linear lesions needed in both atria to prevent atrial fibrillation in a canine model? Circulation 1996;94: I-555. Abstract.
30. Avitall B, Helms RW, Kotov AV, et al. The use of temperature versus local depolarization amplitude to monitor atrial lesion maturation during the creation of linear lesions in both atria. Circulation 1996;94:I-558. Abstract.
31. Wharton JM, Tomassoni G, Pomeranz M, et al. Saline perfused, balloon radiofrequency ablation catheter for creation of linear transmural atrial lesions. Circulation 1996;94:I-493. Abstract.
32. Haïssaguerre M, Jaïs P, Shah DC, et al. Right and left atrial radiofrequency catheter therapy of paroxysmal atrial fibrillation. J Cardiovasc Electrophysiol 1996;7:1132–1144.
33. Haines DE, McRury ID, Whayne JG, Fleischman SD. Atrial radiofrequency ablation: the use of a novel deploying loop catheter design to create long linear lesions. Circulation 1994;90:I-335. Abstract.
34. Avitall B, Hare J, Mughal K, et al. A catheter system to ablate atrial fibrillation in a sterile pericarditis dog model. PACE 1994;17:774. Abstract.
35. Avitall B, Helms RW, Chiang W, Kotov AV. Technology and method for the creation of left atrial endocardial linear lesions to ablate atrial fibrillation. J Am Coll Cardiol 1996;27:400A. Abstract.
36. Riccardi R, Lamberti F, Scaglione M, et al. Vagal atrial fibrillation: atrial mapping and effectiveness of a right atrial catheter ablation. Circulation 1996;94:I-675. Abstract.
37. Cox JL, Jaquiss RD, Schuessler RB, Boineau JP. Modification of the Maze procedure for atrial flutter and atrial fibrillation. II. Surgical technique of the Maze III procedure. J Thorac Cardiovasc Surg 1995;110:485–495.
38. Cox JL, Boineau JP, Schuessler RB, et al. Modification of the Maze procedure for atrial flutter and atrial fibrillation. I. Rationale and surgical results. J Thorac Cardiovasc Surg 1995;110:473–484.
39. Elvan A, Pride HP, Eble JN, Zipes DP. Radiofrequency catheter ablation of the atria reduces inducibility and duration of atrial fibrillation in dogs. Circulation 1995;91:2235–2244.
40. Nakagawa H, Kumagai K, Imai S, et al. Catheter ablation of Bachmanns bundle from the right atrium eliminates atrial fibrillation in a canine sterile pericarditis model. PACE 1996;19:581. Abstract.
41. Jaïs P, Haïssaguerre M, Shah D, et al. Catheter ablation for paroxysmal atrial fibrillation: high success rates with ablation in the left atrium. Circulation 1996;94:I-675. Abstract.

42. Kirchhof CJHJ, Saltman AE, Krukenkamp IB, et al. High density mapping of chronic atrial fibrillation in man. Circulation 1996;94:I-555. Abstract.
43. Jaïs P, Haïssaguerre M, Shah DC, et al. Characteristics of focal atrial fibrillation. PACE 1996;19:650. Abstract.
44. Steiner PR, Kalman JM, Lesh MD. An analysis of spatiotemporal activation patterns to identify local streaming of wavefronts during atrial fibrillation in dogs. Circulation 1996;94:I-351. Abstract.
45. Schoels W, Freigang K, Becker RC, et al. Which type of linear atrial lesion is likely to be arrhythmogenic? PACE 1996;19:651. Abstract.
46. Kotov AV, Brodsky L, Helms RW, Avitall B. The impact of transcatheter generated atrial linear radiofrequency lesions on atrial function and contractility. PACE 1996;19:698. Abstract.
47. Zarse M, Deharo J, Allessie MA. Radiofrequency ablation of anatomical atrial circuits in a rabbit model of atrial fibrillation. Circulation 1996;94:I-676. Abstract.

CHAPTER 19

Radiofrequency Catheter Ablation for Paroxysmal Atrial Fibrillation in Humans:

Elaboration of a Procedure Based on Electrophysiological Data

Michel Haïssaguerre, Pierre Jaïs, Dipen C. Shah,
Jacques Clémenty

Atrial fibrillation (AF) is the most common and recalcitrant form of supraventricular arrhythmia.[1-4] In patients with disabling drug-resistant AF, nonpharmacological management must be considered, including pacemakers,[5-7] catheter ablation of the atrioventricular (AV) junction,[8-11] or surgery.[12-19] The rationale for surgical curative therapies is based on experimental studies that demonstrated the coexistence of several reentrant wavelets in a critical "mass" of atrial tissue perpetuating AF with the corollary that the probability of simultaneous extinction was in inverse proportion to the number of wavelets and atrial mass.[20-29] Recent reports have shown that linear ablative lesions created by application of radiofrequency (RF) energy can be effective in patients with atrial flutter[30-35] and paroxysmal or chronic AF.[36-46] However, scarce electrophysiological data is available on human AF to help us optimize the placement of ablation lines and assess their efficacy.[12,47-51]

In this chapter, we present our electrophysiological data and experience with ablation for paroxysmal AF in 62 patients referred over a period of 30 months.

From *Nonpharmacological Management of Atrial Fibrillation*, edited by F.D. Murgatroyd and A.J. Camm. © 1997, Futura Publishing Co., Inc., Armonk, NY.

Mapping of Human AF: Towards an Electrophysiological Approach

To ascertain the relevance of using electrophysiological data to guide ablation therapy, we have studied patients with paroxysmal AF before and after ablation using multielectrode catheters. Three important electrophysiological characteristics relevant to AF ablation were evidenced: (1) Regional disparities exist in fibrillatory activity during AF (Fig. 1). (2) Arrhythmogenic foci play a significant role in initiating

BIATRIAL CAST : POSTERIOR VIEW

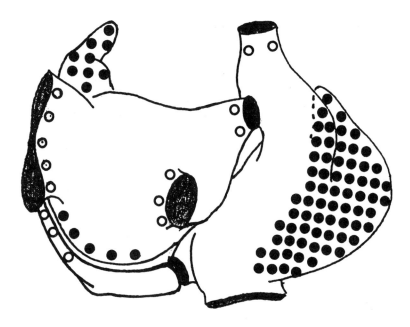

● atrial myocardial ○ venous
ORGANIZED ACTIVITY DURING A FIB

Figure 1. Spatial biatrial distribution of organized electrical activity during AF (see text). Shown here is a drawing of the posterior view of a biatrial cast. The filled-in circles represent atrial myocardium with organized activity; the open circles represent structures of embryologically venous origin also exhibiting such activity. The blank areas represent tissue with disorganized activity, prominent in the left atrium.

or maintaining AF. Such data have not been reported in previous mapping (epicardial) studies because the most arrhythmogenic areas—the atrial tissue of embryological venous origin and the interatrial septum—require endocardial probes for exploration. (3) Electrophysiological criteria can be used to assess linear conduction block.

Regional Disparities in Fibrillatory Activity During Paroxysmal AF

As mentioned above, previous studies have concentrated on limited atrial myocardial mapping, but there is clinical evidence to indicate the concentration of automatic foci around pulmonary veins. Therefore, in the course of our study, we investigated both atrial myocardial and great vein electrical activity.

Atrial Myocardial Activities During AF

Experimental data suggest that wavelets occurring during AF are homogeneously distributed in the atria. We investigated regions showing continuous electrical activity ("fibrillatory activity") during ablation in both atria. This criterion was selected because it was simple to assess (by comparison to fibrillation interval,[47]) and because continuous activity is a reasonable indicator of an area with vulnerable electrophysiological properties. When a baseline was perceived between electrograms, irregular intervals shorter than 100 ms were also considered as continuous activity.

Twenty-five males and two females (mean age, 49 ± 11 years; five with structural heart disease) with paroxysmal AF for 5 ± 6 years underwent atrial mapping. The right atrium was divided into four regions: posterior (intercaval), lateral, anterior, and septal, and the left atrium into three regions (anterior, posterior, septal). A 14-pole catheter (Bard Electrophysiology, Tewksbury, MA, USA) was sequentially positioned in these regions to assess AF time, defined as the duration of continuous electrical activity for 60 seconds (expressed as percent of time). In addition, the left atrium was retrogradely or transseptally explored with a multipolar catheter and its activity compared to that of the coronary sinus (Fig. 2). Lastly, flecainide (2 mg/kg) was infused over ten minutes to assess its effects on fibrillatory activity.

Results: (1) In the right atrium, the intercaval (63 ± 33% of time) and adjacent septal (74 ± 32%) regions were the temporally maximally

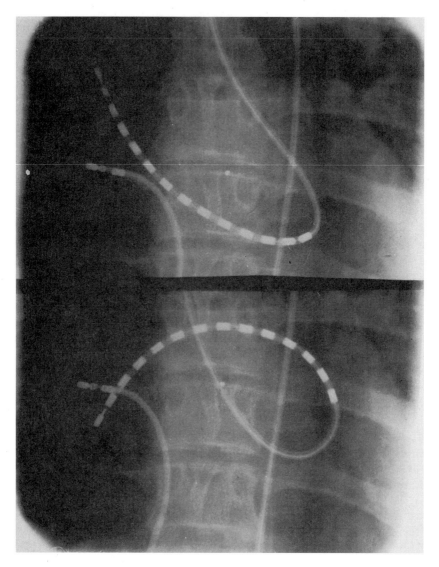

Figure 2. Anteroposterior fluorograms showing the 14-pole dacron catheter (Bard Electrophysiology, Tewksbury, MA, USA) placed retrogradely in the left atrium. In the upper panel, the tip is in the right superior pulmonary vein while in the lower panel, it is in the right lower pulmonary vein.

fibrillatory regions in contrast to lateral (22 ± 23%) and anterior (21 ± 26%) regions which are predominantly trabeculated areas. The AF time differences between the right atrial regions explored were highly significant ($P = 0.008$). The septal ($P = 0.02$) and the posterior ($P = 0.04$) areas (embryologically venous components) were significantly more fibrillatory than the lateral and anterior regions (Fig. 3). Posteriorly, the crista terminalis area separated the organized and fibrillating regions. In patients with fibrillatory activity extending into trabeculated areas, flecainide first regularized these areas before affecting other regions. (2) In the left atrium, a widely fibrillating region was present with the maximally fibrillating area being the septum (65 ±

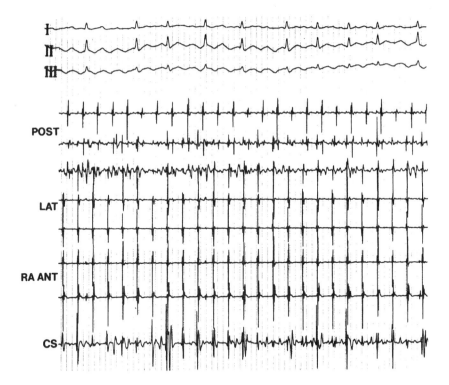

Figure 3. An example of typical right atrial spatial heterogeneity in a patient with paroxysmal AF. Note the markedly disorganized, chaotic, and near continuous activity in the posterior (smooth) right atrium, while the lateral and anterior (trabeculated) right atrium exhibits a stereotypical organized and regular rhythm. Note the fibrillatory activity recorded from the coronary sinus in this patient.

27% of time), the roof and the posterior region (87 ± 11%) between the pulmonary veins (i.e., the "venous component"). In the anterior left atrium, the appendage, again a trabeculated region, frequently exhibited organized electrical activity (AF time: 18 ± 14%). The band of atrial tissue bordering the mitral annulus (and the coronary sinus) was sometimes organized in contrast with the remainder of the left atrium. Whereas the proximal (septal) coronary sinus was usually fibrillating, its posterior and lateral distal part could be organized in spite of fibrillating activity in the neighboring endocardial region, showing that a regular coronary sinus activity is not a reliable indicator of left atrium activity. A widely disorganized coronary sinus was always associated with a similar activity in the left atrium.

In summary, trabeculated areas may represent zones relatively protected from the excitatory influence of multiple neighboring reentrant circuits in contrast to the nontrabeculated areas. Therefore, the atrial tissue exhibiting fibrillatory activity covers a minor area in the right atrium and nearly all the surface of the left atrium. Furthermore, an anatomic boundary—the crista terminalis region—contains the fibrillating area of the right atrium in a "cul-de-sac", whereas there is no such anatomic boundary in the left atrium. These intra- and interatrial spatial disparities may indicate preferential target regions to minimize ablation lines for the prospect of reducing the fibrillating mass.

Great Vein Electrical Activity During AF

Electrical Activity in the Superior Vena Cava (SVC): While performing mapping and ablation for paroxysmal AF, we found dissociated spikelike activity from bipole in the SVC in 15 patients (10 male and 5 female; age range, 26–62 years). Ranging from 0.4–1.2 mV in amplitude, during AF this activity was dissociated in 14 patients and followed the dominant right atrial activity in one patient. During transient sinus rhythm in some patients, this spike formed part of a multicomponent potential—which could be separated and the sequence altered by atrial pacing. Dissociation during sinus rhythm was noted in one patient. The spike activity could be traced superiorly for about 3.5 cm into the SVC. Following ablation it was either markedly attenuated or obscured by fibrillatory activity.

Electrical Activity in the Inferior Vena Cava: Unlike in the SVC, we have been unable to find any local electrical activity in the inferior vena cava. During ascent from the inferior vena cava into the right atrium, an abrupt appearance of electrical activity was noted upon entrance into the right atrium.

Electrical Activity in the Pulmonary Veins: This activity was recorded in 15 patients up to 2.5 cm into the superior veins. In contrast to the SVC activity, the pulmonary vein electrogram followed the major intrinsic deflections of the nearby atrium in one to one fashion in 14 patients and was dissociated in one. Rapid pacing from inside the vein was able to induce AF in some patients. Perhaps because this area represents an electrical "cul-de-sac" receiving impulses from a restricted input, the resulting local electrograms reflect a rapid and regular organized activity unlike the adjoining fibrillating posterior left atrium.

Superior vena cava potentials may therefore represent protected activity from muscle fibers in the proximal SVC as vestigial remnants of the sinus venosus complex. The clinical implication of such activity is at present unknown but including this region in linear longitudinal right atrial ablations may be unnecessary in view of the regional dissociation demonstrated here.

In contrast, pulmonary vein electrograms can track the left atrial activity at a high rate and this region may need to be targeted in left atrial ablation.

Significant Role of Arrhythmogenic Foci

During the study of AF ablation, we encountered a significant incidence of arrhythmogenic foci in patients referred to us for ablation of paroxysmal AF. Arrhythmogenic foci were defined on the basis of a centrifugal pattern of activation during arrhythmia and elimination by localized RF catheter ablation. Two groups could be differentiated: (1) focal AF due to a single primary focus firing rapidly; and (2)) secondary foci which were disclosed only after organization of atrial fibrillatory activity during linear ablation.

Focal Atrial Fibrillation

Very rapid atrial tachycardia originating from a localized substratum can mimic the electrocardiogram (ECG) pattern of coarse AF.[39] Its recognition is important because it can be treated by localized RF catheter ablation. We have encountered seven patients with such a focal origin of AF.

The seven patients, two female and five males, were young (35 ± 6 years) and without structural heart disease. The duration of AF was 1 to 15 years (mean 5 years). Off antiarrhythmic drugs, they had frequent runs of irregular atrial activity at a rate of 320–400 bpm. With antiarrhythmic drugs, extrasystoles or atrial tachycardia with discrete P waves at a rate of 110–260 bpm were discerned with sudden and marked variations in cycle length. Catheter ablation was considered because of drug resistance.

During the electrophysiological study the arrhythmia occurred spontaneously in all patients. It could not be reproduced by programmed stimulation in any patient. Mapping characteristically demonstrated a centrifugal pattern of activation during regular arrhythmia. However when fibrillation was secondarily induced by the atrial tachycardia, an infusion of an antiarrhythmic drug converted this back to the tachycardia, allowing mapping. The ectopic activity was strikingly irregular with shortest cycles of 140 ms. The earliest activity occurred 30 ms to 70 ms before the onset of the ectopic P wave. The abnormal focus was found to be in the right atriun (RA) in three cases, near the upper part of the sinus node in two and at the ostium of the coronary sinus in one. The origin was left-sided for the other four patients—near the right superior pulmonary vein in three patients and at the ostium of the left superior pulmonary vein in one (Fig. 3).

All patients were successfully treated by a mean of 6 ± 6 RF applications. Pacing maneuvers after ablation could not induce sustained atrial arrhythmias in five patients (and produced AF in 2). During a mean follow-up of 9 ± 9 months, all patients were free of clinical arrhythmia without any antiarrhythmic drug.

Patients with such "focal atrial fibrillation" are young, have no structural heart disease and present with frequent episodes of an arrhythmia which is characteristically converted into monomorphic atrial tachycardia or extrasystoles, mostly with drugs but also spontaneously. Localized RF ablation can be curative for this form of AF.

Foci Secondarily Unmasked after Linear Atrial Ablation

Ablation lines as described below yield an organization of atrial activity during AF leading ultimately to sinus rhythm. This facilitates unmasking of right or left atrial foci which would be otherwise inapparent. Such foci could however be suspected in some patients on previous Holter recordings showing frequent extrasystoles or atrial tachycardias.

In a consecutive series of 45 patients having had right ablation lines for paroxysmal AF, foci were unmasked in 12 patients, thus with a prevalence of 27%. The foci appeared as intermittent monomorphic extrasystoles or irregular atrial tachycardia. In these patients, almost all documented atrial extrasystoles originated from the focus which was also the dominant trigger of more sustained atrial arrhythmias. Focal atrial tachycardia was not inducible in any of the patients except one. Figure 4 shows the various locations of foci with most originating near the ostia of great vessels, particularly the left superior pulmonary vein. In only one patient, the focus originated on a previous ablation line suggesting it may have been related to iatrogenic lesions. All foci were eliminated by RF energy resulting also in elimination of atrial

BIATRIAL DISTRIBUTION OF TACHYCARDIA FOCI

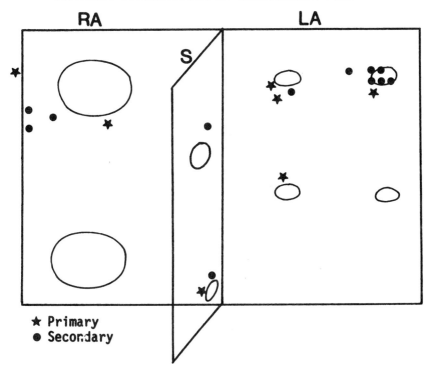

Figure 4. A diagrammatic representation of the distribution of primary and secondary tachycardia foci in both atria. RA = right atrium; LA = left atrium; S = interatrial septum. Circles represent SVC and IVC in the RA, pulmonary veins in the LA and fossa ovalis and coronary sinus in the septum.

bursts and significant symptomatic improvement. One focus reappeared and could not be reablated, yielding numerous atrial bursts which rendered the AF ablation procedure unsuccessful.

Criteria of Linear Conduction Block

In atrial flutter, the creation of an isthmal conduction block is associated with a line of split potentials.[34] There is no clear indicator of efficacy of ablation lines during AF other than restoration of sinus rhythm or noninducibility of atrial arrhythmias.

We therefore analyzed the electrograms of 30 patients who underwent right atrial linear ablation with a multipolar electrode catheter (3 mm interelectrode spacing). Assessment included electrogram recording during pacing near the middle part of the ablation line to produce a perpendicular wave front and maximize conduction delay. A linear conduction block was obviously demonstrated in some patients by the presence of dissociation of atrial electrograms on either side of the line during either right atrial pacing, atrial tachycardia, or AF.

Results: (1) A linear conduction block as defined above was obtained in only four patients either in the intercaval (superior vena cava to inferior vena cava) region or transversely in the right atrium (Fig. 5). Either a local blanking effect or multiple fragmented potentials separated by an isoelectric line was recorded with all the catheter electrodes positioned on the line. The maximum interpotential interval ranged from 20–80 ms. It is important to note that a "single" electrogram could be recorded if all the catheter electrodes were not exactly placed astride the line. (2) In most patients, there was no evidence of such a block. The most common effect of the linear lesions was a diminution in amplitude, fragmentation, and widening of local electrograms with a striking reduction in the dv/dt from unipolar and bipolar recordings. Split and single potentials were unevenly distributed suggesting a patchy line (Fig. 6). Split potentials increased or were evidenced only at shortest cycle lengths in tachycardia indicating functional block. In five patients, conduction times across lines were assessed in comparison to preablation values: a modest prolongation of 10–25 ms was obtained only at the shortest atrial cycle length.

It is therefore difficult to achieve a linear conduction block using current multielectrode catheters. The block obtained is usually functional. The presence of a line of conduction block can be ascertained by

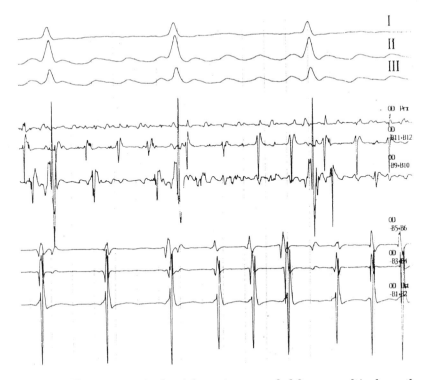

Figure 5. Electrograms in the right atrium recorded from a multipolar catheter placed across an ablation line. During an organized atrial rhythm (on the surface ECG), the upper and lower three bipoles demonstrate a dissociation of electrical activity produced by the intervening ablation line.

analysis of local electrograms on the basis of a blanking effect or noting an interval of electrical silence separating all potentials along the line, particularly during perpendicular activation. This simple assessment may render other sophisticated imaging techniques superfluous for this purpose.

Human Experience of Catheter Ablation Using Ablation Lines

After a series of experimental studies in collaboration with Marcus et al.[44] and Lavergne et al.[36] demonstrating the safety of multielectrode catheter ablation in the atria, we reported a single human case docu-

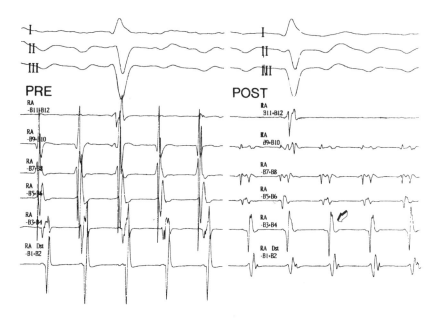

Figure 6. An example of the uneven distribution of resulting double potentials after an RF ablation line. During atrial flutter (which appeared during the previous line) and before ablation, the left panel shows healthy, good amplitude electrograms from multiple bipoles in the right atrium. After ablation, as shown in the panel on the right, double potentials significantly reduced in amplitude are recorded from the bipoles except at B3 B4, where a single potential is recorded (arrow). This is indicative of a gap in the line we attempted to create with sequential RF applications.

menting successful catheter ablation in the right atrium only to prevent paroxysmal AF.[39] This approach was then investigated in 45 consecutive patients.

Paroxysmal AF Treated with an Anatomical and Stepwise Approach Beginning with the RA

Population Study Methods: The patients were 36 males and nine females with a mean age of 51 ± 12 years. They had had paroxysmal AF for 6 ± 6 years despite the use of 5 ± 1 drugs. Several AF episodes occurred each day in 41 patients. Structural heart disease was present in 13 patients (isolated arterial hypertension was excluded). They underwent linear right atrial ablation with each line performed by a single series of energy applications. The catheter used for ablation was either a common 7F deflectable 4 mm tip electrode catheter equipped with a thermocouple (Cordis-Webster, Miami, FL, USA, or Bard Electrophysiology, Tewksbury, MA, USA, catheters) or a specially designed woven dacron multielectrode ablation catheter with 14 electrodes of 4 mm and an interelectrode spacing of 3 mm (Bard Electrophysiology). When the multipolar catheter could not conform to the desired specific locations, energy applications via the usual monopolar ablation catheter were used to perform entire ablation lines or to complete parts of ablation lines previously begun with the multipolar ablation catheter. Using a Medtronic® Atakr (Medtronic, Inc., Minneapolis, MN, USA) or a Stockert® RF (Stockard Gmbh, Freiburg, Germany) generator, a temperature of 55° to 70° C was achieved and maintained at the distal electrode of the thermocouple-equipped catheter. Using the multielectrode ablation catheter, a power setting of 10 W to 20 W was initially used and progressively increased every 10 seconds up to 50 W depending on the impedance displayed during energy delivery and the tolerance to pain experienced by the patient. No intravenous heparin was administered before ablation in the right atrium. A bolus dose of 0.5 mg/kg (body weight) followed by 0.25 mg/kg every 3 hours was administered for ablations in the left atrium. Sedation was generally maintained with IV Midazolam and Nalbuphine.

Ablations lines were always connected to at least one region of block to avoid the constitution of a new reentrant circuit around the line. The region of block was either the AV ring, a vessel insertion, or a previous ablation line. Fifteen patients in group 1 underwent a single septal line. Fifteen patients in group 2 underwent three lines approximately geometrically dividing the right atrial free wall in the longitudinal (1 anterior, 1 posterior) and transverse direction but a 1 centimeter band near the superior vena cava was spared in the anterior line to avoid injuring the sinus node and Bachman bundle. The next 15 patients (group 3) underwent an additional septal line (Fig. 7). In some patients who remained disabled following the right atrial ablation, linear ablations were performed in the left atrium. All patients underwent a transesophageal echocardiography before ablation to check for the absence of thrombi. The multipolar or monopolar ablation catheter was introduced in the left atrium using a retrograde aortic approach through the mitral valve (Fig. 2) or a transeptal approach, both guided by a long introducer sheath. Ablation lines were performed vertically from the two superior pulmonary veins to the mitral annulus including the inferior pulmonary veins in their course. Then a horizontal line connected the superior part of the two vertical lines.

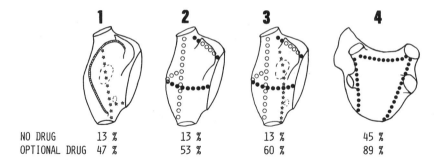

Figure 7. Success rates for paroxysmal AF related to evolving stages of our ablation strategy. 1: Initial 15 patients who underwent only a single septal RA line; 2: Second group of 15 patients with three lines in the RA; 3: Third group of 15 with an additional septal line; 4: Group of nine failures from the above three groups who underwent LA ablation as shown. Corresponding success rates free of drugs and with a drug if necessary are shown below each diagram.

The endpoint of the procedure was the termination of sequential applications for scheduled lines, whether or not sinus rhythm was observed. Patients were discharged without antiarrhythmic drugs or with a single drug that was previously ineffective at the same dosage. The outcome of the procedure was considered a success when the duration of AF after ablation was less than 5% of the preprocedural AF duration as: (a) measured on repeated Holter recordings; and (b) confirmed by the patient diary assessment. The procedure was considered a failure otherwise, even if the patient felt significantly improved. Data were expressed as group mean value ± SD. Quantitative variables were compared using a Student t test and the exact Fisher test was used for qualitative variables. Statistical significance was selected at $P<0.05$.

Results of Right Atrial Ablation: Side effects occurred in three patients (7%) but there was no mortality. The patients, one in group 2 and two in group 3, developed transient asymptomatic sinus node pauses lasting between 2 and 6 seconds. In one patient, such pauses were documented before ablation. In the other two, they occurred after the third postablation day and spontaneously disappeared within 8 days. No thrombus, pericardial effusion or valve damage was observed at the postablation transesophageal echocardiography in 30 patients.

The AF ablation procedure lasted 248 ± 79 minutes including 53 ± 22 minutes of fluoroscopy time. In nearly all patients with previously documented common atrial flutter and 70% of patients without such

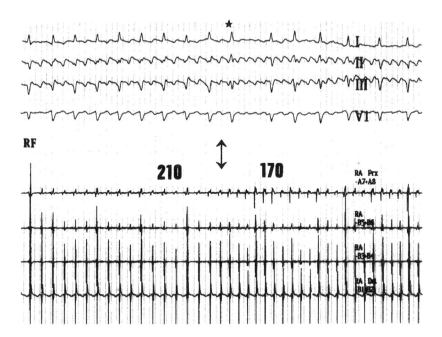

Figure 8. Typical (on the left) and atypical (on the right side after the star) flutter encountered in the course of RF ablation for AF. Note the change in the flutter wave morphology on the surface ECG accompanied by a shortening of the cycle length from 210 ms to 170 ms.

documentation, we observed the conversion of AF to atrial flutter requiring additional ablation in the inferior vena cava-tricuspid isthmus. Two patients also had atypical atrial flutter (Fig. 8) which did not involve the isthmus as shown by resetting technique. RF applications between the tricuspid annulus or the inferior vena cava to the coronary sinus ostium interrupted this new tachycardia circuit. The occurrence of atrial flutter and new atrial focal tachycardias required one (n = 16) and two (n = 3) additional ablation sessions. With a mean follow-up period of 9 ± 3 months (range, 3–21 months) a successful outcome was achieved in 24 patients: seven patients (47%) of group 1, eight patients (53%) of group 2, and nine patients (60%) of group 3. However, only two patients (13%) in each group did not take any antiarrhythmic drugs while the combination of ablation with a drug (flecainide or sotalol) was required in others to achieve success. Three of the unsuccessful patients reported marked attenuation of symptoms despite similar ventricular rates in AF. They were in groups undergoing 3 or 4 lines which may have altered AF perception via a change in local innervation. Lastly, AF became chronic in two patients some weeks after discharge.

Results of Left Atrial Ablation: Nine patients underwent a left atrial ablation procedure including the patients who had converted to chronic AF. AF was interrupted in all patients except one during the session after a progressive organization of local activities. No sustained arrhythmia was inducible after ablation in four patients. AF (n = 2) or left atrial flutter (n = 3) was inducible in other patients using rapid atrial bursts. The atrial flutter circuits involved the perimeter of pulmonary veins propagating probably through gaps in ablation lines (Fig. 9). Two patients required reablation for new atrial focal tachycardias. A hemopericardium without tamponade occurred in one patient. With a mean follow-up of 3 months to 16 months, ablation was successful in seven patients (78%) of whom four (45%) were not taking antiarrhythmic drugs and were relieved of coumadin treatment.

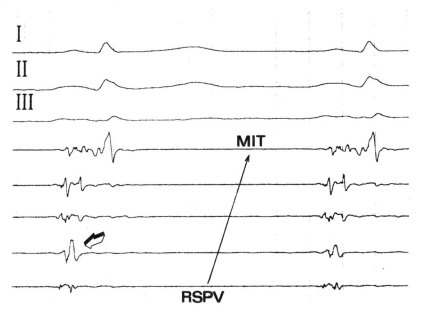

Figure 9. Electrograms recorded from the LA along the line between the right superior pulmonary vein and the mitral annulus after sequential RF applications. Double potentials are recorded during sinus rhythm at four bipoles; however, a single electrogram (arrow) at one bipole indicates a gap in the line.

Prediction of Successful Ablation: Figure 7 shows the success rates obtained with progressively increasing lines either with or without drugs. There was no statistical difference in success rates with 1, 3, or 4 lines in the right atrium. The jump in the success rate from the three right-sided groups to the left ablation group was significant ($P = 0.03$ and 0.048 without drugs and with optional drugs, respectively).

The only variable that was predictive of success without drugs after ablation in the right atrium only (6 patients vs. 39 others) was the presence of an arrhythmogenic focus secondarily ablated (3/6 vs. 7/39, $P = 0.03$). The variables that were predictive of success with or without drugs using a right atrial ablation (24 successes vs. 21 failures) were:

- the presence of arrythmogenic foci (10/24 vs. 0/21, $P<0.01$),
- the noninducibility of sustained atrial arrhythmias with bursts of 300 bpm (5/24 vs. 0/21, $P = 0.04$),
- a shorter duration of fibrillatory activity in the distal coronary sinus (AF time: $13 \pm 14\%$ vs. $35 \pm 27\%$, $P = 0.04$).

The absence of structural heart disease was not a predictive variable.

Elaboration of an Electrophysiologically Guided Procedure

Results of mapping corroborated by those of stepwise ablation, strongly suggest the following electrophysiologically guided approach for AF ablation: (1) Ablation lines centered on the most fibrillating areas (septum, the left atrium rectangle); (2) Linear block assessed by checking the appearance of split potentials during sinus rhythm along the line after ablation; (3) Ablation of secondarily appearing foci and flutter; and (4) An endpoint of either a stable sinus rhythm when the arrhythmia was previously incessant or noninducibility of sustained atrial arrhythmias.

Several comments on the different steps are relevant. First, continuous activity does not necessarily mean that the concerned area is the cause of AF since it may also be generated (fibrillatory conduction) by a rapid regular tachycardia. However, such an area must possess short local wavelengths to sustain high rates and thus is a favorable milieu for AF. The high ablation success rate observed in the left atrium where most of the fibrillating mass is located strongly supports the validity of this target. The selection of lines in the left atrium is centered on the fibrillating mass but they also divide its anatomy geometrically. The vertical lines must connect the pulmonary veins to the mitral annulus whereas the horizontal line can be placed with a certain leeway between the vertical lines. If vertical lines are completely transmural, a gap is necessary in the horizontal line to allow activation of this left atrial quadrilateral from the Bachman bundle. In paroxysmal AF, a line in the left side of the septum is optional connecting the fossa ovalis to either the right pulmonary vein line or the posterior mitral annulus. Second, at the present state of technology, it is difficult to achieve a complete linear block particularly in the left atrium using either a dragging technique or multielectrode ablation catheters despite repeated RF applications. A cycle length-dependent block is usually obtained. Provided an unchanged safety profile is maintained with more complete lines, this allows a significant margin for improvement in results, notably lesser RF applications and procedure duration and less need for antiarrhythmic drugs. The assessment of linear block is easier during a regular rhythm (notably pacing or sinus rhythm with a perpendicular activation wave front) because the ablation lesions can be tracked "on line" with the progressive appearance of split potentials as during isthmal ablation.[34] Third, foci seem to us to be important triggers of paroxysmal AF and they can be eliminated by a limited ablation provided the focal arrhythmia is sufficiently repetitive to be mapped. On the other hand, left atrial flutter ablation is more uncertain with current technologies. Indeed, our experience indicates that fibrillation may be converted ("organized") despite incomplete ablation lines, whereas a higher degree or a total block of conduction is required to prevent atrial flutter. Taking the example of right atrial flutter, it is only when total interruption of the isthmus conduction is achieved that flutter is interrupted (see Fig. 10 in Ref. 35). A successful outcome requires a local conduction block at the tachycardia cycle length even if conduction persists at longer cycle length and in sinus rhythm.[35] Fourth, the endpoints of the procedure must be appreciated individually given the time constraints and inadequacy of current technologies. The noninducibility of atrial arrhythmias is probably the "gold standard" but may lead to more than necessary lesions and it remains to specify a stimulation protocol and criteria of inducibility. In a patient with AF previously incessant or prolonged for hours, the achievement of a stable sinus rhythm may be a reasonable endpoint. Spontaneously terminating left atrial flutter (within a few minutes of induction with an aggressive protocol) may also be satisfactory.

Paroxysmal AF Treated with a Biatrial Electrophysiologically Guided Approach

Method: The study population included 10 patients, seven male and three female, mean age 48 ± 8 years and having several episodes of

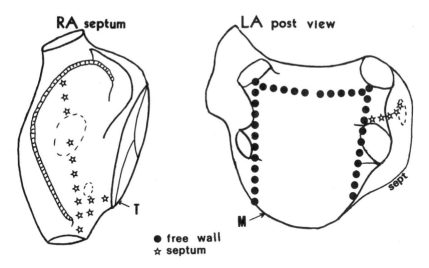

Figure 10. Diagram of the ablation schema used in the LA and RA for the last 10 patients. In the RA, a line extends from the SVC on the septal side to the fossa ovalis down to the IVC, and includes the coronary sinus orifice. In the LA, a line is formed between both superior pulmonary veins, and also from each superior to inferior pulmonary vein, extending down to the mitral valve. Another line is optional connecting the fossa ovalis to either the right pulmonary vein line (as shown by stars) or the posterior mitral annulus.

AF per day. The ablation lines were performed as shown in Figure 10 using a transeptal approach in the left atrium. When possible, lines were performed in sinus rhythm to best follow the creation of linear block. A preset temperature of 55–57°C was selected on a Stockert RF generator using different catheters equipped with a thermocouple. The rest of the protocol and the criteria for success were as defined above.

Results: There was no complication. Ablation lasted 336 ± 113 minutes including 76 ± 34 minutes of fluoroscopic time. In most, but not all, patients a line of split potentials was obtained along the linear lesions connecting the right superior pulmonary vein to the mitral annulus, but this was achieved after multiple repetitions. We were unable to achieve a linear block in the horizontal segments. Additional RF applications were required in four patients to treat arrhythmogenic foci originating from the left side of the septum in one patient and near the left superior pulmonary vein in three. Successful ablation was achieved in nine patients (90%) including six without antiarrhythmic drugs, but with a short follow-up period of 3 months.

Conclusions on Ablation of Paroxysmal AF

Ablation for paroxysmal AF is a relatively safe and promising technique. Subsequent sessions may be required because of residual and unmasked organized atrial arrhythmias. Ablation only in the right atrium provides limited success without drugs. Linear lesions in the left atrium increase the success rate considerably, up to 90% without drug therapy in most. A true linear block is still difficult to achieve using sequential RF applications. We anticipate that the success rate of this procedure may be increased with electrophysiologically better lesion characteristics. A long-term follow-up is required to confirm efficacy and safety of this technique.

References

1. Kerr CR, Chung DC. Atrial fibrillation: fact, controversy and future. Clin Prog Electrophysiol Pacing 1985;3:319–337.
2. Josephson ME. Clinical Cardiac Electrophysiology Techniques and Interpretations. Philadelphia: Lea & Febiger; 1993:117–149.
3. Nattel S. Newer developments in the management of atrial fibrillation. Am Heart J 1995;130:1094–1106.
4. Prystowsky EN, Benson W, Fuster V, et al. Management of patients with atrial fibrillation: a statement for healthcare professionals from the subcommittee on electrocardiography and electrophysiology. American Heart Association. Circulation 1996;93:1262–1277.
5. Coumel P, Friocourt P, Mugica J, et al. Long-term prevention of vagal atrial arrhythmias by atrial pacing at 90/minute. PACE 1983;6:552–560.
6. Rosenquist M. Cardiac pacing in atrial fibrillation. In: Olsson SB, Allessie MA, Campbell RWF, eds: Atrial Fibrillation: Mechanisms and Therapeutic Strategies. Armonk, NY: Futura Publishing Co; 1994:237–250.
7. Daubert JC, Mabo P, Berder V, et al. Atrial tachyarrhythmias associated with high degree interatrial conduction block: prevention by permanent atrial resynchronisation. Eur JCPE 1994;1:35–44.
8. Scheinman MM, Morady F, Hess DS, et al. Catheter-induced ablation of atrioventricular junction to control refractory supraventricular arrhythmias. JAMA 1982;248:855–861.
9. Gallagher JJ, Svenson RH, Kasell JH. Catheter technique for closed chest ablation of the atrioventricular conduction system: a therapeutic alternative for the treatment of refractory supraventricular tachycardia. N Eng J Med 1982;306:194–200.
10. Jackman WM, Wang X, Friday KJ, et al. Catheter ablation of atrioventricular junction using radiofrequency current in 17 patients: comparison of standard and large-tip catheter electrodes. Circulation 1991;83: 1562–1576.
11. Langberg JJ, Chin M, Schamp DJ, et al. Ablation of the atrioventricular

junction with radiofrequency current energy using a new electrode catheter. Am J Cardiol 1991;67:142–147.

12. Cox JL, Canavan TE, Schuessler RB, et al. The surgical treatment of atrial fibrillation: II. Intraoperative electrophysiologic mapping and description of the electrophysiologic basis of atrial flutter and fibrillation. J Thorac Cardiovasc Surg 1991;101:406–426.

13. Williams JM, Ungerleider RM, Lofland GK, et al. Left atrial isolation: new technique for the treatment of supraventricular arrhythmias. J Thorac Cardiovasc Surg 1980;80:373–380.

14. Cox JL, Schuessler RB, D'Agostino HJ, et al. The surgical treatment of atrial fibrillation: III. Development of a definitive surgical procedure. J Thorac Cardiovasc Surg 1991;101:569–583.

15. Cox JL, Boineau JP, Richard B, et al. Five year experience with the Maze procedure for atrial fibrillation. Ann Thorac Surg 1993;56:814–824.

16. Leitch JW, Klein G, Yee R, et al. Sinus node-atrioventricular isolation: long-term results with the corridor operation for atrial fibrillation. J Am Coll Cardiol 1991;17:970–975.

17. Van Hemel NM, Defauw J, Herre Kingma J, et al. Long-term results of the corridor operation for atrial fibrillation. Br Heart J 1994;71:170–176.

18. Shyu KG, Cheng JJ, Chen JJ, et al. Recovery of atrial function after atrial compartment operation for chronic atrial fibrillation in mitral valve disease. J Am Coll Cardiol 1994;24:392–398.

19. Kosakai Y, Kawaguchi AT, Isobe F, et al. Modified Maze procedure for patients with atrial fibrillation undergoing simultaneous open heart surgery. Circulation 1995;92(suppl II):II-359-II-364.

20. Moe GK, Abildskov JA. Atrial fibrillation as a self-sustaining arrhythmia independent of focal discharge. Am Heart J 1959;58:59–70.

21. West TC, Landa JF. Minimal mass required for induction of a sustained arrhythmia in isolated atrial segments. Am J Physiol 1962;202:232–236.

22. Moe GK, Rheinboldt WC, Abildskov JA. A computer model of atrial fibrillation. Am Heart J 1964;67:200–220.

23. Allessie MA, Lammers WJEP, Bonke FIM, et al. Intra-atrial reentry as a mechanism for atrial flutter induced by acetylcholine and rapid pacing in the dog. Circulation 1984;70:123–135.

24. Allessie MA, Lammers WJEP, Bonke FIM, et al. Experimental evaluation of Moe's multiple wavelet hypothesis of atrial fibrillation. In: Zipes DP, Jalife J, eds. Cardiac Electrophysiology and Arrhythmias. Orlando: Grune and Stratton; 1985:265–275.

25. Allessie MA, Rensma PL, Brugada J, et al. Pathophysiology of atrial fibrillation. In: Zipes DP, Jalife J, eds. Cardiac Electrophysiology: From Cell to Bedside. Philadelphia: WB Saunders Co; 1990:548–559.

26. Rensma PL, Allessie MA, Lammers WJEP, et al. Length of excitation wave and susceptibility to reentrant atrial arrhythmias in normal conscious dogs. Circ Res 1988;62:395–410.

27. Le Heuzey J, Boutjdir M, Gagey S, et al. Cellular aspects of atrial vulnerability. In: Attuel P, Olsson SB, Schlepper M, eds. The Atrium in Health and Disease. Mount Kisco, NY: Futura Publishing; 1989:81–94.

28. Ortiz J, Niwano S, Abe H, et al. Mapping the conversion of atrial flutter to atrial fibrillation and atrial fibrillation to atrial flutter: insights into mechanism. Circ Res 1994;74:882–896.

29. Wang Z, Feng J, Nattel S. Idiopathic atrial fibrillation in dogs: Electrophysiologic determinants and mechanisms of antiarrhythmic action of flecainide. J Am Coll Cardiol 1995;26: 277–286.
30. Cosio FG, Lopez-Gil M, Goicolea A, et al. Radiofrequency ablation of the inferior vena cava-tricuspid valve isthmus in common atrial flutter. Am J Cardiol 1993;71:705–709.
31. Lesh MD, Van Hare GF, Epstein LM, et al. Radiofrequency catheter ablation of atrial arrhythmias: results and mechanisms. Circulation 1994;89: 1074–1089.
32. Scheinman MM, Olgin J. Catheter ablation of cardiac arrhythmias of atrial origin. In: Zipes DP, ed. Catheter Ablation of Arrhythmias. Armonk, NY: Futura Publishing Co; 1994:129–149.
33. Fischer B, Haïssaguerre M, Garrigues S, et al. Radiofrequency catheter ablation of common atrial flutter in 80 patients. J Am Coll Cardiol 1995; 25:1365–1372.
34. Fischer B, Jaïs P, Cauchemez B, et al. Double potentials recorded in the cavo-tricuspid isthmus with radiofrequency applications in human atrial flutter. NASPE 1996;19:648. Abstract.
35. Cauchemez B, Haïssaguerre M, Fischer B, et al. Electrophysiological effects of catheter ablation of inferior vena cava-tricuspid annulus isthmus in common atrial flutter. Circulation 1996;93:284–294.
36. Lavergne T, Prunier L, Guize L, et al. Transcatheter radiofrequency ablation of atrial tissue using a suction catheter. PACE 1989;12:177–185.
37. Avitall B, Hare J, Mughal K, et al. Ablation of atrial fibrillation in a dog model. J Am Coll Cardiol 1994;484:276A.
38. Kempler P, Littmann L, Chuang CH, et al. Radiofrequency ablation of the right atrium: acute and chronic effects. PACE 1994;17(Part II):797.
39. Haïssaguerre M, Marcus FI, Fischer B, et al. Radiofrequency catheter ablation in unusual mechanisms of atrial fibrillation: report of three cases. J Cardiovasc Electrophysiol 1994;5:743–751.
40. Haïssaguerre M, Gencel L, Fischer B, et al. Successful catheter ablation of atrial fibrillation. J Cardiovasc Electrophysiol 1994;5:1045–1052.
41. Swartz JF, Pellersels G, Silvers J, et al. A catheter-based curative approach to atrial fibrillation in humans. Circulation 1994;90(4)(Part 2):I-335.
42. Elvan A, Pride HP, Zipes DP, et al. Radiofrequency catheter ablation of the atria reduces inducibility and duration of atrial fibrillation in dogs. Circulation 1995;91:2235–2244.
43. Morillo CA, Klein GJ, Jones DL, et al. Chronic rapid atrial pacing: structural, functional and electrophysiologic characteristics of a new model of sustained atrial fibrillation. Circulation 1995;91:1588–1595.
44. He DS, Mackey S, Marcus FI, et al. Radiofrequency energy for cardiac ablation using a multipolar catheter in sheep. Circulation 1995;92(8)(suppl I):I-265.
45. Jaïs P, Haïssaguerre M, Gencel L, et al. Incidence of common atrial flutter following catheter ablation of atrial fibrillation in the right atrium. Circulation 1995;92(8)(suppl I):I-266.
46. Haines DE, McRury IA. Primary atrial fibrillation ablation (PAFA) in a chronic atrial fibrillation model. Circulation 1995;92(8)(suppl I):I-265.
47. Ramdat Misier AR, Opthof T, Van Hemel NM, et al. Increased dispersion of

"refractoriness" in patients with idiopathic paroxysmal atrial fibrillation. J Am Coll Cardiol 1992;19:1531–1535.

48. Gerstenfeld EP, Sahakian AV, Swiryn S. Evidence for transient linking of atrial excitation during atrial fibrillation in humans. Circulation 1992;86: 375–382.

49. Holm M, Blomström P, Brandt J, et al. Determination of preferable directions of impulse propagation during atrial fibrillation by time averaging of multiple electrogram vectors. In: Olsson SB, Allessie MA, Campbell RWF, eds. Atrial Fibrillation: Mechanisms and Therapeutic Strategies. Armonk, NY: Futura Publishing Co; 1994:67–80.

50. Konings KTS, Kirschhof CJHJ, Smeets JRLM, et al. High-density mapping of electrically induced atrial fibrillation in humans. Circulation 1994;89: 1665–1680.

51. Botteron GW, Smith JM. Quantitative assessment of the spatial organization of atrial fibrillation in the intact human heart. Circulation 1996;893: 513–558.

PART VI

Preventing the Initiation of Atrial Fibrillation

CHAPTER 20

How Might Pacing Prevent Atrial Fibrillation?

Rahul Mehra

The potential role of pacing to prevent atrial fibrillation (AF) has been strongly suggested in the clinical literature. Currently, there are few published studies that support this conclusion because many of the prospective clinical trials have not yet been completed. Published reports in few selected patients suggest that vagally mediated AF can be prevented by atrial pacing. Vagally mediated AF usually occurs at night and is preceded by significant bradycardia or atrial pauses.[1] In another retrospective study, the effect of DDD, VVI and "no pacing" was compared in patients with preexisting AF who also had symptomatic bradycardia.[2] At the end of 6 months, more patients with DDD pacemakers were in sinus rhythm compared to patients with VVI pacemakers or those that were not paced. A multivariate analysis indicated that DDD pacing was associated with a lower risk of recurrent AF. The only prospective randomized comparison of VVI and DDD pacing was conducted by Andersen et al. in patients with sick sinus syndrome.[3] All the patients were in sinus rhythm at the time of randomization and progression into AF over the follow-up period of 5 years was compared in the two groups. The study showed that at the follow-up visits the percentage of patients in AF was lower with DDD pacing but the difference was not statistically significant. The study did not address the question of whether VVI was proarrhythmic or atrial pacing suppressed progression into AF. Although the clinical evidence supporting the role of atrial pacing for prevention of AF is weak, these and many other retrospective studies strongly suggest that pacing may prevent AF.

The primary focus of this chapter will be to analyze how pacing may prevent AF and the electrophysiological mechanisms responsible for it. It is hypothesized that pacing prevents AF by preventing its

From *Nonpharmacological Management of Atrial Fibrillation*, edited by F.D. Murgatroyd and A.J. Camm. © 1997, Futura Publishing Co., Inc., Armonk, NY.

initiation rather than its sustenance. Recent data indicate that even if pacing had a marginal effect on preventing the initiation of AF and thereby increased the duration of sinus rhythm, this could change the electrophysiological properties of the substrate and therefore affect the sustainability of AF. Wijffels et al. have shown that not only does "AF beget AF"' but sinus rhythm may also perpetuate sinus rhythm by altering the electrophysiological properties of the atrium.[4] The effect of pacing could be cumulative and provide greater protection against AF as the duration of sinus rhythm increases. Therefore, prevention of initiation and of sustenance should not be viewed as being totally exclusive of each other but interdependent.

In order to develop a hypothesis of how pacing may prevent AF, this chapter will consist of four sections. First, the mechanisms as well the anatomical sites responsible for initiation of AF will be presented. Since experimental results suggest that AF is initiated when the atrium is activated in a unique manner, the activation sequence of the sinus and premature beats will then be discussed. Finally, these basic concepts will be integrated to develop hypotheses to explain why pacing may prevent AF.

Initiation of Atrial Fibrillation

Most mapping studies indicate that AF is sustained by a reentrant mechanism with multiple wavelets.[5,6] The mechanism of spontaneous initiation of AF can only be speculated on. If the initial beats of AF are reentrant, they can be initiated by one of two mechanisms. The first is that closely coupled ectopic atrial beats from unique atrial sites initiate reentry which degenerates into multiple wavelets of AF. In this case the initiating beat is ectopic, giving rise to reentry. The second mechanism is that a rapid atrial tachycardia such as sinus tachycardia can cause conduction delay and block in the abnormal atrial substrate and the first beat of AF could be reentrant rather than ectopic. This must occur in the presence of an abnormal electrophysiological substrate for it to be sustained since AF cannot be typically sustained in normal healthy atria. A focal mechanism of sustained AF cannot be ruled out completely since some recent mapping studies suggest such a focal origin.[7,8] Holm et al. mapped 13 patients with chronic AF who underwent open heart surgery and found that four of them showed consistent excitation indicative of focal origin. Since AF is a progressive disease, it is possible that in the early stages it is reentrant and ectopy may play a much greater role in chronic AF than in paroxysmal AF.

The results of mapping studies in animals and patients suggest that the most likely mechanism of initiation of AF is due to ectopic atrial beats initiating reentry; these results are discussed below. Significant attention is given to the results on the anatomic sites where this reentry is initiated, i.e., where conduction block and the first reentrant beat occur. It is hypothesized that this information is critically important in order to prevent AF, and this will be discussed in greater detail in the section on how pacing might prevent AF.

Animal Studies

A typical example of an ectopic premature beat initiating reentry and an atrial tachycardia is shown in Figure 1. The left panel shows the distribution of refractory periods in the atrial tissue. The refractory periods were measured at a pacing cycle length of 400 msec, varying from 150 to 210 msec in this canine right atrium. Pacing was conducted from the region of shortest refractory period, i.e., 150 msec. When the

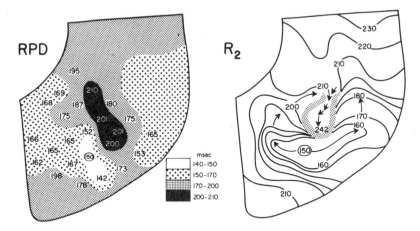

Figure 1. Left panel: The isorefractory period distribution in the canine right atrium. The circled number (150) indicates the site and the timing of the atrial premature beat. Note the high refractory period gradient close to the pacing site. **Right panel:** The activation sequence of the first premature beat R2 constructed from 72 points. Note that the premature beat encounters refractory tissue and travels around a functional arc of block. The latest tissue to be activated is at 242 msec. Although not illustrated, the wave front reenters at the region close to the pacing site. (Reprinted with permission from Boineau et al.[9])

premature beat had a critical coupling interval, reentry was initiated. The conduction of the premature beat and the first reentrant beat is shown in the right panel. Note that an arc of block is created in the right atrial free wall in the region with high gradient of refractory periods and the wave fronts travel around the lines of block. This wave front then reenters at about 242 msec when the tissue proximal to the line of block is excitable again. Although this illustrates the role of dispersion of refractory periods in creating the initial arc of block, anisotropy can also play a critical role in initiation of reentry.[10]

In the studies conducted by Wang et al. in the vagal model of AF, the initial site of reentry was in the region of long refractory period and this occurred in the left atrium around the pulmonary veins.[11] In the sterile pericarditis model of atrial flutter, programmed electrical stimulation typically gave rise to AF which stabilized into atrial flutter. Mapping of the onset of AF indicated that the first spontaneous beat of fibrillation was induced very close to the stimulation site but high resolution mapping of this beat was not presented.[12] In the results of the sterile pericarditis model published by Schoels et al., atrial flutter was induced by programmed electrical stimulation and the first reentrant beat was mapped.[13] Premature stimulation from the posteroinferior aspect of the left atrium resulted in an arc of conduction block in the low right atrium between the inferior vena cava (IVC) and the tricuspid valve. The first spontaneous beat occurred when the conduction time around the region of functional and anatomic block was long enough that tissue proximal to the block between the IVC and tricuspid ring recovered from its refractoriness and activation reentered in that region. Initiation of AF has also been mapped in an acetycholine model of atrial tachyarrhythmias. Mapping was conducted in an isolated canine right atrium and it was observed that most often the initial line of block responsible for reentrant excitation was in the posterior wall and occurred parallel to the crista terminalis.[14] As reentry progressed, the lines of block as well as the site of reentry changed.

In the various models of AF or flutter in which the onset of the first beat has been mapped, the region of initial reentry varies, occuring in the inferior IVC/tricuspid valve junction, along the crista terminalis, or around the left pulmonary veins. Different models of AF seem to give rise to different regions of initial reentry and due to this variability, it is difficult to extrapolate where the initial reentry occurs during onset of AF in patients.

Clinical Studies

Detailed clinical mapping of the initiation of AF has not been conducted. There are a few reports in the literature in which multipolar catheter recordings were made during premature stimulation of the atrium and induction of AF. In patients with a history of atrial flutter or fibrillation, premature stimulation in the high right atrium causes a maximal increase in conduction delay to the coronary sinus (CS) sites, less to the His bundle recording, and least in the high right atrium itself.[15–17] Whether the region of large conduction delay is the site where reentry is initiated is not known. It is also possible that initiation of atrial flutter and fibrillation are similar and analysis of the former may provide critical information regarding initiation of fibrillation. Josephson et al. have observed that during initiation of flutter, an early period of fractionation of electrograms is observed usually at the os of the CS or the atrioventricular (AV) junction.[18,19] They also observed that in patients with atrial flutter, the refractory period at the CS sites was longer, whereas these two refractory periods were comparable in control patients. They found it more difficult to induce flutter from the CS and suggested that the low right atrium is a critical site for the formation of reentrant circuits. Other clinical studies have also shown that when different sites in the atrium are paced at rapid rates, the inferior part of the right atrium experiences 2:1 block at the lowest pacing rate and may be the site with the longest refractory period.[20] It is important to note that in healthy atria, the action potential duration is maximal in the region of the sinus node and decreases down the crista terminalis.[21] Due to this distribution, a premature beat arising in the superior crista terminalis is least likely to experience conduction block because the wave front would encounter tissue of a shorter, not longer, refractory period. In patients with spontaneous AF, this distribution of refractory periods as well as the origin of basic and premature beats may be altered due to pathological changes.

In another study, the mode of onset of AF in 103 episodes in patients with accessory pathways was analyzed.[22] None of these patients had organic heart disease. Programmed electrical stimulation was conducted from the high right atrium. In most episodes of AF, the earliest spontaneous atrial activation occurred in the high right atrium with a high to low activation of the right atrium. In 17% of the episodes, the earliest activation was in the left atrium.

There are several studies in the literature in which the mechanism of induction of atrial "echo beats" has been discussed. It is possible that echo beats and AF may share a common method of initiation although initiation of echo beats degenerates into sustained atrial tachyarrhythmias in very few patients. For example, of the 9 patients studied by Breithardt et al. sustained atrial flutter was induced in only one patient; likewise, AV nodal reentrant tachycardia was also induced in only one.[23] In that study, recordings from 12–15 sites within the right atrium were made during onset of echo beats. During Sl-S2 stimulation from the right atrial appendage, the sequence of atrial activation of the first echo beat was from the high right atrium to low right atrium in eight of the nine patients. In five of these patients, premature atrial stimulation was also performed at the lateral wall of the right atrium; in three of these patients, the activation sequence of the echo beat remained from high to low, and in the other two it was from low atrium to high right atrium. The high to low atrial activation of the echo beats and the morphological analysis of the P wave met the requirements of sinus node reentry. The authors preferred to call it "high right atrial reentry" rather than sinus node reentry since there was no direct evidence for the latter. Although the electrophysiological basis for sinus node reentry has been demonstrated by mapping the isolated rabbit right atrium,[24] its role in initiating sustained AF in patients has not been fully investigated.

Another question has been whether AV nodal reentry or AV reentry could be responsible for initiation of AF. Many investigators have observed that AV reentry can frequently degenerate into AF, and that surgical ablation of the accessory pathway precludes AV reentry and also prevents recurrences of AF.[25] On the other hand, transition of AV node reentry into AF has been a relatively rare observation in the electrophysiological laboratory. It has been hypothesized that this difference may be due to the faster rate of AV reentry. Wathem et al.[26] reported a mean cycle length of 390 ± 75 msec for AV node reentry, whereas the cycle length of AV reentry tends to be approximately 338 ± 70 msec.[27] A faster cycle length of the tachycardia could cause a greater dispersion of refractoriness and predispose to AF. Another possible explanation may be the activation pattern of the atria with the two arrhythmias. During AV reentry, the activation of the right atrium is typically towards the AV node, whereas in AV node reentry it is in the retrograde direction. A retrograde activation of the right atrium may be protective. If the origin of the premature beat is more superior, then the activation of the basic and premature beats would be antidromic to each other. This could "preexcite" the abnormal region which is potentially responsible for block and reentry, and prolong the coupling interval of the premature beat in that region. This would prevent reentry from being initiated and will be discussed in greater detail later. It is also possible that there is no real difference in the incidence of AF in patients with AV reentry and AV node reentry and a greater difference is clinically observed because the patients with AF and Wolff-Parkinson-White (WPW) syndrome have higher ventricular rates and greater hemodynamic compromise, and are therefore more likely to present themselves for medical evaluation. A recent analysis of the incidence of AF in patients with paroxysmal supraventricular tachycardia (PSVT) indicated that 12% of the patients with tachycardia had symptomatic AF during a follow-up of one year and this increased to 19% in about two and one half years.[28] The study showed no difference in the incidence of AF between the patients with AV node reentry and those with AV reentry through an accessory pathway. Although this study documents the prevalence of AF in patients with PSVT, the prevalence of AV nodal reentry in patients with AF has not been evaluated. It is possible that in a subset of patients, AF is initiated by a brief run of AV nodal tachycardia which acts as a trigger.

All these clinical studies suggest that there may not be a consistent site of initiation of reentry in all patients with AF. In different subsets of patients, AF may be initiated around the CS, in the high right atrium, or be due to AV nodal reentry. Since mapping of the left atrium was not conducted in most of these studies, the results could be biased. Detailed clinical mapping needs to be conducted to determine the initial site of reentrant activation in patients with clinical AF. It is also important to establish whether the site of reentry is dependent on the site of premature stimulation or whether it is robust and independent of the site of premature stimulation. The latter would indicate that there are unique areas where conduction block occurs and reentry is consistently initiated.

Activation of the Sinus Beat

Animal studies indicate that AF is initiated when the basic as well as the premature activation of the atrium is unique and this unique activation results in reentrant excitation. For example, in Figure 1, the authors observed that if a premature stimulus was delivered at an area of long refractory period, no reentry was initiated, whereas an earlier premature stimulus delivered to the site of the shortest refractory period in a region of adjacent short and long refractory periods initiated reentry. Similar observations have also been made by other investigators who used a vagal model of induction of AF.[11] They observed that AF was much easier to induce from sites of short than long refractory periods. Morphological analysis of P waves that initiate clinical AF also indicates that premature beats from certain sites may be more proarrhythmic. Based on these observations, it is important to review the normal and premature activation of the atrium before a hypothesis for prevention of AF is formulated.

The normal activation of the atrium as well as its modulation by autonomic and intra-atrial pressure changes has been well documented in animal studies. The normal pacemaker is not localized to a single site and multiple sites within the atria are capable of initiating the impulse. This was demonstrated in animals in which the sinus node was surgically removed and the secondary pacemaker sites were observed between the sinus node and the inferior vena cava.[29,30] Boineau et al. analyzed the relationship between the site of origin of an atrial impulse and its cycle length in dogs.[31,32] They used cardiac nerve stimulation as well as agonist-antagonist infusion to produce changes in cycle length and observed a significant correlation between cycle length and impulse origin. At the shortest cycle lengths, the greatest concentration of origin sites was located at the superior RA-SVC (right atrium-superior vena cava) junction. As the cycle length increased, the site of origin shifted more inferiorly along the sulcus terminalis.

Figure 2 shows the relationship between site of impulse origin and cycle length using a zonal distribution model. The right atrium is divided cranio-caudally into five zones of approximately 10 mm in length. The histograms demonstrate the frequency of impulse origin within

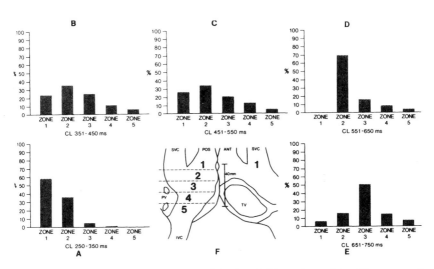

Figure 2. Histograms and zonal model of atrial impulse origin. Figure reads clockwise from bottom left. Right atrium is divided craniocaudally into five zones (**F**). Histograms (**A-E**) represent frequency of impulse initiation in Zones 1–5 expressed as a percentage of total number of observed sites of impulse initiation (Y axis) at each cycle length (CL) range. (Reprinted with permission from Boineau et al.[31])

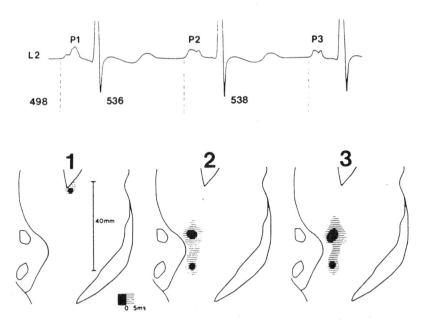

Figure 3. Change in the P wave morphology caused by a shift in the dominant pacemaker site in a dog. Lead 2 ECG is shown on the top. Pl and P2 are two different P wave morphologies that are associated with different cycle lengths. Only the first 5 msec of atrial activation are shown. Note that with lengthening of cycle length, the site of impulse origin shifts inferiorly. (Reprinted with permission from Schuessler et al.[70])

each of the zones for the different cycle lengths. Sites of impulse origin in zone 1 predominated at the shortest cycle lengths (250 to 350 msec) and there was a decreasing frequency of sites of origin in the lower zones 2 to 5. At the cycle lengths between 351 msec and 450 msec, sites within zone 2 predominated. With increasing cycle length, there was a general shift inferiorly in the site of impulse origin. Figure 3 illustrates another example of change in cycle length associated with activation sequence and P wave morphology in a dog. At the cycle length of 498 msec, the activation began at the junction of right atrial appendage and the SVC. As the cycle length increased to 536 msec and 538 msec, the site of earliest activation shifted inferiorly 2 cms to the intracaval band and was associated with a change in the P wave morphology. A dual origin of the atrial impulse where the two sites are more than 1 cm apart and are activated within 10 msec to 15 msec was also frequently observed at different cycle lengths. Mapping of pacemaker location has also been conducted with cardiac nerve stimulation and demonstrates a similar cranial shift in pacemaker location with sympathetic stimulation and a caudal shift with parasympathetic stimulation.[33] Changes in blood pressure by phenylephrine and nitro prusside can also affect heart rate and pacemaker location. In an animal study, an inverse relationship between blood pressure and heart rate was observed.[34] The maximum heart rate occurred at low arterial pressures and this in turn was associated with a cranial shift in the site of origin of the sinus impulse.

Mapping of the human right atrium also demonstrates that the origin of sinus beats is clustered posteriorly along the sulcus terminalis and anteriorly at the RA-SVC junction, a region approximately 1.5 cm wide and 7.5 cm long.[35] This was mapped in 14 patients with WPW undergoing surgery of their bypass tracts. Brody et al.[36] were the first to systematically document that normal patients may demonstrate multiple P wave morphologies and these differences may be due to a change in the site of the atrial pacemaker. Spontaneous or artificial modulation of the autonomics such as stress testing, tilting, or Valsalva maneuvers may modify the cycle length and alter the activation sequence of the atrium. The effect of organic heart disease and atrial dilatation on the origin of the atrial impulse in humans is not known.

Origin of Premature Beats

It has been well documented by Capucci et al. that closely coupled premature beats are much more likely to initiate AF than beats of long coupling intervals.[37] Onset of AF in 20 patients was analyzed and the premature beats that initiated AF had a shorter coupling interval than the isolated premature beats (412 ± 68 msec vs. 470 ± 67 msec; $P<.01$), whereas the basal rates were the same under the two conditions. It is hypothesized that not only is the coupling interval important, but also the site of origin of the premature beat. This is supported by the animal studies discussed previously in which AF could only be initiated when premature stimulation was conducted from certain unique sites.[9,11] Analysis of the morphology of the premature P waves that initiate clinical AF also indicates that they frequently have a morphology that is identical to that of the sinus beat.[38] This suggests that these beats may originate along the sinus node/crista terminalis region, similar to that of the sinus complex. The sites of origin of ectopic atrial tachycardias (EAT) in patients are indicators of sites with abnormal ectopy and it is also possible that these sites are similar to the sites from which premature beats arise. EAT is a relatively uncommon form of supraventricular tachycardia that is resistant to pharmacological therapy and is treated with radiofrequency (RF) ablation. The majority of the ectopic atrial tachycardias are localized to the right atrium and predominantly along the crista terminalis and the right atrial appendage, although sites along the superior pulmonary veins have also been observed infrequently.[38–40] Schuessler et al. analyzed the site of origin of atrial premature beats that initiate spontaneous atrial tachyarrhythmias in an acetycholine-infused preparation of the canine right atrium.[41] They showed that not only could a reentrant tachycardia be initiated by closely coupled beats, the site of origin of these premature beats was also typically along the crista terminalis.

All of these results indicate that the site of impulse origin is under the dynamic control of the autonomic nervous system and can vary significantly, primarily along the crista terminalis. Variability in the site of origin of the sinus beat may sometimes set up unique patterns of activations, which when coupled with closely coupled premature beats from the crista terminalis could initiate AF. In patients with paroxysmal AF (PAF) who have frequent atrial premature beats (APBs), this may explain why only some of the premature beats initiate AF. It is hypothesized that unique activation of the basic and premature beats needs to exist in an abnormal substrate to initiate the arrhythmia. Based on these observations, the effect of atrial pacing on activation sequence can be assessed. In patients with sick sinus syndrome and bradycardia, the site of atrial pacing would tend to dominate the activation sequence. However, in patients with minimal bradycardia, the site of origin of the atrial impulse is most likely to vary between the site of pacing and the superior aspect of the crista terminalis which would tend to be the site of origin of higher spontaneous rates. Variability in the site of origin of the the basic beat increases the probability that premature beats originating from unique sites may initiate reentry in an abnormal substrate. One approach for prevention of AF is to reduce the degree of variability of the origin of the sinus beat and initiate atrial activation from a region where premature beats are least likely to induce AF. Although such a unique pacing site is not yet known, the goal would be to always have a consistent pattern of atrial activation. This can be achieved by pacing the atrium at a higher rate than the intrinsic rate. If this pacing rate is too high and clinically unacceptable, one can also suppress the sinus node by blocking agents or ablation of the sinus node region and then overdrive pace the atrium at an acceptable rate. Another alternative would be to develop pacing algorithms that ensure continuous pacing of the atria. Multisite triggered pacing may also achieve this provided the sensing electrodes are close to the origin of the atrial impulse.

Mechanisms for Prevention of Atrial Fibrillation

Based on the previous discussion, pacing may prevent AF by: (1) Prolonging the coupling interval of the premature beats in the abnormal substrate where reentry is initiated by pacing from unique atrial sites; (2) Suppressing the premature beats; or (3) Altering the electrophysiological properties of the substrate so that even if premature beats occurred, they would be less likely to initiate AF.

Prolongation of the Coupling Interval of Premature Beats in the Abnormal Substrate

Mapping studies indicate that reentry is initiated when the coupling interval of the premature beat is short enough to cause block in the abnormal substrate. At longer coupling intervals, slow conduction and block could occur but are insufficient to facilitate reentrant excitation. The abnormal substrate is the tissue with long refractory periods and high refractory period gradients or with significant anisotropy where reentry is initiated. It is hypothesized that AF can be prevented by increasing the coupling interval of the premature beat in this abnormal substrate. This can be done by pacing the abnormal region itself or pacing at a site that is antidromic to the activation of the abnormal substrate by the premature beat. Both of these concepts tend to "preexcite" the abnormal substrate and increase the coupling interval of a spontaneous premature beat and will be discussed below. The first method requires that the location of the abnormal substrate be known; the second method requires less precise information regarding the location of the abnormal substrate, but the site of origin of the premature beats that initiate AF should be known.

Pacing from the Abnormal Substrate

When pacing is done from the abnormal substrate responsible for initial line of block and reentry, it activates this tissue before any other part of the atrium is activated and is termed "preexcitation". Since the

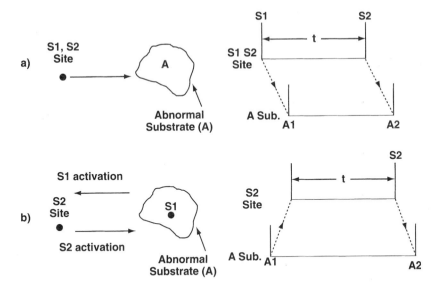

Figure 4. In **a**, the site of pacing Sl and premature beat S2 are orthodromic to each other. The coupling interval of the premature beat at the site of stimulation is "t". This results in activation of the abnormal substrate at a coupling of Al-A2 which is not significantly prolonged. In **b**, the Sl stimulation is from the abnormal substrate and the site as well as the coupling interval of S2 does not change. Now the activation of the Sl and S2 beats are antidromic to each other resulting in a long Al-A2 coupling in the abnormal substrate.

activation of the premature beat is antidromic to the activation of the basic beat, the coupling interval of activation in the abnormal substrate is prolonged, as is illustrated in Figure 4. In order to implement this, we need to know the region where reentry is initiated and it is assumed that there is only one critical region where block occurs. For example, in the case illustrated in Figure 1, the region where reentry was initiated was the region with long refractory periods. If that region was paced, its effect would be to prolong the coupling interval of the premature activation in the abnormal substrate provided the premature beats originated from some other site and their coupling interval at the site of origin of the premature beats did not change. A longer coupling of the premature activation in the abnormal substrate would reduce the probability of initiating AF. This concept has been well documented for the prevention of ventricular tachyarrhythmias.[42–44] With detailed isochronal mapping, the region of reentry was defined and it was shown that if that tissue was preexcited, reentrant excitation could be prevented. As discussed previously, the region where reentry is initiated and progresses to AF is not well documented in patients and therefore the optimal pacing site cannot be determined yet. Some of the regions that have been suggested are the high right atrium, the coronary sinus region, and the AV node itself. It is also possible that the substrate is so heterogeneous that block as well as reentry can be initiated at various sites in the left and right atria. In such a case, all these sites would need to be paced and preexcited to prevent AF. If there are two such sites this may be possible, but with multiple sites it may not be practicably implementable.

Pacing Antidromic to the Activation of the Premature Beat

If the exact location of the substrate for reentrant excitation cannot be determined, it is still possible to preexcite that region by pacing at a site such that the abnormal substrate is activated antidromic to the activation by the premature beat.[38] This requires that the site of origin of the premature beats is known as well as the general region where block occurs. One would pace from a site opposite to the site of origin of the premature beats such that the abnormal substrate is located between the basic and premature beat activation as illustrated in Figure 5. Pacing in this manner will increase the shortest Al-A2 coupling interval in the abnormal region and reduce the probability of block and reentrant excitation. This hypothesis assumes that the site of origin of the premature beats responsible for AF initiation does not vary significantly. As discussed previously, the crista terminalis may be the most consistent site for initiation of atrial premature beats. Therefore, pacing should be done from a region such that the abnormal substrate is straddled between this pacing site and the crista terminalis. Clinically, since it is not known if there is a consistent site of the abnormal substrate where conduction block occurs across patients, the optimal site of pacing cannot be determined yet.

Dual-Site Pacing

If the optimal site cannot be determined because the location of the abnormal substrate and/or the location of premature beats is not known clinically, the probability of preventing AF can be increased by pacing at two sites rather than one because it is likely that one of those two sites could meet the criteria. It is important to note that dual site-pacing will not result in a longer Al-A2 than the "optimal" single site.[38]

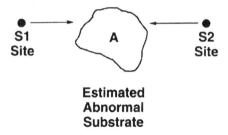

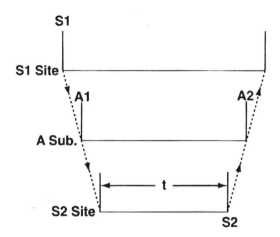

Figure 5. The site of pacing (Sl) and the site of origin of the premature beat are on the opposite sides of the abnormal substrate. The Sl beat activates the abnormal substrate and then the site of origin of the premature beat. Since the coupling interval of the premature beat is "t", its antidromic activation results in a significantly longer Al-A2 coupling interval in the abnormal substrate.

This is because pacing from the second site could result in orthodromic conduction of the premature beat and could only shorten the Al-A2 time in the abnormal substrate. Therefore, if there is one region of block and reentry, pacing from two sites cannot be more protective than pacing from the single "optimal" site. However, if the optimal pacing site is not known, dual-site pacing could increase the probability of prevention of AF. There are other conditions which could make dual atrial pacing more beneficial. If there are two regions rather than a single one where reentry is most likely to be initiated, then pacing and preexcting both these sites directly would be important to prevent initiation of AF at either of the sites. Some recent clinical as well as animal studies indicate that dual-site atrial pacing may provide a greater protection against AF and flutter than single-site pacing.[45-49] Dual-site pacing may also improve cardiac hemodynamics and provide indirect electrophysiological benefits for prevention of AF.

Suppression of Premature Beats

An alternative strategy to prevent AF is to suppress the atrial premature beats (APBs) that initiate AF. Suppression of APBs may not be a sufficient condition to suppress AF but if all APBs were suppressed, AF could only be initiated as a result of sinus tachycardia where the first beat of AF is reentrant rather than ectopic. ECG tracings of the onset of AF in certain cases indicate that premature beats that initiate AF are preceded by bradycardia.[38] This was observed in patients with vagally mediated AF[1] as well as in other clinical reports.[50] In such patients, the clinical results indicate that increasing the pacing rate can suppress ectopy and induction of AF. There is, however, an upper pacing rate which can be tolerated by patients without eliciting undesirable symptoms. An alternative approach is to avoid pacing at a high rate continuously. New pacing algorithms have been developed which pace at a high rate transiently following sensed premature beats. The pacing rate is then gradually decelerated over time. A clinical test with an algorithm that resulted in a 12.5% increase in atrial pacing rate following a sensed APB was conducted in 70 patients with frequent atrial ectopy.[51] The increased rate was maintained for 20 beats if no further APBs were sensed and then the pacing cycle length was increased by 63 msec every 20 beats until the lower rate or sinus rhythm was reached. The algorithm reduced the number of APBs but there was no statistical reduction in the number of AF episodes. However, in patients with frequent AF episodes, fewer episodes occurred when the algorithm was active. The authors noted that efficacy of the algorithm may have been limited by a precautionary feature of the algorithm which was designed to be deactivated by two or more APBs occurring in succession. The pacemaker statistics indicated that this occurred frequently. This study also shows the possibility of discordance between a reduction in the frequency of APBs and AF. The two may not always be correlated and a reduction in premature beats may not result in prevention of AF.

Another pacing algorithm that may reduce atrial ectopy is termed "rate stabilization".[52] It has been well documented that onset of tachyarrhythmias is frequently preceded by short/long sequences.[38] Pacing at a fixed cycle length would prevent the long pause and reduce the maximum cycle length of the atrial beat. It has been observed that at least for prevention of ventricular arrhythmias, pacing at a fixed cycle length is sometimes insufficient to prevent the tachyarrhythmias.[53] An alternative approach is to transiently increase the pacing rate following a spontaneous premature beat using the "rate stabilization" algorithm (Fig. 6). The coupling interval of the premature beat is measured and the next pacing escape interval is set equal to coupling interval of the premature beat plus an incremental interval "T". The interval of the following beat is further incremented by "T" and so on until the escape interval is reached. The typical values of "T" may range from 50 msec to 200 msec. The desired effect of this algorithm is to overdrive/suppress the atrium following an atrial premature beat. Rate stabilization may also prevent tachyarrhythmias by reducing the dispersion of refractory periods due to the higher pacing rates. Clinical efficacy of this algorithm for suppression of atrial tachyarrhythmias has not been determined yet.

The mechanism by which an increase in atrial rate suppresses atrial ectopy can be due to the direct electrophysiological effects or due to electromechanical feedback effects. Intracellular recordings from diseased human atrial tissue frequently show partially depolarized cells and the existence of "abnormal automaticity".[54] This abnormal automaticity may be suppressible by overdrive pacing at higher rates. Although triggered activity caused by early afterdepolarizations (EADs) is bradycardia-dependent and can be suppressed by pacing, there is no experimental evidence of its presence in atrial tissue as of yet. Overdrive suppression of atrial pacemaker tissue has also been well documented in awake normal animals as well as after excision of the sinus node and it is greatly exaggerated in animals with an excised sinus node.[30]

Changes in pacing rate may also alter the frequency of atrial ectopic beats due to the effect of rate on atrial pressure which in turn affects atrial ectopy. An increase in the ventricular pacing rate increases atrial pressure and this might be a direct mechanoelectrical effect or a reflex neuromechanism.[55,56] In canine experiments, an increase in atrial pressure has been correlated with an increase in the incidence of APBs.[57] In these animals, the incidence of APBs was 2% at atrial pressures of 1–6 mm, while at pressures of 43 mm or more it was 11%. Therefore, a reduction in atrial pressure caused by a change

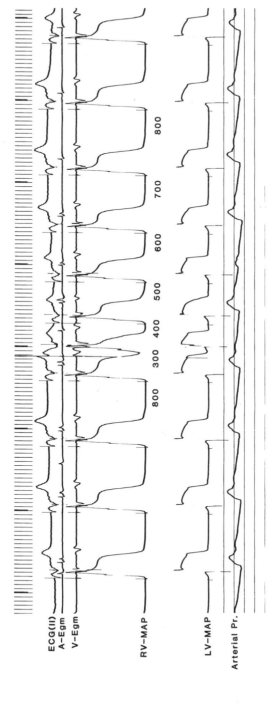

Figure 6. Illustration of the rate stabilization algorithm for ventricular pacing. Surface ECG, atrial and ventricular electrograms as well as monophasic action potential (MAP) recordings are shown. During ventricular pacing at 800 msec, a premature beat at 300 msec is simulated. The next pacing interval is 400 msec (300 + 100), followed by 500 msec (400 + 100) and so on until the lower escape interval of 800 msec is reached. The incremental interval (100 msec in this case) can be varied.

in the pacing rate could prevent premature beats and the ability to induce AF.

Effect of Atrial Pacing on the Electrophysiological Substrate

Another mechanism by which atrial pacing may prevent initiation or sustenance of AF is by altering the electrophysiological substrate itself. Animal studies indicate that an increase in pacing rate reduces the dispersion of refractory periods[58] and a high dispersion is associated with an increased likelihood of induction of tachyarrhythmias. As shown in Figure 1, conduction block and reentry tends to occur where the refractory period gradients are high. An increase in atrial pacing rate would reduce the dispersion of refractory periods in the atrium in such a manner that even in the presence of premature beats, they may be less likely to induce AF. It should be noted that although animal studies have shown a relationship between pacing rate and dispersion, this has not been observed in the clinical studies[59] and may be related to the limited number of sites where the refractory period measurements were made clinically.

Atrial pacing may also have a more cumulative chronic effect on prevention of AF. Recent animal studies by Wijffels et al. have shown that when AF is sustained over long periods of time, it alters the electrophysiological properties of the atrial tissue and facilitates the sustenance of AF, i.e., "atrial fibrillation begets atrial fibrillaton".[4] The electrophysiological changes are primarily related to alteration in the rate adaptation of refractory periods. In control animals, the atrial refractory periods prolong with longer atrial pacing cycle lengths, whereas in the animals in chronic AF, the rate adaptation of refractory periods is blunted and the refractory periods become relatively constant at long cycle lengths. This observation has also been made in patients with inducible AF, by Attuel et al.[60] Wijffels et al. also showed that when the animals were maintained in sinus rhythm for a short period of time, it was much more difficult to induce AF, suggesting that sinus rhythm begets sinus rhythm. Not only was AF difficult to induce but the rate adaptation in refractory periods became closer to that observed in the control animals. This indicates that even if pacing does not prevent all AF episodes but only decreases the total time the patient is in AF, the increased presence of sinus rhythm could alter the electrophysiological substrate and make AF less sustainable.

The effect of rate adaptation of refractory periods on the ability to sustain arrhythmias was recently investigated in a computer model of cell activation. In this "automata model",[61] reentry was initiated in a matrix of 900 units with each unit representing an aggregate of cardiac cells. Each element, following excitation by its neighbor, underwent time-dependent changes in excitability and the refractory period of each element was dependent on the previous cycle length. The slope of the curve that defines the relationship between cycle length and refractory periods was varied between 0.15 and 0.9. A low slope indicates that there is a very small increase in refractory period with an increase in cycle length. It was observed that the reentry was stable and sustained at slopes less than 0.6, whereas at higher slopes, the induced reentrant tachycardias were unstable with continuously varying cycle lengths that terminated spontaneously. These computer modeling results validate the animal and clinical results which indicate that sustained tachyarrhythmias are associated with minimal adaptation of refractory period with cycle length.

Atrial pacing at different rates or changes in the AV interval can also change the intra-atrial pressure and thereby alter the electrophysiological properties of the atrial tissue. There are conflicting data on the effect of an increase in atrial pressure on atrial refractoriness. Some studies indicate that an increase in pressure increases refractoriness[62-64] as well as the dispersion of refractoriness and inducibility of AF.[65] Other studies have shown no change[66] or even a decrease in the atrial refractory periods.[67] Some of these differences may be due to differences in species or methodology of measurement of these parameters. In most of these studies the increase in pressure was associated with an increased inducibility of atrial tachyarrhythmias. Spontaneous and induced atrial arrhythmias increased remarkably in canine hearts with left atrial dilatation caused by a balloon catheter.[68] Whether the increase in spontaneous episodes was due to an increase in atrial ectopy or changes in the electrophysiological substrate is not known. Preliminary results also indicate that an elevation of right atrial pressure within normal limits in patients with PAF has a profibrillatory effect.[69]

Summary

There are many clinical studies which suggest that atrial pacing can prevent AF. It is hypothesized that pacing prevents AF primarily by preventing the initiation of the arrhythmia although it may also have some effects on arrhythmia sustainability by altering the electrophysiological properties of the tissue. If AF is initiated by a spontaneous ectopic beat causing reentry, pacing should be conducted in a manner that prolongs the prematurity of the ectopic beat in the abnormal substrate so that conduction block and reentry do not occur and AF is prevented. This can be done by pacing at an "optimal" location which would be within the abnormal substrate or by pacing at a site so that the activation of the abnormal substrate is antidromic to its activation by the premature beat. Determining this optimal site requires information regarding the anatomic location of the abnormal substrate or the site of origin of the premature beats that initiate reentry. There are some clinical data that suggest that the location of the abnormal substrate where reentry occurs may vary among patients and could be in the high right atrium or near the coronary sinus. More clinical data are needed to define the initial location of reentry and to determine whether it is robust or varies as the site of the premature beat is varied. If the initial site of reentry is robust, then pacing could prevent AF as a result of this mechanism.

Pacing the atrium may also prevent AF by suppressing the premature beats by overdrive suppression or by the electromechanical feedback effects. An increase in pacing rate can also alter the dispersion of refractory periods or alter atrial hemodynamics which can permanently affect the electrophysiological properties of the tissue. This may also provide a protective effect against the initiation and sustenance of AF.

In the future, more studies need to be conducted to define the basic mechanism of initiation of AF in patients. This, along with the delineation of the site of initial reentry and the location of the origin of premature atrial beats that initiate reentry will help us optimize pacing for prevention of AF and aid in our understanding of why pacing prevents AF.

Acknowledgment: The author wishes to thank Diane Knaeble for her assistance in the preparation of this chapter.

References

1. Coumel P, Friocourt P, Mugica J, et al. Long-term prevention of vagal atrial arrhythmias by atrial pacing at 90/minute: experience with six cases. Pace 1983;6:552–560.
2. Reimold SC, Lamas GA, Cantillon CO, et al. Risk factors for the development of recurrent atrial fibrillation: role of pacing and clinical variables. Am Heart J 1995;129:1127–1132.
3. Andersen HR, Thuesen L, Bagger JP, et al. Prospective randomised trial

of atrial versus ventricular pacing in sick-sinus syndrome. Lancet 1994; 344:1523–1528.

4. Wijffels M, Kirchhof C, Dorland R, et al. Atrial fibrillation begets atrial fibrillation: a study in awake chronically instrumented goats. Circulation 1995;92:1954–1968.

5. Allessie MA, Lammers WJEP, Bonke F, et al. Experimental evaluation of Moe's multiple wavelet hypothesis of atrial fibrillation. In: Zipes DP, Jalife J, eds. Cardiac Electrophysiology and Arrhythmias. Orlando, FLA: Grune & Stratton; 1985:265–275.

6. Konings KTS, Kirchhof CJHJ, Joep SRLM, et al. High-density mapping of electrically induced atrial fibrillation in humans. Circulation 1994;89: 1665–1680.

7. Jaïs P, Haïssaguerre M, Shah DC, et al. Characteristics of focal atrial fibrillation. Pace 1996;19:650.

8. Holm M, Blomstrom P, Brandt J, et al. Documentation of atrial areas with a consistent excitation pattern in patients with chronic atrial fibrillation. Pace 1994;17:750.

9. Boineau JP, Schuessler RB, Mooney CR, et al. Natural and evoked atrial flutter due to circus movement in dogs: role of abnormal atrial pathways, slow conduction, nonuniform refractory period distribution and premature beats. Am J Cardiol 1980;45:1167–1181.

10. Spach MS, Josephson ME. Initiating reentry: the role of nonuniform anisotropy in small circuits. J Cardiovasc Electrophysiol 1994;5:182–209.

11. Wang J, Liu J, Feng J, et al. Regional and functional factors determining induction and maintenance of atrial fibrillation in dogs. Am J Physiol 1996; 71:H148-H158.

12. Shimizu A, Nozaki A, Rudy Y, et al. Onset of induced atrial flutter in the canine pericarditis model. JACC 1991;17:1223–1236.

13. Schoels W, Gough WB, Restivo M, et al. Circus movement atrial flutter in the canine sterile pericarditis model: activation patterns during initiation, termination, and sustained reentry in vivo. Circ Res 1990;67:35–50.

14. Schuessler RB, Grayson TM, Bromberg BI, et al. Cholinergically mediated tachyarrhythmias induced by a single extrastimulus in the isolated canine right atrium. Circ Res 1992;71:1254–1267.

15. Buxton AE, Waxman HL, Marchlinkski FE, et al. Atrial conduction: effects of extrastimuli with and without atrial dysrhythmias. Am J Cardiol 1984; 54:755–761.

16. Cosio FG, Palacios J, Vidal JM, et al. Electrophysiologic studies in atrial fibrillation: slow conduction of premature impulses. A possible manifestation of the background for reentry. Am J Cardiol 1983;51:122–130.

17. Papageorgiou P, Boyle N, Monahan K, et al. Site-dependent intra-atrial conduction delay: relationship to initiation of atrial flutter/fibrillation. JACC 1995;169A.

18. Josephson ME. Atrial flutter and fibrillation. In: Bussy RK, Klass FM, eds. Clinical Cardiac Electrophysiology. Philadelphia: Lea & Febiger; 1993: 275–310.

19. Watson RM, Josephson ME. Atrial flutter. I. Electrophysiologic substrates and modes of initiation and termination. Am J Cardiol 1980;45:732–741.

20. Franz M, Moore H, Zabel M, et al. Action potential alternans and slow

conduction provoked by overdrive pacing in the "substrate" area in atrial flutter. JACC 1994;458A. Abstract.

21. Spach MS, Dolber PC, Anderson PAW. Multiple regional differences in cellular properties that regulate repolarization and contraction in the right atrium of adult and newborn dogs. Circ Res 1989;65:1594–1611.

22. Fujimura O, Klein GJ, Yee R, et al. Mode of onset of atrial fibrillation in the Wolff-Parkinson-White syndrome: how important is the accessory pathway? J Am Coll Cardiol 1990;15:1082–1086.

23. Breithardt G, Seipel L. Sequence of atrial activation in patients with atrial echo beats. In: Bonke F, ed. The Sinus Node. The Hague, Netherlands: Martinus Nijhoff Medical Division; 1978:389–408.

24. Allessie MA, Bonke F. Re-entry within the sinoatrial node as demonstrated by multiple micro-electrode recordings in the isolated rabbit heart. In: Bonke F, ed. The Sinus Node. The Hague, Netherlands: Martinus Nijhoff Medical Division; 1978:389–408.

25. Prystowsky EN. Tachycardia-induced tachycardia: a mechanism of initiation of atrial fibrillation. In: DiMarco JP, Prystowsky EN, eds. Atrial Arrhythmias: State of the Art. Armonk, NY: Futura Publishing Co; 1995: 81–95.

26. Wathem M, Natale A, Wolfe K, et al. An anatomically guided approach to atrioventricular node slow pathway ablation. Am J Cardiol 1992;70: 886–889.

27. Jackman WM, Beckman KJ, McClelland JH, et al. Treatment of supraventricular tachycardia due to atrioventricular nodal reentry by radiofrequency catheter ablation of slow-pathway conduction. N Engl J Med 1992; 327:313–318.

28. Hamer ME, Wilkinson WE, Clair WK, et al. Incidence of symptomatic atrial fibrillation in patients with paroxysmal supraventricular tachycardia. JACC 1995;25:984–988.

29. Euler DE, Jones SB, Gunnar WP, et al. Cardiac arrhythmias in the conscious dog after excision of the sinoatrial node and crista terminalis. Circulation 1979;59:468–475.

30. Randall WC, Rinkema LE, Jones SB, et al. Overdrive suppression of atrial pacemaker tissues in the alert, awake dog before and chronically after excision of the sinoatrial node. Am J Cardiol 1982;49:1166–1175.

31. Boineau JP, Schuessler RB, Roeske WR, et al. Quantitative relation between sites of atrial impulse origin and cycle length. Am. J Physiol 1983; 245:H781-H789.

32. Boineau JP, Schuessler RB, Mooney CR, et al. Multicentric origin of the atrial depolarization wave: the pacemaker complex: relation to dynamics of the atrial conduction, P-wave changes and heart rate control. Circulation 1978;58:1036–1048.

33. Schuessler RB, Boineau JP, Wylds AC, et al. Effect of canine cardiac nerves on heart rate, rhythm, and pacemaker location. Am J Physiol 1986;19: H630-H644.

34. Schuessler RB, Canavan TE, Boineau JP, et al. Baroreflex modulation of heart rate and initiation of atrial activation in dogs. Am J Physiol 1988; 24:H503-H513.

35. Boineau JP, Canavan TE, Schuessler RB, et al. Demonstration of a widely

distributed atrial pacemaker complex in the human heart. Circulation 1988;77:1221–1237.

36. Brody DA, Woolsey MD, Arzbaecher RC. Application of computer techniques to the detection and analysis of spontaneous P wave variations. Circulation 1967;36:359–371.

37. Capucci A, Santarelli A, Boriani G, et al. Atrial premature beats coupling interval determines lone paroxysmal atrial fibrillation onset. Int J Cardiol 1992;36:87–93.

38. Mehra R, Hill M. Prevention of atrial fibrillation/flutter by pacing techniques. In: Saksena S, Luderitz B, eds. Interventional Electrophysiology: A Textbook. Armonk, NY: Futura Publishing Co; 1996:521–540.

39. Shenasa H, Merrill JJ, Harner ME, et al. Different characteristics of left and right atrial ectopic tachycardias. Pace 1994;17:II-750.

40. Shenasa H, Merrill JJ, Harner ME, et al. Distribution of ectopic atrial tachycardias along the crista terminalis: an atrial ring of fire? Circulation 1993;88:I-29.

41. Schuessler RB, Rosenshtraukh LV, Boineau JP, et al. Spontaneous tachyarrhythmias after cholinergic suppression in the isolated perfused canine right atrium. Circ Res 1991;69:1075–1087.

42. Mehra R, Gough WB, Zeiler R, et al. Dual ventricular stimulation for prevention of reentrant ventricular tachyarrhythmias. JACC 1984;2:272.

43. Mehra R, Santel D. Electrical preexcitation of ischemic tissue for prevention of ventricular tachyarrhythmias. Pace 1986;9:282.

44. Restivo M, Gough WB, El-Sherif N. Reentrant ventricular rhythms in the late myocardial infarction period: prevention of reentry by dual stimulation during basic rhythm. Circulation. 1988;77:429–444.

45. Prakash A, Hill M, Lewis C, et al. Comparative efficacy of high right atrial, coronary sinus and dual site right atrial pacing in prevention of atrial fibrillation. Pace 1996;19(Part II):634.

46. Prakash A, Saksena S, Giorgberidze I, et al. Arrhythmias recurrence patterns during atrial pacing. JACC 1996;27:74A.

47. Hill M, Mongeon L, Mehra R. Prevention of atrial fibrillation: dual site atrial pacing reduces the coupling window of induction of atrial fibrillation. Pace 1996;19(Part II):630.

48. Daubert C, Mabo P, Berder V. Arrhythmias prevention by permanent atrial resynchronisation in advanced interatrial block. Eur Heart J 1990;11:237.

49. Daubert C, Mabo P, Berder V, et al. Atrial tachyarrhythmias associated with high degree interatrial conduction block: prevention by permanent atrial resynchronisation. Eur JCPE 1994;4:35–44.

50. Goel BG, Han J. Atrial ectopic activity associated with sinus bradycardia. Circulation 1970;42:838–853.

51. Murgatroyd FD, Nitzsche R, Slade AKB, et al. A new pacing algorithm for overdrive suppression of atrial fibrillation. Pace 1994;17:1966–1973.

52. Mehra R. Rate Stabilization Pacemaker. U.S. Patent # 4,941,671. 1990.

53. Leclerq JF, Zimmerman M, Coumel P. Is it possible to prevent ventricular tachyarrhythmias by pacing? In: Breithardt G, Borggrefe M, Zipes D, eds. Nonpharmacological Therapy of Tachyarrhythmias. Mount Kisco, NY: Futura Publishing Co; 1987:395–407.

54. Kimura T, Imanishi S, Arita M, et al. Two different mechanisms of automaticity in diseased human atrial fibers. Jap J Physiol 1988;38:851–867.

55. Burnett JC Jr, Osborn MH, Hammill SC. The role of frequency of atrial contraction versus atrial pressure in atrial natriuretic peptide release. J Clin Endocrinol Metab 1989;69:881–884.
56. Cohen TJ, Veltri EP, Lattuca JJ, et al. Hemodynamic responses to rapid pacing: a model for tachycardia differentiation. Pacing Clin Electrophysiol 1988;11(Part I):1522–1528.
57. Sideris DA, Toumanidis ST, Tselepatiotis E, et al. Atrial pressure and experimental atrial fibrillation. Pace 1995;18:1679–1685.
58. Han J, Millet, Chizzonitti B, et al. Termporal dispersion of recovery of excitability in atrium and ventricle as a function of heart rate. Am Heart J 1966;71:481.
59. Michelucci A, Padaletti L, Porciani MC, et al. Dispersion of refractoriness and atrial fibrillation. In: Olsson SB, Allessie MA, Campbell RWF, eds. Atrial Fibrillation: Mechanisms and Therapeutic Strategies. Armonk, NY: Futura Publishing Co; 1994:81–108.
60. Attuel P, Childers R, Cauchemz B, et al. Failure in the rate adaptation of the atrial refractory period: its relationship to vulnerability. Int J Cardiol 1982;2:179–197.
61. Mehra R, Ruetz L. Effect of refractory period changes with cycle length on stability of a reentrant tachycardia. Pace 1996;19(Part II):560.
62. Sideris DA, Kontoyannis DA, Michalis L, et al. Acute changes in blood pressure as a cause of cardiac arrhythmias. Eur Heart J 1987;8:45–52.
63. Klein LS, Miles WM, Zipes DP. Effect of atrioventricular interval during pacing or reciprocating tachycardia on atrial size, pressure, and refractory period. Circulation 1990;82:60–68.
64. Kaseda S, Zipes DP. Contraction excitation feedback in the atria: a cause of change in refractoriness. J Am Coll Cardiol 1988;11:1327–1336.
65. Isobe F, Schuessler RB, Mitsuna M, et al. High atrial pressure directly affects the dispersion of refractoriness and the inducibility of atrial fibrillation. Circulation 1993;88:I326.
66. Calkins J, El-Atassi R, Leon AN. Effect of the atrioventricular relationship on atrial refractoriness in humans. Pace 1992;15:771–778.
67. Ravelli F, Allessie MA. Atrial stretch decreases refractoriness and induces atrial fibrillation in the isolated rabbit heart. Circulation 1995;92:1754–1755.
68. Soliti F, Vecsey T, Kekesi V, et al. The effect of atrial dilatation on the genesis of atrial arrhythmias. Cardiol Res 1989;23:882–886.
69. Antonian A, Kanakakis J, Milonas J, et al. Contraction excitation feedback in the atrium in the lone atrial fibrillation. Pace 1993;16:1112.
70. Schuessler RB, Boineau JP, Bromberg BI, et al. Normal and abnormal activation of the atrium. In: Zipes DP, ed. Cardiac Electrophysiology: From Cell to Bedside. Philadelphia: WB Saunders; 1995.

CHAPTER 21

Detection of Atrial Fibrillation by Pacemakers and Antiarrhythmic Devices

Steven Swiryn, Adam T. Schoenwald, Alan V. Sahakian

Detection of atrial fibrillation (AF) is an important capability in the areas of bradycardia pacing, devices for ventricular arrhythmia therapy, and newer devices for the treatment of AF itself. This chapter will review the need for such a capability, the properties of AF which may provide opportunities for its detection, and properties which may be a source of difficulties. We will offer comments on accuracy and time requirements for detection algorithms and give some examples of already proposed, and often successful, solutions to detection. Finally, we will offer some caveats about data used to develop such algorithms.

For bradycardia pacemakers, there are a number of needs that a detection algorithm for AF can address. Atrial pacing will fail to capture in the presence of AF, and should therefore be inhibited. Furthermore, the pacemaker may not only continue to pace in the atrium, but may trigger ventricular pacing at irregular or inappropriately rapid rates. Automatic mode switching or conversion (i.e., the ability to change the operational mode of pacing in response to a change in rhythm) can avoid this by changing, for example, from the DDDR mode to VVIR or DDIR with the onset of AF and reverting to DDD with the return of sinus rhythm.

For ventricular antiarrhythmic devices, the detection of AF can prevent inappropriate or even occasionally dangerous delivery of ventricular therapy. Because most such devices use ventricular rate as the main criterion for ventricular tachyarrhythmia detection, a rapid ventricular response to AF is a common cause of inappropriate pacing

This work was supported in part by the Hartman Family Fund.
From *Nonpharmacological Management of Atrial Fibrillation*, edited by F.D. Murgatroyd and A.J. Camm. © 1997, Futura Publishing Co., Inc., Armonk, NY.

or shocks.[1] There are reports of cases where such inappropriate therapy can even induce a ventricular tachyarrhythmia.[2]

Newer devices designed to treat AF itself with cardioversion, drug delivery,[3] or pacing are in various stages of development. Obviously, such devices require accurate detection of AF. The specific requirements for such an algorithm are likely to be different from those for bradycardia pacemakers or devices for management of ventricular tachyarrhythmias. An initial decision must be made for each specific application as to whether it will be adequate to detect any atrial tachyarrhythmia and respond to it as "atrial fibrillation", or if it will be required that AF be detected specifically and differentiated from other atrial tachyarrhythmias. Clearly, algorithms for the former situation are much simpler (though not simple) and for many clinical situations may be all that is required. On the other hand, detection of AF itself may be desirable for certain newer applications and presents a somewhat different and more complex set of issues.

Atrial Fibrillation as a Signal to Be Detected

It is commonly taught that an irregularly irregular ventricular rate is a central criterion for AF. Given this teaching, an algorithm for the detection of AF starts and ends with the most easily detected feature of a rhythm strip, the QRS complex. The failure of this algorithm can be demonstrated by considering the case of an older patient with hypertension, recent heart failure, mitral valve disease, and a recent embolic event, who has complete heart block and a VVIR pacemaker and asking whether such a patient requires anticoagulation. Thus, while an irregularly irregular ventricular response is a common (but not universal) *consequence* of AF and may be a helpful clue to its presence, it is not a *criterion* for AF. Atrial flutter, multifocal atrial tachycardia, sinus rhythm with frequent premature atrial complexes, sinus arrhythmia, and a number of other rhythms also commonly produce an irregularly irregular ventricular response.

Though the need for attention to atrial signals in order to detect AF seems obvious, the above is intended to illustrate the choices that face a designer of an AF detection algorithm. On the one hand are the large events, readily understood, detectable with "off the shelf" hardware and software solutions borrowed from problems we have already solved, with many of the bugs already discovered and removed, using low power consumption, and requiring only standard lead designs. There is tremendous attraction and practicality in these features.

Table 1
Potentially Detectable Features of Atrial Fibrillation

Features Not Quintessential to Atrial Fibrillation
Ventricular irregularity
Atrial rate
Rate itself
Probability density function
Baseline crossings
Features Quintessential to Atrial Fibrillation
Variability in atrial electrogram morphology
Variability in atrial activation direction
Variability in multisite atrial activity
Variability in atrial activation timing
Global versus local activity comparisons
Variability in atrial signal amplitude
Power spectrum
"Percent power"
Magnitude-squared coherence

For many applications, such an algorithm may not only be acceptable but preferable. However, the greater the requirement for specificity in an AF detection algorithm, the more one is pushed to detect features which are quintessential to AF. This may require newer thinking, with more complex software and hardware solutions. Table 1 lists potentially detectable features of AF, divided into those which are quintessential to this rhythm and those which are not but may still serve in less specific detection algorithms.

Having dismissed ventricular irregularity above (even ventricular fibrillation may not be well differentiated from ventricular tachycardia by ventricular irregularity[4]), the immediate attraction for the algorithm developer is atrial rate.[5,6] It can be expected that rate or some of its close correlates, e.g., amplitude probability density function,[6,7] or "quiet interval",[8] or baseline crossings,[8] will be an important part of many practical algorithms. Classically, atrial rate in AF is defined as greater than 350 bpm and, for atrial flutter, less than 350 bpm. Our group has recorded AF in the presence of class I antiarrhythmic drugs with local atrial rates below 200 bpm,[9] and atrial flutter with rates greater than 400 bpm has been well described.[10] One can argue that mistaking flutter for fibrillation is not a major difficulty, just as early defibrillators treated ventricular tachycardia and ventricular fibrillation (VF) quite successfully with a single therapy. However, many patients now benefit from third generation automatic defibrillators with antitachycardia pacing designed for ventricular tachycardia and high-energy shocks designed for VF. Even in such third generation defibrillators, there may be some opportunities for antitachycardia pacing which are lost because of the inability of any currently available device to detect VF specifically. Given the less immediately threatening nature of atrial arrhythmias, and until shocks can be asymptomatic, there may be an advantage in exploring more specific algorithms so that pacing may be used for rapid, but nonfibrillatory rhythm. There are a number of difficulties with the measurement of atrial rate during AF, some of which are discussed below.

Most of the quintessential features of AF are reflections of its variability in space and time (Fig. 1).[11,12] Many of these provide opportunities for detection algorithms with the potential for increased specificity, although some may be more practical than others given current device and lead technology. Variability in electrogram morphology,[5] local activation direction,[13,14] signal amplitude,[15] and comparison of global versus local activity,[16] magnitude-squared coherence,[17] and frequency content[6] have all been proposed as potential detection algorithms. Whether any of these algorithms provide enough increase in accuracy to justify their difficulties in implementation remains to be seen.

Difficulties with the Atrial Fibrillation Signal

There is a substantial loss in signal amplitude when comparing sinus rhythm with atrial fibrillation.[5] There is, however, a correlation between signal amplitude during sinus rhythm and that during AF at the same recording site in the same patient.[18] In addition, the signal varies greatly in amplitude from moment to moment.[19] Upstroke velocity and electrogram morphology are also variable. There may be considerable variability in the signal at different atrial locations.[19,20]

Because the atria are not being activated coherently, globally recorded signals are very different from local signals.[16] Thus, lead configuration is a determinant of signal characteristics during AF to a much greater degree than for organized rhythms.[21,22] Closely spaced bipoles in contact with the atrial endocardium tend to record discrete electrograms with slower rates, compared with more "fibrillatory" appearing signals at faster apparent "rates" for wider bipoles in the blood pool.

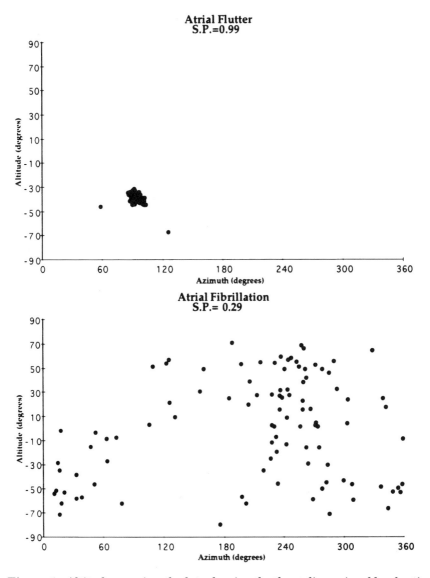

Figure 1. Altitude vs. azimuth plots showing the three-dimensional local activation directions for 100 consecutive activations of atrial flutter (**top**) and AF (**bottom**) in the same patient; each point represents the direction of one activation. The value for spatial precision (S.P.), a dimensionless number ranging from 0 to 1 which quantifies the degree of consistency of a series of direction measurements, is indicated under the rhythm designation. Atrial flutter, which is characterized by regular activation patterns, has high spatial precision, while AF, characterized by irregular activation patterns, has low spatial precision.

Accuracy and Time Considerations

When detecting VF, the strategy has always been to err on the side of sensitivity, since the clinical cost of missing VF is unacceptable. Clearly, if AF detection were ever used to inhibit therapy for a ventricular defibrillator, one would have to be certain that this would not impair this sensitivity to VF. Further, any such detection algorithms could not be allowed to delay VF therapy to any appreciable degree.

For other applications, however, the lack of immediate danger from AF allows a more balanced approach between sensitivity and specificity. A much longer time period in order to accomplish detection might be acceptable. As with any other decision making, Baye's theorem applies, and the pretest likelihood of a true positive result has a great influence on the predictive accuracy of any algorithm. As an example, if a patient has one episode of AF per month, and one has an algorithm which evaluates a 4-second segment of data, then the pretest likelihood of a true positive for AF is approximately 1:600,000. Therefore, even an algorithm with a specificity of 99.5% will still falsely label almost 3,000 segments of sinus rhythm per month as AF. As a consequence, specificity results from a study data set which seem impressive at first glance may be inadequate in practice. A patient who is having a mix of sinus rhythm and AF comparable to most study data used for algorithm development will require some prophylactic antifibrillatory therapy before strategies (e.g., antifibrillatory devices) for dealing with sporadic episodes become clinically appropriate.

Accuracy requirements are also dependent on the relative discomfort and risk of inappropriate therapy. Clearly, an inappropriate shock (at least with present technology) must be avoided more assiduously than inappropriate atrial pacing.

At first glance, sensitivity to AF seems less important than specificity, since this rhythm is not immediately life-threatening. However, for mode-switching applications, it may be that detection immediately after the onset is more desirable since it is the change in rhythm to which patients are often most sensitive. For devices designed to treat AF, there also may or may not be an advantage in more immediate detection. Recent data elegantly show that AF itself changes the electrophysiological milieu to make further episodes of longer duration more likely.[23] The time course of this "electrophysiological remodeling" on a scale of hours to days has been characterized, but the details of this time course on a scale of seconds to a minute or two have not yet been scrutinized. If it should turn out that significant electrophysiological remodeling occurs in the first few seconds or minutes after the onset of AF, it may be that immediate detection and effective therapy will be relatively more desirable, and could conceivably prevent further episodes.

Sources of Test Data

A number of factors must be considered in collecting a database of signals with which proposed algorithms may be developed and tested. First, although a number of animal models have been proposed and signals from such models are qualitatively similar to those recorded during human AF, there are quantitative differences. Furthermore, acetylcholine administration, or other cholinergic interventions are often used in such models. In the presence of acetylcholine, the signal characteristics of AF can change dramatically, both in terms of rate and morphology.[24]

Human AF recordings often consist of induced AF, for example, in patients with Wolff-Parkinson-White syndrome or other substrates for supraventricular tachycardia. Such patients usually have otherwise structurally normal hearts. It is not yet known with certainty whether induced fibrillation is comparable in mechanism or signal characteristics to spontaneous fibrillation.[25] Other databases contain recordings from established (i.e., chronic) AF in patients of varying degrees and etiologies of heart disease. However, signals from the onset of spontaneous AF are not generally available. A variety of transitional rhythms has been described at the onset of spontaneous AF[26,27] and, depending on how rapidly detection is required, it may be that these transitional rhythms, and not established AF, need to be the object of a detection algorithm. Such data may only become available as devices capable of recording electrograms during spontaneous episodes come into initial use. Thus, there may be a "bootstrapping" process for algorithm development, with improvements based on data made available from first generation devices.

In addition to considerations of induced versus spontaneous fibrillation, acute versus chronic fibrillation, and the underlying substrate of organic heart disease, lead systems used to record test data have a substantial influence on signal characteristics (see below). Data recorded from permanently implanted leads are not readily available and this imposes a further limitation on algorithm development.

Leads

Lead configuration is a major determinant of signal characteristics for all rhythms, but much more so for fibrillatory rhythms.[21] Therefore, it is possible that some algorithms may only function well for particular lead systems and not for others. Such considerations as bipolar or unipolar sensing, with endocardial contact or "floating" in the blood pool, can be expected to have considerably more influence on the detection algorithms for fibrillation per se than for detection merely of rapid atrial activity of any mechanism.

Because of the nature of fibrillation[17,25,28] lead systems capable of multisite atrial sensing may have a great advantage.[17,25] Alternatively, the ability to compare local to global activity[16] or to detect changes in local activation direction[13,20,29,30] can greatly advance detection of AF, although these capabilities are probably not necessary for certain applications. The practicality of these more sophisticated algorithms remains to be demonstrated. Whether certain applications will require new and innovative lead designs specifically for the detection of AF remains to be seen.

Summary

In general, simpler algorithms, perhaps those using atrial rate or derivatives of rate for detection, will prove the most practical for many applications. However, it may turn out that, for certain more sophisticated applications, and especially as various components of this technology improve, more sophisticated algorithms that detect quintessential features of AF will be needed. Since it involves careful scrutiny of the signal generated by AF, the study of algorithms provides many opportunities for an improved understanding of the nature of AF. Therefore, the development of such algorithms can be looked at in the context of this broader purpose. Furthermore, as devices for the management of AF come into use, data recorded from these devices about AF in the clinical setting will certainly further our understanding of this important arrhythmia. Finally, since the similarities between both the signal and the mechanism of AF and VF are many, an understanding of the problems involved in detection as well as mechanism translate at least in part from one chamber of the heart to the other.

References

1. Nunain SO, Roelke M, Trouton T, et al. Limitations and late complications of third-generation automatic cardioverter-defibrillators. Circulation 1995; 91:2204–2213.
2. Manz M, Gerckens U, Luderitz B. Erroneous discharge from an implanted

automatic defibrillator during supraventricular tachyarrhythmia induced ventricular fibrillation. Am J Cardiol 1986;57:343.

3. Arzbaecher R, Bump T, Munkenbeck F. An algorithm for automatic infusion of procainamide in acute management of paroxysmal atrial fibrillation. In: Computers in Cardiology Conference. Los Angeles: IEEE Computer Society Press; 1984:57.

4. Ropella KM, Baerman JM, Sahakian AV, et al. Differentiation of ventricular tachyarrhythmias. Circulation 1990;82:2035–2043.

5. Jenkins J, Noh KH, Guezennec A, et al. Diagnosis of atrial fibrillation using electrograms from chronic leads: evaluation of computer algorithms. Pacing Clin Electrophysiol 1988;11:622–631.

6. Slocum J, Sahakian A, Swiryn S. Computer discrimination of atrial fibrillation and regular atrial rhythms from intra-atrial electrograms. Pacing Clin Electrophysiol 1988;11:610–621.

7. Langer A, Heilman M, Mower M. Considerations in the development of the automatic implantable defibrillator. Biomed Inst 1973;10:163–167.

8. Kim J, Bocek J, White H, et al. An atrial fibrillation detection algorithm for an implantable atrial defibrillator. In: Computers in Cardiology Conference. Los Angeles: IEEE Computer Society Press; 1995:48.

9. Ropella KM, Sahakian AV, Baerman JM, et al. Effects of procainamide on intra-atrial electrograms during atrial fibrillation: implications for detection algorithms. Circulation 1988;77:1047–1054.

10. Wells JL, MacLean WA, James TN, et al. Characterization of atrial flutter: studies in man after open heart surgery using fixed atrial electrodes. Circulation 1979;60:665–673.

11. Allessie MA, Lammers WJEP, Bonke FIM, et al. Experimental evaluation of Moe's multiple wavelet hypothesis of atrial fibrillation. In: Zipes DP, Jalife J, eds. Cardiac Electrophysiology and Arrhythmias. Orlando, FL: Grune and Stratton; 1985:265–275.

12. Winfree AT. Electrical turbulence in three-dimensional heart muscle. Science 1994;266:1003–1006.

13. Schoenwald AT, Sahakian AV, Swiryn S. Detecting atrial fibrillation using spatial precision: measuring local activation direction variability using short segment lengths to quickly differentiate fibrillation from regular rhythms. IEEE Engineering Med Biol 1996;15:45–51.

14. Holm M, Blomstrom P, Brandt J, et al. Determination of preferable directions of impulse propagation during atrial fibrillation by time averaging of multiple electrogram vectors. In: Olsson SB, Allessie MA, Campbell RW, eds. Atrial fibrillation: Mechanisms and Therapeutic Strategies. Armonk, NY: Futura Publishing Company; 1994:67–80.

15. Bloem D, Arzbaecher R, Guynn T, et al. Detection of atrial fibrillation via pacemaker threshold scanning. In: Computers in Cardiology Conference. Los Angeles: IEEE Computers Society Press; 1994:69–72.

16. Ropella K, Sahakian A, Baerman J, et al. Coherence estimation from a single intra-cardiac lead with two electrode elements. In: IEEE Engineering in Medicine and Biology Society Conference. IEEE Press; 1990: 586–587.

17. Ropella KM, Sahakian AV, Baerman JM, et al. The coherence spectrum: a quantitative discriminator of fibrillatory and non-fibrillatory cardiac rhythms. Circulation 1989;80:112–119.

18. Wood MA, Moskovljevic P, Stambler BS, et al. Comparison of bipolar atrial electrogram amplitude in sinus rhythm, atrial fibrillation, and atrial flutter. Pacing Clin Electrophysiol 1996;19:150–156.

19. Wells JL, Karp RB, Kouchoukos NT, et al. Characterization of atrial fibrillation in man: studies following open heart surgery. Pacing Clin Electrophysiol 1978;1:426–438.

20. Gerstenfeld EP, Sahakian AV, Swiryn S. Evidence for transient linking of atrial excitation during atrial fibrillation in humans. Circulation 1992;86: 375–382.

21. Baerman JM, Ropella KM, Sahakian AV, et al. Effect of bipole configuration on atrial electrograms during atrial fibrillation. Pacing Clin Electrophysiol 1990;13:78–87.

22. Allessie M, Kirchhof C, Scheffer GJ, et al. Regional control of atrial fibrillation by rapid pacing in conscious dogs. Circulation 1991;84:1689–1697.

23. Wijffels MC, Kirchhof CJ, Dorland R, et al. Atrial fibrillation begets atrial fibrillation: a study in awake chronically instrumented goats. Circulation 1995;92:1954–1968.

24. Sih H, Sahakian A, Arentzen C, et al. Epicardial maps of very short wavelength, acetylcholine modulated, swine atrial fibrillation. Pacing Clin Electrophysiol 1995;18:804. Abstract.

25. Botteron GW, Smith JM. Quantitative assessment of the spatial organization of atrial fibrillation in the intact human heart. Circulation 1996;93: 513–518.

26. Pagé PL, Hassanalizadeh H, Cardinal R. Transitions among atrial fibrillation, atrial flutter, and sinus rhythm during procainamide infusion and vagal stimulation in dogs with sterile pericarditis. Can J Physiol Pharmacol 1991;69:15–24.

27. Killip T, Gault JH. Mode of onset of atrial fibrillation in man. Am Heart J 1965;70:172–179.

28. Konings KTS, Kirchhof CJHJ, Smeets JRLM, et al. High-density mapping of electrically induced atrial fibrillation in humans. Circulation 1994;89: 1665–1680.

29. Goldreyer BN, Olive AL, Leslie J, et al. A new orthogonal lead for P synchronous pacing. PACE 1981;4:638–644.

30. Gerstenfeld EP, Sahakian AV, Baerman JM, et al. Detection of changes in atrial endocardial activation with use of an orthogonal catheter. J Am Coll Cardiol 1991;18:1034–1042.

CHAPTER 22

What Can Pacemakers Tell Us About Atrial Fibrillation?

Philippe Ritter, Stéphane Garrigue, Serge Cazeau, Arnaud Lazarus, Daniel Gras, Jacques Mugica

In the late 1970s, investigators involved in cardiac pacing reported memory functions that could provide information about the occurrence of various events such as arrhythmias.[1-3] A decade later, a limited amount of stored data was available in a small number of pacemakers, and the recognition of atrial tachyarrhythmias (AT) was beginning to be seriously addressed.[4-11] Today, the most recent generations of dual chamber pacemakers are of definite value in identifying AT.[12] Apart from event counting, data on AT episodes are stored in the RAM memory of the pacemaker, and then retrieved by telemetry and displayed on the programmer screen. These diagnostic functions are useful tools for improved determination of the real incidence of AT in the paced population.

The conditions that allow the diagnosis of AT by the pacing system include the following: high sensitivity with short refractory periods in the atrial channel; a large random access memory (RAM) capacity with reliable data storage; and reliable analysis with comprehensible presentation of Holter data.

Atrial Sensing

Adequate atrial sensitivity is the primary condition, without which a diagnosis cannot be made. Several physiological and pathological situations can greatly influence the atrial signal amplitude (e.g., respiration, eating, exercise, arrhythmia). Eighty-three consecutive patients who had been implanted with a DDDR pacemaker 2 months previously

From *Nonpharmacological Management of Atrial Fibrillation*, edited by F.D. Murgatroyd and A.J. Camm. © 1997, Futura Publishing Co., Inc., Armonk, NY.

were asked to exercise on a treadmill after a programming session performed at rest, with an atrial sensing safety margin above 100%. Thirty-eight percent of patients experienced atrial sensing deficiencies at maximal exercise (unpublished data). These were solved by reprogramming the atrial sensitivity setting at its minimum value, in all but two patients. Therefore, it is our practice to routinely program the maximum sensitivity available. An additional reason for proposing this principle is the reduction of atrial signal amplitude during ATs (especially AF). In order to avoid or minimize the risk of far-field potentials, we systematically use the bipolar sensing configuration. These rules could be applied to VDD pacing systems. Some reports show similar reliability of atrial sensing during sinus rhythm with VDD systems. However, during ATs it is our experience that atrial sensing is more frequently ineffective with VDD pacemakers as compared to DDD systems (even if atrial sensitivity is set higher in the former), thus compromising arrhythmia diagnosis.

Programming a short atrial refractory period allows detection of fast atrial rates. In older pacemaker generations, the atrial sensing window is equal to ventricular cycle length minus total atrial refractory period (TARP); TARP is equal to atrioventricular (AV) delay plus postventricular atrial refractory period (PVARP).[13] Consequently, ATs can be sensed only when these two parameters are programmed short. Atrial sensing can even be compromised during DDDR pacing as the AV delay applied on paced P waves may be extended (to allow for the relative delay in atrial conduction compared with sensed P waves). Additionally, the AV delay programmed in patients with spontaneous AV conduction is frequently long in order to allow normal ventricular activation where possible and save energy.[14,15] Thus, the only option that is left (to achieve the objective of a short TARP to optimize atrial sensing) is to program a very short PVARP. However, the problem of protection against endless loop tachycardia (pacemaker-mediated tachycardia) related to retrograde conduction then arises. This is well managed with algorithms analyzing the stability of retrograde conduction (ELA Medical, Le Plessis Robinson, France; Diamond, Vitatron Medical, Dieren, The Netherlands; Medico, Rubceno, Italy).[16] With other models the principle of a short PVARP cannot be used.

Manufacturers therefore developed pacemakers that were able to sense atrial signals within refractory periods for diagnostic purposes. The aim of AT recognition is the triggering of mode switching. The purpose of this function is to prevent the "runaway" ventricular rate that occurs when the pacemaker attempts to track an AT. In fact, the diagnostic functions of pacemakers are closely related to their mode-switching ability.

To shorten the absolute atrial refractory period, manufacturers divide the PVARP into two parts. The first part is an absolute PVARP, the so-called "atrial blanking period", which has a duration of 100–150 ms. The second part of the PVARP is a relative refractory period. A P wave that falls within this period does not initiate an AV delay and ventricular spike. In other words, P waves falling within this part of the PVARP are not associated with the ventricles: this period is used for diagnostic purposes only, and extends the atrial sensing window considerably. Furthermore, some pacemakers allow atrial sensing after a first period of blanking during AV delay (different from the ventricular blanking of paced P waves). However, this can give rise to problems with far-field detection, and consequent mode-switching. In other words, the pacemaker senses twice the actual sinus rate and establishes the erroneous diagnosis of AT. Then the pacemaker activates the function intended to avoid runaway ventricular pacing, i.e., DDIR or VDIR mode (mode-switching).[17-19] The only manufacturer that has attempted to prevent this specific problem is Vitatron; their device forces the automatic extension of atrial blanking when the pacemaker repeatedly senses an event, just after atrial blanking, that might be a far-field potential (the so-called "atrial refractory period after ventricular pacing"). Alternatively, crosstalk can be eliminated by the extension of the duration of atrial blanking in devices that have this capability, or by diminishing the atrial sensitivity (although the latter will decrease the ability of the pacemaker to sense ATs). Consequently, all fast atrial rhythms can be detected and induce mode switching. The AT episodes can then be stored in the RAM of the pacemaker.

RAM Capabilities and Data Storage

The precision and quantity of information stored by a pacemaker depend on its RAM capacity. Consequently, some pacemakers provide only a duration of pathological atrial rates, but it is not possible to discriminate between frequent premature atrial complexes (PACs) and sustained AT. Other devices can store a single atrial rate histogram that provides cumulative data between two visits. Again, one can see that a great number of short atrial cycles has occurred, without being able to differentiate between frequent PACs and sustained AT.

Today, two series of pacemakers can provide detailed, reliable, and chronologically labeled information on ATs (the ELA Chorus® series, ELA Medical, Le Plessis Robinson, France; and the Medtronic Thera® series, Medtronic, Inc., Minneapolis, MN, USA). With the Medtronic devices, the Holter function can be programmed to one of two settings.

If rate histograms are selected, the information is cumulative and the detail in the stored data is low. If mode-switching storage is selected, the information relating to ATs becomes much more interesting. The stored data depend on the reliability of the mode-switching function. When mode switching has occurred, the date and timing of occurrence are displayed and a zoom function allows retrieval of an atrial timing diagram that shows the onset and termination of episodes. A short atrial electrogram is also shown for one of the episodes.

The ELA system has existed since 1988. Three different sets of histograms are available. Each can be assigned to one type of event (atrial intervals, ventricular intervals, AV intervals, ventricular premature complexes, etc.). These events are classified according to their intervals, and distributed accordingly into eight successive bins with programmable boundaries. The data are stored over programmable periods of time (15 minutes to 6 months) in successive tables. This makes the mixing of data between two successive periods of time impossible. One histogram represents all successive stored tables[20] for one type of event. It is possible to assign the three histograms to the same family of events, e.g. atrial intervals. These histograms will only differ by the programmed period of time, e.g., 1 hour, 1 day, and 1 week (Tables 1–4).

Table 1

Statistics

Date of last reset:		5/30/1995
V paced	357071	14%
V sensed	2115902	86%
PVCs	113	
Safety pacing	2	
A paced	7023	
A sensed	403839	16%
PACs	2912	
Programmations	0	
Cardiac cycles	2472973	
ELTs	0	
Fallback	255	
Time in fallback	56360100	ms
Wenckebach	35	
Minimum PP interval	109	

This table shows the statistics retrieved from the pacemaker. The number of fallback operations (Mode switching) is 255. The patient was asymptomatic. The atrial rhythm responsible for at least one of those fallback operations was probably atrial fibrillation because the minimal PP interval was measured at 109 ms (Chorum® RM).

Table 2

Histogram Summary Table
A Int Duration = 3 Hours

Range (ms)	<203	≥203 <313	≥313 <422	≥422 <500	≥500 <641	≥641 <781	≥781 <922	≥922
min-1	>295	≤295 >192	≤192 >142	≤142 >120	≤120 >94	≤94 >77	≤77 >65	≤65
1	0	0	0	0	1	14399	0	0
2	0	0	0	0	1	14399	0	0
3	0	0	0	0	0	14400	0	0
4	0	0	0	0	0	14400	0	0
5	0	0	0	0	3	14397	0	0
6	0	0	0	0	0	14420	0	2
7	1	0	0	0	0	14386	0	7
8	4	3	0	0	0	14362	0	19
9	1	1	0	0	0	14378	0	11
10	0	0	0	1	1	14386	0	6
11	0	0	0	0	0	14384	0	8
12	0	0	0	0	0	14394	0	3
13	0	0	0	0	1	14385	0	7
14	0	1	0	1	2	14368	1	26
15	1	1	1	1	0	14384	1	7
16	0	2	1	2	3	14419	3	10
17	0	2	0	0	1	14395	0	2
18	0	0	0	0	0	14400	0	0
19	3	3	0	0	1	14377	0	11
20	1	1	0	0	3	14396	1	12
21	1	0	8	2	8	14569	6	26
22	3938	1269	2792	307	18	11675	6	24
23	22620	6263	13724	1274	86	15	0	1
24	21409	6829	13444	1310	197	42	9	5
25	15178	9442	10410	1910	1387	466	150	139
26	13872	9650	9852	1887	1706	606	209	186
27	11105	8162	8706	1770	2107	1071	430	659
28	17368	7330	13126	1705	637	186	44	21
29	18645	7205	13592	1564	290	95	20	5
30	14562	10455	11497	2538	492	129	54	68

The columns define the ranges of atrial (A) intervals stored on a 3-hour basis. Thirty sets of 3-hour duration each are stored. The patient obviously had an atrial tachyarrhythmia from row 22 to row 30. The patient was then paced at the programmed basic rate.

Table 3

Histogram Summary Table
V Int Duration = 3 Hours

Range (ms)	<281	≥281 <359	≥359 <422	≥422 <500	≥500 <641	≥641 <781	≥781 <922	≥922
min-1	>213	≤213 >167	≤167 >142	≤142 >120	≤120 >94	≤94 >77	≤77 >65	≤65
1	0	0	0	1	4	14386	9	0
2	0	0	0	0	3	14393	4	0
3	0	0	0	0	0	14397	3	0
4	0	0	0	0	2	14393	5	0
5	0	0	0	1	5	14388	6	0
6	0	0	0	0	5	14386	8	1
7	0	0	0	0	10	14381	9	0
8	0	0	0	0	29	14368	27	0
9	0	0	0	0	18	14366	16	0
10	0	0	0	0	15	14371	14	0
11	0	0	0	0	12	14376	12	0
12	0	0	0	0	3	14390	7	0
13	0	0	0	0	9	14380	11	0
14	0	0	0	1	35	14355	33	0
15	1	0	0	1	9	14370	19	0
16	0	0	0	2	24	14394	28	0
17	0	0	0	0	7	14380	13	0
18	0	0	0	0	1	14396	3	0
19	0	0	0	0	19	14359	22	0
20	0	0	0	4	21	14352	23	0
21	2	1	2	19	29	14523	88	0
22	1	184	1037	1399	1578	11829	124	0
23	0	470	4073	6142	8758	2010	99	0
24	0	552	3744	5843	8486	2402	212	1
25	4	61	2511	4666	8556	3647	475	0
26	6	77	2461	4455	8446	3889	461	5
27	13	140	3074	5013	8483	3379	297	1
28	2	969	5071	7344	7727	1361	62	0
29	1	997	5382	7071	7744	1340	49	0
30	1	329	4600	6257	8594	1818	121	0

The ventricular (V) intervals table, corresponding to the atrial (A) intervals table shown in Table 2, shows similar data. The patient was not dependent on the pacemaker and AV conduction was still present during fallback operation. However, the number of very short V cycles is much lower than for the atrium in the rows corresponding to fallback operation.

Table 4

Histogram Summary Table
A Int Duration = 2 Days

Range (ms)	<203	≥203 <313	≥313 <422	≥422 <500	≥500 <641	≥641 <781	≥781 <922	≥922
min-1	>295	≤295 >192	≤192 >142	≤142 >120	≤120 >94	≤94 >77	≤77 >65	≤65
1	124126	56154	85647	11733	6446	129480	880	1134
2	177082	130611	146850	33221	19492	18575	5482	11475
3	63	28357	122	27585	111997	129840	46	84
4	0	87151	1	53067	238268	3	0	0
5	0	260121	0	2839	189455	0	1	0
6	0	310178	5	2	156770	0	0	0
7	0	221236	0	0	203365	0	0	0
8	0	66424	1	1110	282304	4	2398	2
9	0	9871	0	38765	292157	2	0	0
10	0	150697	104	7140	241444	2	3	0
11	0	363321	2307	1	123399	0	1	5
12	0	272350	321	1	179193	0	30	12
13	0	103644	1	2762	278422	0	0	0
14	0	40770	1	207021	127095	0	1	2

A intervals recording on a 2-day basis. There are two distinct periods. From row 4 to row 14, the probability for an atrial flutter is high because A cycles were recorded mostly in two different rate ranges. From row 1 to row 3, the probability for atrial fibrillation is high because A intervals are distributed all over the rate ranges.

During follow-up, the interrogation of the Holter memories through the telemetry provides all atrial events sorted among the programmed bins that occurred during the last 30 hours in the first histogram, during the last 15 days in the second, and during the last 14 weeks in the third.

Data Analysis and Presentation

We conducted a series of studies to analyze the value of pacemaker internal Holter data regarding atrial tachyarrhythmias.[20-23]

As a first step, we assessed the reliability of this internal Holter function in comparison with the current "gold standard": surface ECG Holter monitoring over short periods of time.[20] Six patients (mean age 57 ± 2 years) who were implanted for complete AV block with a DDD pacemaker (Chorus model 6234) were asked to perform three or four exercise tests separated by a 10-minute rest period; the tests involved repeated step-ups. The overall duration of each procedure was 15 minutes. For a given patient, the internal Holter histograms were programmed according to basic rate, upper rate limit, and refractory periods. Successive tables were stored every 15 minutes. Atrial and ventricular events were recorded. The surface ECG was simultaneously recorded on a Holter tape. At the end of each 15-minute period, pacemaker statistics were printed out. At the end of the protocol, internal Holter histograms were printed and the Holter tape was analyzed (ELATEC® analyzer, ELA Medical). Artifacts and erroneous ventricular events on the automated analysis of the surface Holter recordings were excluded by a beat-by-beat manual analysis. Then, for each 15-minute period, ventricular events were ranked according to the internal Holter histogram channel boundaries in order to make the comparisons possible between surface Holter and internal Holter histograms. One hundred seventy-six ventricular surface Holter and internal Holter histograms were gathered in 22 tests (two patients exercised three times, and four patients four times each) and were highly correlated (R = 0.97, P<0.0001). Rate profiles of the histograms provided by the surface Holter and the corresponding internal Holter were similar.

Sinus rhythm and AT are diagnosed according to the initial prematurity of the first atrial event of the tachycardia. Three or four tests were performed by each patient in order to trigger mode-switching and to analyze the typical profiles of internal Holter in patients with complete AV block during mode-switched operation. In the short intervals range, the number of atrial events exceeds the number of ventricular events. In the long intervals range, the number of atrial events is less than the number of ventricular events. Mode switching is counted in the pacemaker statistics.

The presence of mode switching in the statistics of the device may facilitate AT assessment, but it is not a necessary and sufficient condition. The diagnosis of AT requires the combination of different criteria extracted from the Holter tables[21]: (1) in all cases, a great number of short atrial intervals recorded in the atrial table, with bipolar sensing to exclude artifacts or myopotentials; (2) in the presence of AV block, ventricular intervals stored between basic rate and upper rate limit or fallback rate; (3) in the absence of AV block, ventricular intervals stored between basic rate and the AV node refractory period; (4) in cases of mode switching (VVI functioning), no memorized AV intervals; and (5) in the absence of mode switching, a great variability of AV intervals (Wenckebach functioning).

In accordance with these findings, we evaluated the internal Holter criteria found during investigation for the diagnosis of AF. In ten patients, surface Holter recording was made in patients having AT after implantation of the Chorus 6234 model. AT diagnosis was made with the internal Holter and verified with the surface Holter. Not one diagnostic error was made during this second study.

These principles were then applied to determine the incidence of AT in our paced population (Tables 5–8).[22] Of the 2,050 patients implanted at our center during the 40 months of the study, 262 were implanted with the Chorus series models. Two-hundred thirteen patients (aged 70 ± 13 years, 62% female) were followed for 361 ± 281 days (3 to 1,020). Forty patients were totally or partially lost during follow-up and nine died of noncardiac causes. The indications for pacemaker implantation were typical of our overall pacemaker population: permanent high degree AV block (30%), trifascicular block with long HV interval (21%), brady-tachy syndrome (21%), sinus node dysfunction (10%), carotid sinus syndrome (6%), other indications (12%). Clinical, echocardiographic, and electrophysiological data were recorded as well as pacing parameters.

Twenty-eight percent of patients had a history of AT before implan-

Table 5

Statistics

Date of last reset:		3/24/1994
V paced	5817431	96%
V sensed	216144	4%
PVCs	13868	
Safety pacing	25	
A paced	50184	1%
A sensed	5840046	97%
PACs	868	
Programmations	18	
Cardiac cycles	6033578	
ELTs	0	
Fallback	5	
Time in fallback	51498520	ms
Wenckebach	38	
Minimum PP interval	109	

Five fallback operations occurred since last follow-up.

Table 6

Histogram Summary Table
A Int Duration = 3 Hours

Range (ms)	<203	≥203 <266	≥266 <328	≥328 <391	≥391 <500	≥500 <688	≥688 <859	≥859
min-1	>295	≤295 >226	≤226 >183	≤183 >154	≤154 >120	≤120 >87	≤87 >70	≤70
1	0	0	0	0	3	1990	12474	194
2	0	0	1	0	0	152	11909	1161
3	0	0	0	0	0	8	12829	362
4	4203	1512	1243	3247	2654	1158	8332	93
5	14956	2302	5327	9224	4029	1699	321	160
6	15135	1878	4291	10629	3594	1483	350	253
7	11484	1894	3451	8066	3247	2211	2348	185
8	0	0	0	0	3	6858	8610	79
9	0	0	0	0	1	4259	8938	1704
10	0	0	0	1	1	159	4131	8236
11	0	0	0	0	0	10	11668	1617
12	0	0	0	0	1	57	13335	334
13	0	0	0	0	0	1161	12744	153
14	0	0	0	0	2	3357	9758	1348
15	0	0	0	1	1	322	11009	2296
16	0	0	0	1	0	84	11660	1833
17	0	0	0	2	3	4284	10834	157
18	0	0	0	0	1	15	4133	8402
19	0	0	0	0	2	4	9961	3185
20	0	0	0	0	1	30	12918	609
21	0	0	0	0	0	581	12208	1056
22	0	0	0	0	1	1312	8712	3665
23	0	0	0	0	0	1969	8847	3167
24	0	0	0	0	0	2251	10077	1879
25	0	0	1	1	1	1624	12898	138
26	0	0	0	0	0	122	11195	2123
27	0	0	0	0	0	49	14128	6
28	0	10	7	1	5	1749	12677	6
29	0	0	0	3	7	2034	12705	102
30	0	0	0	0	2	743	13247	216

A intervals table recorded on a 3-hour basis. The patient had an atrial arrhythmia (rows 4–7).

Table 7

Histogram Summary Table
V Int duration = 3 Hours

Range (ms)	<250	≥250 <297	≥297 <344	≥344 <391	≥391 <500	≥500 <688	≥688 <859	≥859
min-1	>240	≤240 >202	≤202 >175	≤175 >154	≤154 >120	≤120 >87	≤87 >70	≤70
1	0	0	0	1	5	1997	12451	210
2	0	0	0	0	2	154	11913	1155
3	0	0	0	0	2	11	12848	339
4	0	4	24	75	7006	2582	8374	31
5	9	112	552	1105	19124	4099	146	5
6	13	223	1058	1870	19389	3181	110	4
7	17	275	1161	1931	15153	3330	2103	6
8	0	0	0	0	10	6835	8633	74
9	0	0	0	0	6	4246	8952	1700
10	0	0	0	0	3	159	4139	8227
11	0	0	0	0	1	12	11653	1630
12	0	0	0	1	8	53	13356	310
13	0	0	0	0	5	1176	12728	155
14	0	0	0	3	13	3349	9758	1349
15	0	0	0	1	5	316	11033	2277
16	0	0	0	1	6	75	11688	1814
17	0	0	1	3	9	4293	10820	162
18	0	0	0	0	1	17	4072	8438
19	0	0	0	0	2	9	9973	3192
20	0	0	0	0	1	35	12906	618
21	0	0	0	0	6	568	12239	1035
22	0	0	0	0	12	1287	8798	3607
23	0	0	0	0	5	1942	8896	3149
24	0	0	0	0	1	2215	10082	1886
25	0	0	1	1	3	1650	12897	136
26	0	0	0	0	0	123	11172	2145
27	0	0	0	0	0	48	14130	6
28	0	0	0	1	10	1766	12660	11
29	0	0	5	4	3	2020	12687	113
30	0	0	0	1	4	763	13229	211

The V intervals table was recorded during the same period of observation as the A intervals table shown in Table 6.

Table 8

Histogram Summary Table
A Int Duration = 2 Days

Range (ms)	<234	≥234 <375	≥375 <500	≥500 <609	≥609 <719	≥719 <828	≥828 <922	≥922
min-1	>256	≤256 >160	≤160 >120	≤120 >98	≤98 >83	≤83 >72	≤72 >65	≤65
1	0	1	5	1306	39693	88930	79696	8575
2	0	2	12	70	12238	94960	71106	30938
3	0	3	11	1885	37227	110853	52940	16085
4	0	4	6	1412	34528	61656	74891	38284
5	0	0	10	2372	44795	74157	53099	40239
6	0	1	8	2274	46465	67030	71112	28835
7	23428	9530	12065	5358	51574	76393	55773	16498
8	1	4	16	2607	33512	66283	70133	38816
9	0	3	18	2294	42924	90545	69622	13304
10	0	1	12	1488	36544	95939	70540	13384
11	0	4	19	1071	46531	61226	81092	24633
12	0	0	16	5343	74266	83765	59043	5343
13	0	1	15	2781	51539	64869	77478	21246
14	39197	20578	17051	20960	63325	63485	46240	9687

A intervals recorded on a 2-day basis. The patient had two more episodes one month and 14 days before interrogation.

tation. Forty-eight and one-half percent of patients experienced AT during follow-up. AT duration was less than 24 hours and largely asymptomatic in 31.1% of the patients (81.5% of the episodes); AT duration was less than 8 days in 10.3% of patients; a permanent arrhythmia occurred in only 7%, and always followed a period of paroxysmal episodes. Forty-three percent of patients without AT prior to implantation presented at least one episode after 207 ± 203 days of follow-up. In patients with a history of AT prior to implantation, the disorder recurred more often (62%, P = ns) and much earlier (127 ± 113 days, $P<0.01$).

Multivariate analysis identified the presence of AV block ($P<0.02$), frequent atrial premature beats (P = 0.004), and male gender (P = 0.008) as independent risk factors for atrial arrhythmias after pacing. Implantation for trifascicular block was independently associated with a lower incidence (P = 0.008) of AT. Age, the existence of structural heart disease, atrial size, ejection fraction, pacing and sensing thresholds, and antiarrhythmic drug therapy were not predictive factors in this population.

In a subgroup of 65 patients (aged 73 ± 10 years, 48% female, 52% male) presenting with a documented brady-tachy syndrome (BTS) (70% of this subgroup) or isolated sinus node disease (SND) without a history of AT (30%), the mean follow-up was 389 ± 284 days. Sixty percent of this group, 10 SND and 29 BTS, (*P* = ns) experienced AT recorded after 310 ± 296 and 174 ± 170 days (*P* = ns), respectively. The incidence of AT episodes was inversely related to the proportion of atrial pacing (as opposed to spontaneous atrial rhythm), (*P* = 0.01). Unlike in the general population, age, the existence of structural heart disease, atrial size (47 ± 12 mm), ejection fraction (65 ± 10%), pacing and sensing thresholds, and the presence or absence of antiarrhythmic drugs were not predictive factors for AT occurrence during follow-up, but hypertension was an independent risk factor (*P*<0.03). Fifteen percent of patients (5 sinus node disease and 5 BTS) presented with nonsignificant AT, requiring no treatment. At 334 ± 191 days of follow-up, 15% (9 BTS and 1 SND) presented with symptomatic prolonged AT. The nine BTS patients had 2 ± 0.5 episodes lasting more than 7 days, and 4.6 ± 2.3 episodes lasting less than 7 days. The patient with SND had 16 short and one prolonged episode of AT. The difference between the number of prolonged episodes is significant (*P*<0.05). Five percent of patients presented with chronic AT after 360 ± 142 days.

The long-term information obtained from the pacemaker memory paints a very different picture from previous studies based on surface Holter monitoring. The discrepancy is probably explained by increased sensitivity compared to the traditional evaluation as well as the continuous acquisition of data, and it modifies our perception of the natural history of AT in the population of patients with DDD pacing systems. Despite the absence of morphological information on electrograms, the superiority of this method is obvious as compared to surface Holter in the long term. It was interesting to note that atrial pacing was associated with relatively infrequent AT episodes, but that antiarrhythmic drug therapy was not. The overall high prevalence of AT during follow-up in DDD pacing, even among patients without a history of atrial arrhythmias, indicates the importance of effective mode switching in all DDD pacemakers.

Finally, we analyzed the incidence of AT in a prospective study on a selected population of patients with SND or BTS.[23] Twenty-one patients, 10 male and 11 female aged 68 ± 14 years, were all implanted for sinus node disease (17 with documented AT prior to implantation) with a pacemaker providing internal Holter. Follow-up was based on documentation of symptoms, ECG, 24-hour surface Holter, and pacemaker interrogation at 6 weeks, and 4, 8, 12, 16, and 20 months. At every follow-up visit, pacemaker operation was checked and the statistics were reset. During follow-up, (14.2 ± 6.1 months), six patients (mean follow-up, 6.2 ± 5.5 months) did not present any AT: they had no symptoms, complication, or occurrence of AT in the surface or internal Holter. Fifteen had AT diagnosed in the surface or internal Holter (mean follow-up, 14.2 ± 6.1 months). The mean delay of an occurrence was 6.8 ± 5.5 months. In 5 of the 15 patients, AT was diagnosed only by the internal Holter. Two other patients had AT episodes revealed by the internal Holter before the diagnosis was made with the surface Holter (4 months vs. 12 months and 6 weeks vs. 4 months). In conclusion, the incidence with which AT was detected was 75.4% (15/21) with the internal Holter, versus 47.6% (10/21) with the classical criteria for AT diagnosis (history and surface Holter).

Today, data memorized in the RAM program of the device can be relied upon with even more confidence. Due to an improvement in the algorithm that regulates mode switching during AT, the pacemaker remains in VDIR mode as long as AT is sustained. In the past, because of intermittent atrial sensing dropout and consequent multiple mode switches during a single episode, a pacemaker could mistakenly count several episodes of AT. The most recent generation of pacemakers takes into account the possibility of intermittent atrial sensing. This behavior explains the capability of the pacemaker to remain in mode switching for a long period of time, although it is likely that the pacemaker cannot detect all atrial events during AT, and multiple arrhythmic episodes separated by only a beat or so of sinus rhythm may be counted as one episode. Event marker chains provide another tool that allows the verification of the stored information.

Nineteen patients (aged 63 ± 17 years, 9 females, 10 males) were implanted with the Chorum® device (ELA Medical) for AV block (n = 6) or sinus node disease (n = 13) (unpublished data). A comparison was made between internal Holter data and surface Holter recording, prior to hospital discharge. At 1 month, 12 patients underwent an exercise test. Before discharge, five patients had one AT episode that was properly recognized by the pacemaker with appropriate triggering of mode switching. At 1 month follow-up, internal Holter showed mode switching in six patients (Figs. 1 and 2). No mode switching was induced during exercise.

In the near future, because of the availability of stored atrial electrograms in addition to atrial event histograms at the moment of diagnosis, the gold standard technique to assess the efficacy of antiarrhythmic therapies may well become telemetric data stored by implanted devices rather than surface ambulatory monitoring. We have already learned that the incidence of atrial tachyarrhythmia in paced patients is much higher than previously expected. It also appears that antiarrhythmic therapy has limited efficacy for atrial tachyarrhythmias. This information will reinforce the development of the antiarrhythmic prevention function of the pacemaker itself (e.g., atrial resynchronization, overdriving, or algorithms avoiding postextrasystolic pauses). The same tools can then be used to evaluate the benefit or adverse consequences of these new treatment concepts.

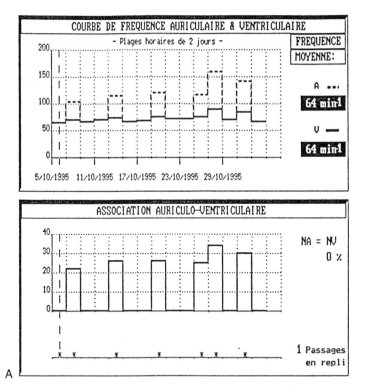

Figure 1. A. The upper panel shows the mean atrial (dotted line) and ventricular (black line) curves recorded during the last month before interrogation. Mean atrial rate is intermittently higher than the mean ventricular rate suggesting the occurrence of AT. The lower panel confirms that several episodes of AV dyssynchrony occurred. On the bottom line, stars indicate that an event marker chain has been recorded.

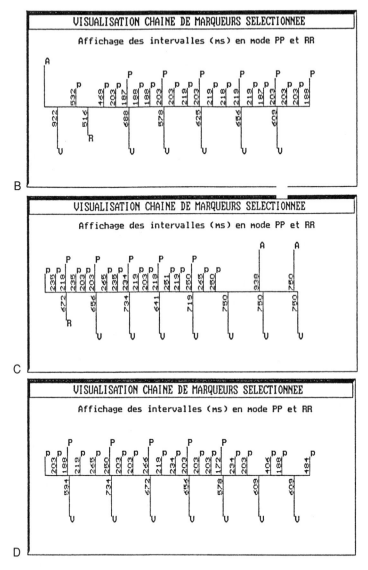

Figure 1. B. This event marker chain was recorded on October 19, 1995 at 7: 14 p.m. and shows the onset of an AT episode. The AV association is of the 3: 1 type. **C.** A few seconds later, the termination of AT is also shown. The pacemaker did not trigger the mode switching because the episode was not sustained. **D.** One minute later, AT resumes and is sustained, triggering the mode switching.

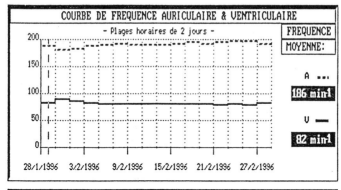

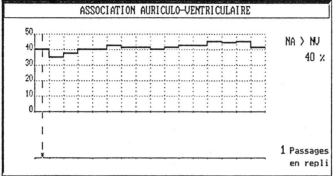

Figure 2. The diagrams show the persistence of a high atrial rate (**upper panel**, dotted line) throughout the follow-up period (1 month) and a permanent AV dissynchrony (**lower panel**). Only one fallback operation was triggered at the moment of the first pacemaker programming just after implantation.

References

1. Edhag O, Vallin H. An implantable bradycardia indicating pacer. 1st European Symposium on Cardiac Pacing. London, May 1978.
2. Attuel P, Mugica J, Buffet J. The diagnostic pacemaker. 1st European Symposium on Cardiac Pacing. London, May 1978.
3. Ripart A, Jacobson P. Memory technology and implantable Holter systems. In: Barold S, Mugica J, eds. The Third Decade of Cardiac Pacing. Mount Kisco, NY: Futura Publishing Co; 1982:353–364.
4. Mugica J, Coumel P, Attuel P. Holter implantable, concept de stimulation cardiaque avec fonction Holter incorporée. Arguments cliniques. In: Mugica J, ed. Cardiostim 80-SEPFI, Paris, 1981:23–30.
5. Ripart A, Jacobson P, Dalmolin R. Clinical value of a microcomputer in an implantable pacemaker. In: Quetglas GM, et al., eds. The Applications of

Computers in Cardiology. Amsterdam: Elsevier Science Publishers; 1984: 57.

6. Levine PA. Holter and pacemaker diagnostics. In: Aubert AE, Ector H, Stroobandt R, eds. Cardiac Pacing and Electrophysiology. Dordrecht, The Netherlands: Kluwer Academic Publishers; 1994:309–324.

7. Berkhof MMJ, Snoek JP, Goethals MPN, et al. Clinical relevance of histograms in the follow-up of DDDR pacemakers. In: Aubert AE, Ector H, Stroobandt R, eds. Cardiac Pacing and Electrophysiology. Dordrecht, The Netherlands: Kluwer Academic Publishers; 1994:325–331.

8. Ripart A. Holter and telemetry in pacemakers and ICDs: new developments. In: Aubert AE, Ector H, Stroobandt R, eds. Cardiac Pacing and Electrophysiology. Dordecht, The Netherlands: Kluwer Academic Publishers; 1994:333–346.

9. Sanders R, Martin R, Frumin H, et al. Data storage and retrieval by implantable pacemakers for diagnostic purposes. PACE 1984;7:1228–1233.

10. Hayes DL, Higano ST. Utility of rate histograms in programming and follow-up of a DDDR pacemaker. Mayo Clin Proc 1989;64:495–502.

11. Lascault G, Frank R, Barnay C, et al. Clinical usefulness of a "diagnostic" dual chamber pacemaker PACE 1993;16:918A.

12. Cazeau S, Ritter P, Limousin M, et al. What is the reliability of the Holter function of a new DDD pacemaker compared to the gold standard surface ECG Holter recording? PACE 1993;16:931A.

13. Lau CP. The follow-up of dual chamber rate-adaptive pacemakers. In: Barold SS, Mugica J, eds. New Perspectives in Cardiac Pacing. Mount Kisco, NY: Futura Publishing Co; 1993:425–455.

14. Rosenqvist M, Isaaz K, Botvinik EH, et al. Relative importance of activation sequence compared to atrioventricular synchrony in left ventricular function. Am J Cardiol 1991;67:148–156.

15. Harper GR, Pina IL, Kutalek SP. Intrinsic conduction maximizes cardiopulmonary performances in patients with dual chamber pacemakers. PACE 1991;14:1787–1791.

16. Girodo S, Limousin M, Ritter P, et al. New algorithm for prevention and termination of pacemaker endless-loop tachycardia. In: Barold SS, Mugica J, eds. New Perspectives in Cardiac Pacing. Mount Kisco, NY: Futura Publishing Co; 1988:405.

17. Barold SS. Automatic mode switching during antibradycardia pacing in patients without supraventricular tachyarrhythmias. In: Barold SS, Mugica J, eds. New Perspectives in Cardiac Pacing. Mount Kisco, NY: Futura Publishing Co; 1993:455–481.

18. Ritter P, Cazeau S, Kojoukharov Y, et al. Critical analysis of the different algorithms designed to protect the paced patient against atrial tachyarrhythmias in dual chamber pacing. In: Aubert AE, Ector H, Stroobandt R, eds. Cardiac Pacing and Electrophysiology. Dordrecht, The Netherlands: Kluwer Academic Publishers; 1994:355–362.

19. Sutton R. Mode switching in DDDR pacing. In: Aubert AE, Ector H, Stroobandt R, eds. Cardiac Pacing and Electrophysiology. Dordrecht, The Netherlands: Kluwer Academic Publishers; 1994:363–370.

20. Ritter P, Henry L, Cazeau S, et al. Reliability of the implantable Holter function of a new DDD pacemaker. Eur JCPE 1992;2(suppl 1A):A23. Abstract.

21. Cazeau S, Ritter P, Nitzsché R, et al. Diagnosis of atrial arrhythmia using the Holter function of a new DDD pacemaker. PACE 1994;17(Part II): 2106–2114.
22. Cazeau S, Garrigue S, Ritter P, et al. Atrial arrhythmias in DDD pacing: a continuous prospective evaluation. Eur JCPE 1996;6(suppl 5):46. Abstract.
23. Ritter P. The 24-hour Holter is not the gold standard technique to assess the efficacy of antiarrhythmic therapies in the brady-tachy syndrome. Eur JCPE 1995;6(suppl 5):208. Abstract.

CHAPTER 23

Prevention of Atrial Fibrillation with Single and Multisite Atrial Pacing

Sanjeev Saksena, Atul Prakash, Ryszard B. Krol,
Anand N. Munsif, Irakli Giorgberidze, Philip Mathew,
Raj R. Kaushik

Introduction

From a description of "Delirium Cordis":

"I cannot therefore see that extra-systoles are the cause of this irregular pulse, and believe that, until we acquire more experience, we are bound to assume in this case a great irregularity in the rhythm of the heart, together with marked chronotropic and bathmotropic variations. Whether the changes in these cases are of a myogenic or neurogenic character must still remain an open question."

K.F. Wenckebach.
In: *Arrhythmia of the Heart: Excessive Irregularity—Delirium Cordis*
S 81, Groningen, 1903

Since the observations and conjectures offered by Wenckebach in 1903 as to the nature of atrial fibrillation (AF), therapeutic efforts directed at the causes, associations and consequences of AF have been widely studied in this century. In considering nonpharmacological electrical therapies directed at prevention of AF, certain observations have particular relevance. AF often coexists or develops *de novo* in patients

From *Nonpharmacological Management of Atrial Fibrillation*, edited by F.D. Murgatroyd and A.J. Camm. © 1997, Futura Publishing Co., Inc., Armonk, NY.

with symptomatic bradyarrhythmias requiring cardiac pacemaker implantation. It is therefore not surprising that the occurrence and frequency of AF in these patients has been widely examined. Reduced AF recurrence rates during long-term surveillance have been reported in paced patients with either vagally mediated bradycardia-dependent AF or in sick sinus syndrome patients implanted with atrial or dual chamber pacemakers.[1-5] In the former instance, elimination of bradycardia, which is necessary for arrhythmogenesis, has been widely suggested as the mechanism of AF prevention.[1,2] In the latter instance, while the data are suggestive of an antiarrhythmic effect of atrial pacing, due to the small or retrospective nature of most reports, it is not conclusive. Comparative populations exposed to ventricular pacing alone are either frequently absent or poorly matched.[6] This has prompted discussion of the need for a large prospective trial which has now become a reality.[7] Clinical studies have also introduced new multisite atrial pacing modes and pilot experiences attest to their beneficial antiarrhythmic effects for AF prevention.[8,9] Recent attention has been focused as well on the mechanisms of AF initiation and maintenance. The interaction of pacing modes with these arrhythmogenic mechanisms is, however, poorly delineated.

This chapter will review: (1) The electrophysiological effects of acute and chronic atrial pacing modes on potential arrhythmogenic mechanisms for AF; (2) The clinical data available for evaluation of the role of atrial pacing in AF prevention; (3) Potential guidelines for patient selection and management; and (4) Future directions for device therapy and investigation.

Atrial Pacing Modes and Electrophysiological Aspects

Atrial pacing with single- and dual-site stimulation is currently in use. Simultaneous dual-site stimulation is usually performed though sequential stimulation may be considered. Single-site stimulation has usually been performed from the lateral high right atrium or the right atrial appendage, infrequently from the distal or mid-coronary sinus and most recently, at the coronary sinus ostium. In congenital heart disease, left atrial stimulation sites have been employed, usually with epicardial leads.

Atrial activation patterns in high right atrial, coronary sinus ostial and distal coronary sinus pacing, and induced atrial flutter/fibrillation have been studied in our laboratory.[10,11] Global atrial activation time reflected in P wave duration shows minimal differences in single-site pacing as compared to sinus rhythm. However, regional atrial activation differences can be striking. A comparison of sinus rhythm and right *atrial appendageal pacing* shows earlier excitation of the atrioventricular (AV) nodal-His and adjoining septal regions with the latter mode. The coronary sinus ostial region is, however, rapidly activated during sinus rhythm perhaps due to proximity to posterior atrial inputs into the AV nodal region. *Coronary ostial pacing* activates the low septal right atrium, including the AV junctional tissues and the inferior right atrium, more rapidly than the inferior left atrium. Conduction delay in propagation along the coronary sinus is also seen. *Distal coronary sinus pacing* results in similar conduction delay in the reverse direction, yet activation of the AV nodal-His regions precedes the proximal coronary sinus in this pacing mode. These pacing data suggest an important role for preferential atrial propagation based either on anatomic obstacles or anisotropic conduction resulting in important regional differences in atrial activation. Consequently, recovery of excitability is altered in a similar fashion. This may potentially result in elimination of sites of conduction delay that may be involved in reentrant arrhythmogenesis.

Dual-site stimulation has hitherto been largely performed by simultaneous stimulation of the high right atrium and either coronary sinus ostium (dual-site right atrial) or distal coronary sinus (biatrial) sites. In contrast to single-site pacing, both modes abbreviate global atrial activation which is reflected in P wave duration. In *dual-site right atrial pacing*, right atrial activation is advanced in virtually all regions including the crista terminalis, AV junction, and interatrial septum. Wave front collison occurs in the mid- to high-interatrial septum. While left atrial activation is also advanced, terminal activation occurs in the superolateral left atrium and distal coronary sinus. In *biatrial pacing*, left and superior right atrial activation is advanced with wave front collision now occurring in the vicinity of the coronary sinus ostium or low interatrial septum. Terminal activation is in the lateral right atrium or superior interatrial septum.[12]

The thesis that atrial conduction delays are not introduced and may be eliminated by these pacing modes merits study. Luck and Engel noted that dispersion of atrial refractoriness in right atrial sites is not ameliorated by overdrive single-site atrial pacing at different rates, though rate adaptation at each site can be seen.[13] Propagation of fixed coupled high right atrial premature beats with coupling intervals of 300 ms to 400 ms in these different pacing modes is unaltered in patients with and without spontaneous AF or flutter, indicating that new areas of delay are not introduced by different atrial activation patterns.[14] Only very premature beats, coupled 10–20 ms beyond refractory period, exhibit conduction delay. Alternatively, premature beats arising contralateral to the pacing site exhibit conduction delay at long coupling intervals. Triggered pacing could also alter propagation patterns of such premature beats resulting in collision of dual atrial wave fronts with the ectopic wave front after its initial inscription. The lines of conduction block that may develop could both hinder or, in some instances, promote reentry. Further studies on other sites of origin for such beats and more careful scanning of coupling intervals with respect to sinus rhythm are in progress.

Another approach to assess antiarrhythmic effects has been to examine the impact of the pacing train on induced AF. Reproducibly induced AF using single to triple extrastimuli during high right atrial drive could be suppressed in 56% of patients using a dual-site right atrial drive train.[15] This suppression was seen in patients exhibiting a greater dispersion of refractoriness between the high right atrial and coronary sinus ostial pacing sites, suggesting that a potential mechanism may lie in elimination of this dispersion by altering recovery of excitability. More detailed mapping of atrial regions involved in the initial reentrant wave front in AF and the subsequent "daughter" wavelets that develop are needed.

Other potential mechanisms for suppression of spontaneous AF include effects on triggers such as atrial ectopic beats. Investigators have extensively documented that atrial premature beats that initiate AF are more premature than those that fail to do so, implying the importance of critical delay in reentrant excitation.[16] Others have suggested that a large atrial cycle length variability of >200ms occurring in 45% of patient recordings may be critical to some patients.[17] Sudden changes in refractoriness and subsequent recovery of excitability due to changes in cycle length may be important in these patients. Overdrive pacing could alter atrial premature beat propagation as discussed above, directly suppress automaticity in diseased atrial fibers, or avoid cycle length variability involved in arrhythmia initiation. Another potential mechanism would involve the impact of atrial stretch/distension on atrial conduction and automaticity. Daubert et al. have applied biatrial pacing in patients with hypertrophic cardiomyopathy and atypical atrial flutter presumably of left atrial origin.[18] The use of biatrial pacing to resynchronize the atria has been associated with favorable effects on atrial transport potentially reducing atrial wall stretch. Altering myocardial wall stretch has been associated with alterations in both automaticity and conduction.[19] Initial hypotheses of benefits of atrial pacing involved hemodynamic benefits which could reduce AF recurrences.[20] Dual-site right atrial pacing has been recently reported by Vardas et al. to improve atrial contribution to ventricular filling above single-site pacing.[21] Hemodynamic benefit can mediate atrial mechanical and, secondarily, electrophysiological remodeling.

Electrical remodeling of the atrium has been strongly implied by experiments conducted by Allessie and co-workers in a chronic goat model.[22,23] This remodeling may mediate development of persistent AF as well as progressive reestablishment of sinus rhythm depending on the direction taken by the intervention.[22] Thus, it is conceivable that the electrophysiological remodeling induced by multisite atrial pacing may be of greatest value in reestablishment of sinus rhythm at onset but this may be subsequently maintained by less aggressive or other interventions, e.g., single-site pacing, drugs, etc. However, the important caveat here is that the extent of remodeling feasible in a human atrium with organic disease may be considerably different than human or animal atria without organic disease.

Clinical Experience with Atrial Pacing in AF Prevention

A large number of retrospective analyses and two prospective studies have examined the value of single-site atrial pacing.[4–6,20,24–29] Figure 1 is a meta-analysis of a large number of reported studies that compared ventricular and atrial-based pacing modes in patients with sick sinus syndrome. An overall picture of two to four times increased incidence of recurrent AF in ventricular pacing in follow-up periods of 3 to 5 years emerges. What is unclear is whether this is a proarrhythmic effect of ventricular based pacing, i.e., an increase over untreated patients, a true antiarrhythmic effect of atrial based pacing, or both. In either case, the use of ventricular pacing alone does not seem desirable. Reimold and co-workers, in a nonrandomized study of sick sinus syndrome patients, noted that 40% of patients in the VVI mode were in sinus rhythm at 6 months as compared to 55% of unpaced patients in their study.[30] Eighty percent of patients with DDD pacing were in sinus rhythm, but this cannot be compared with the unpaced group since this latter group did not have coexisting bradycardia. However, this study does raise the possibility that the reduced AF recurrence rates seen in retrospective data (Fig. 1) may, in part, be due to antiarrhythmic effects of atrial pacing and, in part, due to proarrhythmia of ventricular pacing.

Two prospective studies on single-site atrial pacing with moderate

Pacing in Sick Sinus Syndrome
Incidence of Chronic AF

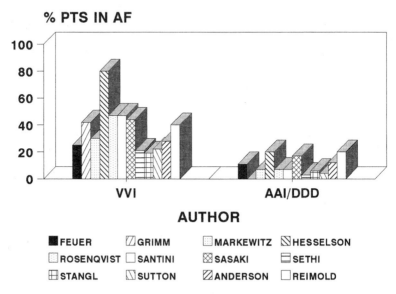

Figure 1. Incidence of chronic AF in patients undergoing cardiac pacing for sick sinus syndrome as reported in different series.[4–6,20,24–31,39] Note that the incidence of chronic AF is significantly higher in the VVI pacing mode as compared to the AAI/DDD pacing mode. Only one report (Andersen et al.[31]) is a prospective study, while the remainder are retrospective analyses. None are randomized trials. (See text for critical analysis.) AF = atrial fibrillation; PTS = patients.

patient enrollment confirm this difference in AF recurrence rates. One nonrandomized prospective study by Andersen et al., which compared the different pacing modes applied at two different institutions in the same geographical area, showed a 12% incidence of AF during single-site AAI pacing as compared to 28% with VVI pacing.[31] Lamas et al. noted a reduced incidence of AF in a prospective randomized multicenter trial at 1 year with AAI or DDD pacing as compared to VVI pacing. This study is serving as a pilot for a large national multicenter prospective trial[32] referred to as the Mode Optimization Survival Trial (MOST). In all of these studies, the atrial stimulation site has not been standardized, with most trials permitting any high right atrial site. While the comparative efficacy of different single atrial stimulation sites in AF prevention has not been formally examined, Seidl et al. reported a higher AF recurrence rate with the lateral high right atrial pacing site as compared to the right atrial appendage.[33]

Multisite atrial pacing studies are largely reported in pilot experiences. Daubert et al. performed biatrial pacing in 19 patients with advanced interatrial block and drug-refractory atrial flutter and AF.[8] Eight patients had atypical atrial flutter, two patients had AF, and nine patients had both arrhythmias. Triggered pacing in the DDDR mode was used. Sixteen patients had arrhythmia suppression initially but instability of the pacing site in the distal coronary sinus occurred in over one-third of patients with loss of pacing and relapses. Lead repositioning usually at a more proximal location was often performed. Absence of a prospective study design and any comparison arm were limitations of this analysis.

We have compared the clinical efficacy and safety of single-site pacing and dual-site right atrial pacing in a prospectively designed cross-over clinical experience.[34-46] At the time of this report, 29 patients have received such systems. Two right atrial screw-in pacing leads placed at the high right atrium and the coronary sinus ostium were cross-connected with a Y connector to the atrial output of a DDDR pacemaker. Continuous atrial overdrive pacing was established by a high lower rate limit and aggressive rate-response with concomitant drug therapy. Drug therapy was directed at sinus rate control as well as antiarrhythmic effects on the atrial substrate, and was individualized to each patient. Drug selection was determined by prior drug history, with all patients receiving a previously ineffective drug. Lack of drug tolerance or AF relapses during drug titration or in-hospital resulted in changes in therapy. This process resulted in a drug optimization period in many patients which ranged from 1 to 40 days. After drug optimization, patients were initially assigned to dual-site right atrial pacing for 90 days (phase 1) and consenting patients were switched to a single-site pacing mode for 90 days (phase 2). In 16 patients, this has been high right atrial pacing, while in 13 patients it is coronary sinus ostial pacing. A second period of switching back to dual-site (phase 3) and later again to single-site pacing (phase 4)for 180-day periods in consenting patients has been planned.

Data on AF recurrence intervals derived from ECG recordings and symptoms in patients with documented arrhythmia correlation in the past, obtained in the 3 months preceding pacemaker implant, were used as control data. Arhythmia-free intervals in the first 20 patients

DUAL SITE RA PACING

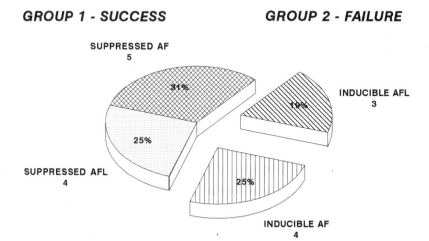

N = 16 PTS

Figure 2. Success of acute dual-site pacing in suppression of induced atrial flutter and fibrillation in patients with spontaneous atrial flutter and fibrillation. Note that 56% of all patients with reproducibly inducible atrial flutter and fibrillation from the high right atrium were suppressed with dual-site drive preceding the high right atrial extrastimulus(Group 1). Seven of these patients went on to chronic dual-site pacing with good results. AF = atrial fibrillation; AFL = atrial flutter; PTS = patients; RA = right atrium.

completing 6 months of follow-up are shown in Figure 2. Note that this analysis shows significant benefit in arrhythmia-free intervals of all atrial pacing modes over the control period. By this study design, the maximum permissible arrhythmia-free interval was 90 days. The two single-site modes cannot yet be compared due to unequal sample sizes arising from sequential use of the modes in the study. In contrast, the dual-site mode shown has incremental benefit over both single-site modes. One-year freedom from frequent recurrent relapsing or chronic AF approximates 80%. This has been accompanied by a marked decline in antiarrhythmic drug use from a mean of 3.5 drugs preoperatively to 1.4 drugs during pacing ($P<.05$).

Lead dislodgement at the coronary sinus ostial site is not usually seen. Only one patient experienced dislodgement in the operating room requiring repositioning, and this patient has remained stable after hospital discharge. Acute and chronic pacing thresholds are higher at the coronary sinus ostial site but remain within acceptable limits for atrial pacing. Additional complications observed in this experience include a rise in ventricular thresholds without lead dislodgement, requiring lead repositioning in two patients with screw-in leads, probably related to lead tunneling. This has not been seen after switching to steroid eluting tine-tipped leads in the ventricle. High right atrial lead dislodgement occurred in one patient in-hospital with recent open heart surgery and required lead repositioning. Late pacemaker pocket infection due to unrelated sepsis required system explant in one patient. There have been 1–4 (mean of 2.1) AF recurrences in eight patients. Seven of eight recurrences occurred initially in the single-site high right atrial pacing mode. Two patients had AF recurrences related to acute congestive heart failure, one due to acute pneumonitis, and three due to either drug withdrawal or reduction of lower rate with loss of overdrive pacing. Four of these seven patients who had their initial recurrence in the single-site high right atrial pacing mode had recurrences in the dual-site mode with two eventually progressing to chronic AF. Many of these recurrences were transient and resolved with resolution of the triggering event but cardioversion was required in four patients.

These pilot data suggest a benefit of both single and dual-site atrial pacing modes in AF prevention. Pacing in either mode increased arrhythmia-free periods and dual-site pacing offered increased benefit. The suitability of the coronary sinus ostium as a location for long-term atrial pacing is established by this study. A large multicenter prospective randomized study is now planned to compare support atrial pacing with single and dual-site pacing.

Patient Selection for Multisite Atrial Pacing

Clear guidelines for patient selection are still under investigation. Based on early clinical data, certain patient groups or arrhythmias can be identified as being susceptible to such intervention.

(1) Daubert et al. have reported use of biatrial pacing in patients with the clinical constellation of advanced intratrial block, with manifest atypical atrial flutter alone or in combination with AF.[8] This unique patient group has responded well to pacing with and without drug therapy in their experience. Hemodynamic transport benefit with decrease in atrial stretch may be of particular importance here. Of some impor-

tance is the consideration that atrial flutter initiates AF and preexcitation of the atrial flutter substrate in the left atrium may be of benefit due to collision of wave fronts in critical areas of flutter initiation. Similar concepts have been applied by us to atrial tachycardia circulating around an anatomic obstacle. In one of our patients, incessant atrial tachycardia circulated around the septal patch of an atrial septal defect repair. This patient had failed five antiarrhythmic drug trials and prior catheter ablation. After initiation of dual-site pacing, this arrhythmia was suppressed as long as continuous overdrive pacing was maintained in conjunction with beta-blocker therapy during a follow-up period of 13 months. Similarly, this concept can be considered when a polymorphic atrial flutter precedes AF. We have noted that such rhythms are associated with regions of discrete and fragmented chaotic electrogram activity.[10,11] Such fragmented activity is located in coronary sinus ostial locations more frequently than in high right atrial sites, and may be vulnerable to local paced preexcitation.

(2) In patients with reproducibly initiated AF with single-site pacing, we have tested dual-site drive trains with successful suppression in 56% of patients (Fig. 3). Several such patients have undergone implantation of chronic dual-site right atrial pacing systems with good results. Of seven patients with acute suppression, none had a recurrence in the first 90 days of dual-site pacing; three of these patients had recurrences when mode switched to high right atrial pacing.

(3) We have also applied the multisite atrial pacing technique to unselected patients with AF and atrial flutter. Initiation of AF was never bradycardia-dependent and drug-induced bradycardia during the treatment of AF was the basis for pacing in most patients. AF was the initial rhythm in 19 patients, atrial flutter in three patients, and both coexisted in seven patients. Eighty-two percent of patients were maintained in sinus rhythm at 1 year. Patients maintaining sinus rhythm with single and dual-site atrial pacing were characterized by paroxysmal arrhythmia, near normal left atrial (LA) diameter, and well preserved left ventricular function. Underlying heart disease was present in 19 patients and no definite relation to the etiology of the disease could be noted. In patients requiring one cardioversion shock, two of five have maintained sinus rhythm for 6 months to 13 months.

Future Directions for Device Therapy

Our data would suggest that occasional cardioversion in the first year in expectation of electrophysiological and possibly anatomic re-

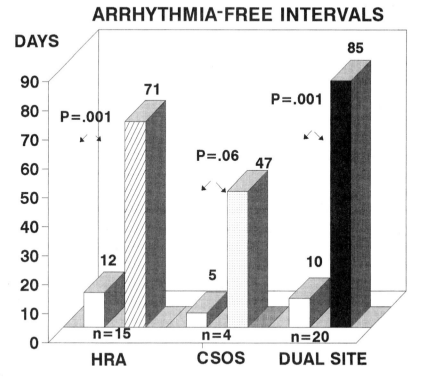

Figure 3. Arrhythmia-free intervals after institution of atrial pacing at different sites in phases 1 and 2 of the clinical experience.[35,36,38] Note that the prepacing arrhythmia-free interval on drug therapy alone is shown for each pacing site in the left bar and the postpacing interval by the right bar. The actual values are shown above each bar with significance of the comparison with the control period. All atrial pacing modes combined also had significantly longer arrhythmia-free intervals than the control period. By study design, the longest interval possible was 90 days. CSOS = coronary sinus ostium; HRA = high right atrium.

modeling is an important adjunctive therapy. Backup atrial defibrillllation with catheter-based techniques will be a critical component of treatment approaches directed at prevention and management of AF. Adjunctive roles for drug therapy and even catheter-based ablative therapy directed at modifying the electrophysiology of the atrial substrate and the consequent impact of pacing methods can be argued. Most current patient data have been obtained in patients with paroxysmal arrhythmia, with much less data on chronic AF. This group must still be considered more speculative with respect to efficacy unless converted by drug or other techniques to a paroxysmal arrhythmia. For the present, paroxysmal AF offers a window of opportunity for electrical intervention.

Future Directions for Investigation

A rather large number of avenues for fruitful investigation is emerging from our early studies. Fundamental mechanistic studies of the effects of different pacing modes and sites on atrial electrophysiology in humans need expansion. Detailed mapping studies to evaluate the effect on atrial substrates for AF as well as spontaneous triggers appear imminent.[37] The role of combined therapy and the contribution of complementary therapies needs delineation. The combination of pacing and defibrillation therapies in a single device appears to warrant pilot investigation.[38] Large prospective multicenter studies, now in progress, on the value of atrial rate-responsive versus demand-support pacing, and single versus dual site pacing, should further delineate this issue. More extensive studies on defined patient populations and carefully classified clinical arrhythmias such as chronic AF or atrial flutter will be needed. The time window for electrical interventions is still unclear in the natural history of AF. Whether one or more windows exists is still a subject for conjecture and hypothesis testing. Finally, the extent of electrical remodeling feasible in humans as a function of their disease states is a long-term objective of clinical investigation. This brief summary serves only to outline the myriad of research issues that surround this most prevalent of cardiac arrhythmias as recognized by Wenckebach.

References

1. Attuel P, Pellerin D, Mugica J, et al. DDD pacing: an effective treatment modality for recurrent atrial arrhythmias. PACE 1988;11:1647–1654.
2. Coumel P, Friocourt P, Mugica J, et al. Long-term prevention of vagal atrial arrhythmias by atrial pacing at 90/minute: experience with six cases. PACE 1983;6:552–560.
3. Boccadamo R, Toscano S. Prevention and interruption of supraventricular tachycardia by antitachycardia pacing. In: Luderitz B, Saksena S, eds. Interventional Electrophysiology. Mount Kisco, NY: Futura Publishing Co; 1991:213–223.
4. Stangl K, Seitz K, Wirtzfeld A, et al. Differences between atrial single chamber pacing and ventricular single chamber pacing with respect to

prognosis and antiarrhythmic effect in patients with sick sinus syndrome. PACE 1990;13:2080–2085.
 5. Sgarbossa EB, Pinski SL, Maloney JD, et al. Chronic atrial fibrillation and stroke in paced patients with sick sinus syndrome: relevance of clinical characteristics and pacing modalities. Circulation 1993;88:1045–1053.
 6. Rosenqvist M, Brandt J, Schuller H. Long-term pacing in sinus node disease: effect of stimulation mode on cardiovascular mortality and morbidity. Am Heart J 1988;116:16–22.
 7. Lamas GA, Ellenbogen KA, Griffin JJ, et al. for the PASE Investigators. Quality of life and clinical events in DDDR versus VVIR paced patients: design and preliminary results of a randomized trial. Circulation 1995; 92(suppl):I-533. Abstsract.
 8. Daubert C, Mabo P, Berder V. Arrhythmia prevention by permanent atrial resynchronization in advanced interatrial block. Eur Heart J 1990;11:237.
 9. Prakash A, Saksena S, Hill M, et al. Dual site atrial pacing for the acute and chronic prevention of atrial fibrillation: a prospective study. J Am Coll Cardiol 1995;25:230A. Abstract.
10. Giorgberidze I, Munsif AN, Krol R, et al. Correlation of electrocardiographic and intracardiac right and left atrial electrogram findings during "atypical" type 2 atrial flutter. PACE 1996;19(II):711. Abstract.
11. Prakash A, Saksena S, Kaushik R, et al. Right and left atrial activation patterns during dual site atrial pacing in man: comparison with single site pacing. PACE 1996;19(II):697. Abstract.
12. Munsif AN, Prakash A, Krol RB, et al. Crista terminalis, atrial septal and coronary sinus activation during single and dual site atrial pacing. PACE 1996;19(II):578. Abstract.
13. Luck JC, Engel TR. Dispersion of atrial refractoriness in patients with sinus node dysfunction. Circulation 1979;60:404–411.
14. Prakash A, Hill M, Giorgberidze I, et al. Propagation of atrial premature beats during atrial pacing: insights from regional atrial mapping. PACE 1996;19(II):642. Abstract.
15. Prakash A, Saksena S, Krol RB, et al. Electrophysiology of acute prevention of atrial fibrillation and flutter with dual site right atrial pacing. PACE 1995;18:803. Abstract.
16. Capucci A, Santarelli A, Boriani G, et al. Atrial premature beats coupling interval determines lone paroxysmal atrial fibrillation onset. Int J Cardiol 1992;36:87–93. Abstract.
17. Mehra R, Hill M. Prevention of atrial flutter/fibrillation. In: Saksena S, Luderitz B, eds. Interventional Electrophysiology. 2nd edition. Armonk, NY: Futura Publishing Co; 1996:521–540.
18. Daubert C, Gras D, Leclercq C, et al. Biatrial synchronous pacing: a new therapeutic approach to prevent refractory atrial tachyarrhythmias. J Am Coll Cardiol 1995;25:230A. Abstract.
19. Ong JJC, Lee JJ, Hough D, et al. Mechanisms of termination of reentrant wave fronts in the atrium: implications for prevention of atrial fibrillation. J Am Coll Cardiol 1996;27:60A. Abstract.
20. Feuer JM, Shandling AH, Messenger JC, et al. Influence of cardiac pacing modes on the long term development of atrial fibrillation. Am J Cardiol 1989;64:1376–1379.
21. Vardas PE, Simantirakis EM, Manios EG, et al. Acute and chronic hemody-

namic effects of bifocal vs. unifocal right atrial pacing. J Am Coll Cardiol 1996;27:74A. Abstract.

22. Wijffels MCEF, Kirchhof CJHJ, Dorland RD, et al. Atrial fibrillation begets atrial fibrillation: a study in awake chronically instrumented goats. Circulation 1995;92:1954–1968.

23. Allessie MA. Electrophysiological sequelae of atrial fibrillation. In: Kulbertus HE, Wellens HJJ, Bourgeois IMGP, Sutton R, eds. Atrial Fibrillation: Facts From Yesterday—Ideas For Tomorrow. Armonk, NY: Futura Publishing Co; 1994;74–76.

24. Hesselson AB, Parsonnet V, Bernstein AD, et al. Deleterious effect of long term single chamber ventricular pacing in patients with sick sinus syndrome: the hidden benefits of dual chamber pacing. J Am Coll Cardiol 1992; 19:1542–1549.

25. Santini M, Alexidou G, Ansalone G, et al. Relation of prognosis in sick sinus syndrome to age, conduction defects and modes of permanent cardiac pacing. Am J Cardiol 1990;65:729–735.

26. Sutton R, Kenny RA. The natural history of sick sinus syndrome. PACE 1986;9:1110.

27. Sasaki Y, Shimotori M, Akahane K, et al. Long-term follow-up of patients with sick sinus syndrome: a comparsion of clinical aspects among unpaced, ventricular inhibited paced, and physiologically paced groups. PACE 1988; 11:1575–1583.

28. Sethi KK, Bajaj V, Mohan JC, et al. Comparison of atrial and VVI pacing modes in symptomatic sinus node dysfunction without associated tachyarrhythmias. Indian Heart J 1990;42:143.

29. Markewitz A, Schad N, Hemmer W, et al. What is the most appropriate stimulation mode in patients with sinus node dysfunction? PACE 1986;9: 1115–1120.

30. Reimold SC, Lamas GA, Cantillon CO, et al. Risk factors for the development of recurrent atrial fibrillation: role of pacing and clinical variables. Am Heart J 1995;129:1127–1132.

31. Andersen HR, Thuesen L, Bagger JP, et al. Prospective randomized trial of atrial versus ventricular pacing in sick sinus syndrome. Lancet 1994; 344:1523–1528.

32. Lamas GA, Estes NM, Schneller S, Flaker GC. Does dual chamber or atrial pacing prevent atrial fibrillation?: the need for a randomized controlled trial. PACE 1992;15:1109–1113.

33. Seidl K, Hauer B, Schwick N, et al. Is the site of atrial lead implantation in dual chamber pacing of importance for preventing atrial fibrillation? The hidden benefits of lead implantation in the right atrial appendix. PACE 1995;18:810. Abstract.

34. Saksena S, Prakash A, Hill M, et al. Efficacy of atrial pacing for atrial fibrillation prevention: role of atrial and ventricular bradycardia. Circulation, 1995:92(I):I-532. Abstract.

35. Saksena S, Prakash A, Hill M, et al. Prevention of recurrent atrial fibrillation with chronic dual site right atrial pacing. J Am Coll Cardiol 1996;28: 687–694.

36. Prakash A, Hill M, Lewis C, et al. Comparative efficacy of high right atrial, coronary sinus and dual site right atrial pacing in prevention of atrial fibrillation. PACE 1996;19(II):634. Abstract.

37. Hashuba K, Centurion OA, Shimizu A. Electrophysiologic characteristics of human atrial muscle in paroxysmal atrial fibrillation. Am Heart J 1996; 131:778–789.
38. Saksena S, Prakash A, Madan N, et al. Prevention of atrial fibrillation by pacing. PACE 1997. In press.
39. Grimm W, Langenfeld H, Maisch B, et al. Symptoms, cardiovascular risk profile and spontaneous ECG in paced patients: a five-year follow-up study. PACE 1990;13:2086–2090.

PART VII

Termination of Atrial Fibrillation: The Basics

CHAPTER 24

Insights into the Mechanisms of Atrial Fibrillation:

Role of the Multidimensional Atrial Structure

José Jalife, Richard A. Gray

Introduction

Atrial fibrillation (AF) is probably the most frequently occurring cardiac rhythm disturbance, next to premature atrial and ventricular systoles.[1,2] Overall, about two million Americans have chronic AF.[3] In addition, AF is the most common cardiogenic cause of stroke,[4] which makes it a major clinical problem. Yet, despite the magnitude of the problem and almost 120 years of intense research and speculation, the detailed cellular and pathophysiological mechanisms of AF remain poorly understood.

After the studies of Moe et al.[5-7] in the late 1950s and 1960s, electrophysiologists have agreed that the stability of fibrillation is a function of several factors, including a nonuniform distribution of refractory periods; a sufficiently large area of tissue; and a relatively brief refractory period and/or relatively slow conduction velocity of the impulse. Such considerations are consistent with the fact that vagal stimulation, which leads to an inhomogeneous abbreviation and thus dispersion of refractory periods, increases the probability of sustained fibrillation. All these concepts are based on Moe's "multiple wavelet" hypothesis of fibrillation[6] which he derived from a computer model of a two-dimen-

Supported in part by grant P01-HL39707 from the National Heart, Lung and Blood Institute, National Institutes of Health, and by a grant from InControl, Inc., Redmond, WA.
From *Nonpharmacological Management of Atrial Fibrillation*, edited by F.D. Murgatroyd and A.J. Camm. © 1997, Futura Publishing Co., Inc., Armonk, NY.

sional atrial sheet. The model underwent self-sustained turbulent activity: temporal dispersion of refractory periods gave rise to irregular and tortuous impulse propagation. In addition, there was fractionation of wave fronts with aperiodic local activity and numerous reentrant circuits. Thus, the simple two-dimensional model gave rise to activity which, at least superficially, resembled fibrillation. According to that model, fibrillation was certainly reentrant; it was almost certainly not a simple circus movement. Moreover, once initiated, fibrillatory activity in the model was independent of the initiating event.

In 1985, Allessie et al.[8] mapped the spread of excitation in the atria of a dog heart during acetylcholine-induced AF, and provided the first demonstration in vivo of multiple propagating wavelets giving rise to turbulent atrial activity. These investigators estimated that sustainment of fibrillation in the canine atrium required a critical number of four to six wavelets, which was supported by subsequent experiments.

To date, most of the studies on the mechanism of AF have been based on the simplifying assumption that the atria behave like a smooth and homogeneous sheet of cardiac muscle. Yet it is well known that the mammalian atria are highly complex multidimensional structures interrupted by natural orifices. In addition, the atria are composed of an intricate and heterogeneous branching network of subendocardial muscular bundles forming multiple ridges and pectinate muscles that line and/or bridge the thinner atrial free walls and appendages. The major orifices of the atria have long been suspected to be involved in the initiation and maintenance of reentrant arrhythmias.[9-11] However, only relatively recently, a handful of studies have focused attention on the role of the naturally occurring complexities of the atrial subendocardial structures in the mechanisms of cardiac arrhythmias.[12-17] The importance of atrial structure in clinical arrhythmias is also beginning to be recognized in the clinic, for example in the studies on atrial flutter in the Lesh laboratory.[18] Spach's studies[13-15] have greatly advanced our understanding of the role of such structural complexities in wave propagation. In fact, Spach et al.[14] were first in bringing attention to the fact that "macroscopic" discontinuities (i.e., at size scale of 1 mm or greater) play an important role in discontinuous propagation, in the establishment of unidirectional block, and in the initiation of reentry. We have taken advantage of the knowledge gained from Spach's experiments and from the study of the dynamics of wave propagation in excitable media to design computer simulations and experiments aimed at answering several specific questions regarding wave propagation. These questions include: (a) What is the role played by the heterogeneous network of pectinate muscles and trabeculae that line the subendocardium in propagation throughout the atria during sinus rhythm, atrial pacing and AF?; (b) What is the frequency dependence of propagation at such networks, particularly at branching points and points of connection with the underlying atrial free wall?; and (c) What is the effect of the complex three-dimensional structure of the subendocardium on the stability of reentrant patterns initiated on the epicardial surface of the right or left atrium?

In this chapter, we present our initial studies attempting to address such questions. We have used three different approaches: First, the Langendorff-perfused heart preparation[19] which enables us to map optically the patterns of wave propagation on the epicardial surface of the right atrium of the sheep heart. Second, the superfused right atrial preparation, for which two video cameras are used to record simultaneously from the endocardial and epicardial surfaces of the right atrium. The idea is to establish the precise origin of epicardial breakthroughs secondary to discordant endocardial/epicardial activation. Third, in computer simulations, we have begun to address the question of whether propagation from the pectinate muscles to the atrial free wall is responsible for destabilization of reentrant vortices in the underlying atrial free wall, and whether asynchronous propagation through the three-dimensional network of pectinate muscles plays a role in AF.

Langendorff-Perfused Right Atrium

A diagram of the Langendorff-perfused heart preparation is shown in Figure 1. After excision, the sheep heart was perfused with Tyrode's solution at a rate of about 200–300 ml/min. Temperature was 37–38° C and control recordings were taken to ensure that the heart was in sinus rhythm and contracting forcefully and rhythmically. This was followed by a bolus coronary injection of 30 ml of the voltage sensitive dye Di-4-ANEPPS (15 μg/ml), which resulted in a very large level of fluorescence (for further details see refs. 19–22). To stop the heart's contraction, we continuously perfused it with 10 mM diacetyl monoxime (DAM). DAM is an electromechanical uncoupler which has very small effects on action potential characteristics.[19] We used a tungsten halogen lamp to excite the fluorescence of the dye and a charged coupled device (CCD) camera for recording.[20–23] Both the excitation light and CCD camera were focused on the anterior epicardial surface of the right atrial wall. In all experiments presented here, time resolution was 240 frames/sec (i.e., one frame every 4.16 msec). In five preliminary experiments, the average cycle length during sinus rhythm was 603 ± 50 ms

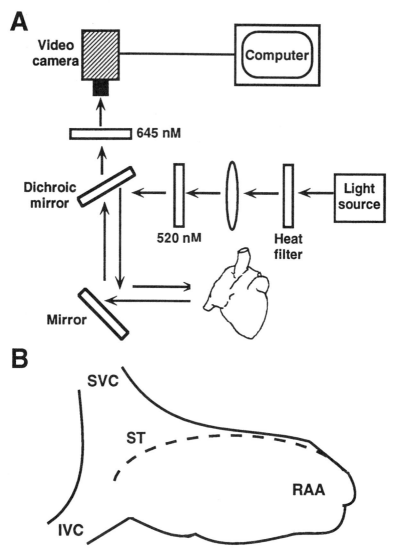

Figure 1. A. Diagram of experimental setup. The Langendorff-perfused heart was loaded with Di-4-ANEPPS (15 μg/ml) by bolus intracoronary injection and then placed in front of the optical system for video imaging. **B**. Diagram of the epicardial surface of the anterior wall of the right atrium as viewed by the video camera. SVC = superior vena cava; IVC = inferior vena cava; ST = sulcus terminalis; RAA = right atrial appendage. See text for further details. (Reprinted from Gray RA, Pertsov AM, Jalife J,[23] with permission from the American Heart Association, Inc.)

(mean ± standard deviation) in control and 680 ± 120 ms after the addition of the DAM and dye. This difference was not significant. In some experiments (N = 4) coronary perfusion of acetylcholine (ACh) prolonged sinus cycle length from control to 753 ± 143 ms (P<0.05 by Student's t-test).

Normal Sequence of Activation

In Figure 2, we present epicardial patterns of wave propagation in the right atrium as 4-msec isochrone bands on the next slide for sinus rhythm (A) and pacing at basic cycle length (BCL) = 500 ms (B) and BCL = 150 ms (C) in the same heart. During sinus rhythm at a cycle length of 550 ms, conduction was nonuniform, with a breakthrough site in the right atrial appendage near the right border (light gray). Pacing from the sulcus terminals at a rate similar to the sinus rate exhibited a much different pattern of propagation. The conduction velocity (CV) was slower and more uniform (panel B). The elliptical wave of excitation propagated from the stimulating electrode with uniform local CV and no evidence of breakthrough activity. Pacing at a faster rate (BCL = 150 ms) showed slower and more heterogeneous conduction patterns (panel C). Notice that the vertical conduction velocity exhibited a greater reduction at fast pacing rates compared to horizontal velocity. The fact that a breakthrough pattern was observed during sinus rhythm but there was a uniform epicardial pattern during pacing suggests that preferential propagation was occurring through the subepicardial pathways.

Initiation of Reentry by Programmed Stimulation

Reentry was frequently initiated in the epicardium as a result of heterogeneity in conduction away from the pacing site. In Figure 3, we show an isochrone map of beat 8 in an episode where reentry was initiated by burst pacing using a sequence of 10 pulses (BCL = 220 ms). In this case, pacing caused the wave to block below and to the left of the stimulating electrode leading to a wave propagating in the counterclockwise direction that collided with the next paced beat. When the stimulator was turned off, the counterclockwise wave continued rotating unimpeded, leading to a reentrant arrhythmia. This is illustrated in panel B, which shows individual pixel recordings from five different sites on the surface of the right atrium (RA) (panel A) during three consecutive rotations.

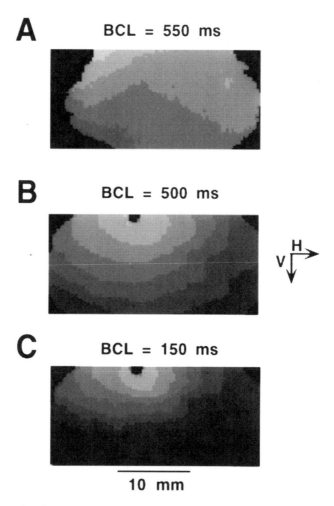

Figure 2. Isochrone maps (4 ms) of sequence of activation of the anterior epicardial surface of the right atrium. In all panels, gray levels denote activation times (white, earliest activation; dark gray, latest activation). **A**: During sinus rhythm, the first epicardial activation site is near sulcus terminalis (top left) and the wave front moves rapidly throughout the wall; a small breakthrough site occurs near the right atrial appendage (light gray), suggesting preferential propagation through subepicardial pathways. **B**: Epicardial stimulation through a bipolar electrode near the sulcus terminalis (black spot near top center) at a basic cycle length (BCL) of 550 ms results in a completely different activation sequence. **C**: Stimulation at a BCL of 150 ms results in a slower and more complex activation sequence. H = horizontal; V = vertical. (Modified from Gray RA, Pertsov AM, Jalife J,[23] with permission from the American Heart Association, Inc.)

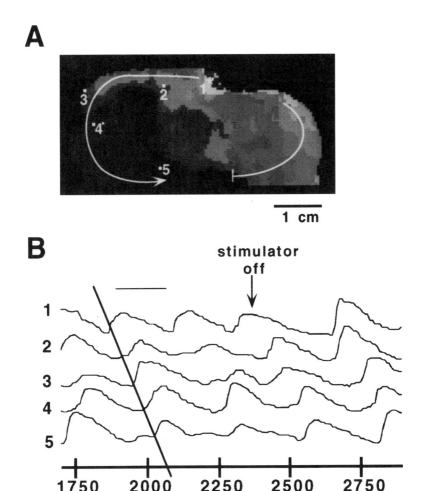

Figure 3. Initiation of reentry by burst epicardial pacing (train of 10 pulses; BCL = 220 ms) near the top center. **A**: 4-ms isochronal map of two counter-rotating waves initiated sequentially during pacing (time of activation is indicated by the gray level, white being the earliest site). The wave initiated by pulse number 8 blocked unidirectionally on the right but conducted to the left and began to rotate in the counterclockwise direction until it collided with the wave initiated by pulse number 9, which propagated in the opposite direction. **B**: Individual pixel recordings from sites 1—5 demonstrate that reentrant activity persisted after the stimulator was turned off. (Modified from Gray RA, Pertsov AM, Jalife J,[23] with permission from the American Heart Association, Inc.)

Incomplete Reentry

Although reentrant patterns were observed transiently during the initiation of AF, we never observed more than one rotation of a reentrant circuit exhibiting continuous propagation on the epicardial surface.[22] As shown in Figure 4, isochrone maps calculated from video recordings obtained during the transition to AF showed reentry around a line of functional block. In seven experiments, lines of functional block were almost always oriented in the horizontal direction with respect to the right atrial free wall (see Fig. 2 for coordinates). We estimated the length of these reentrant sites as two times the length (~1.8 cm) of the lines of functional block drawn by hand in the isochrone maps exhibiting reentry (either one or two straight lines were used to calculate the length of block). The average length of these reentrant pathways was 3.7 cm (n = 7). The average difference between latest and earliest activations within one beat was about 168 ms, which was shorter than the arrhythmia period due to noncontinuous wave propagation. The conduction velocity around these lines of block was calculated from the difference of earliest and latest activations and the length of the functional circuit. The value obtained (24.4 ± 8.8 cm/s) was different from the horizontal conduction velocity and the vertical velocity at BCL = 160 ms. Moreover, activation was not continuous along the reentrant circuit. There was a long interval in which the wave front was not observed on the epicardial surface. In seven experiments, the average value for this interval was about 78 ms. We hypothesize that propagation through the pectinate muscles attached to the right atrial free wall was responsible for the apparent discontinuity observed in this preparation.

Optical Mapping of Atrial Fibrillation

Thus far, we have analyzed 15 episodes of AF from 6 Langendorff-perfused hearts. We studied the patterns of activation from the epicardial surface of the right atrial free wall. The average period of activation was 138 ± 25 ms and complete reentrant pathways were never observed on the epicardium. The propagation patterns were characterized by a combination of incomplete reentry, breakthrough patterns and collisions of waves. A series of sequential 4-msec isochrone maps in a 600 ms interval (panels A-E) is presented in Figure 5. A pseudo-horizontal ECG, obtained by integrating the transmembrane signal on both the right and left sides of the image and taking the difference is shown

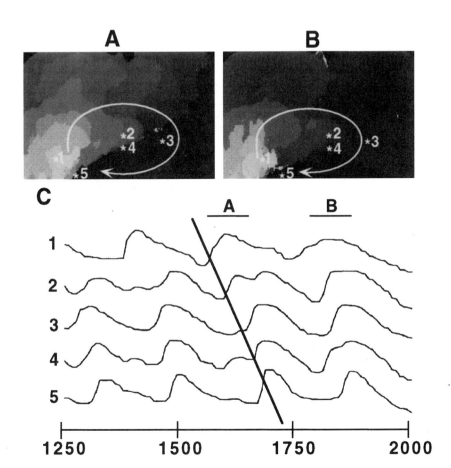

Figure 4. Incomplete reentry. **A and B**: 4-ms epicardial isochrone maps of two sequential wave rotations of incomplete reentry at the onset of AF. Note that the line of block drifts from A to B, but remains orientated along the horizontal axis of the right atrial free wall. Note also that reactivation of the earliest site (1) in panel B is preceded by a 70 ms interval during which no epicardial depolarization was manifest after activation of the latest site (5) in panel A. **C**: Individual pixel recordings from sites 1—5 show characteristic reentrant activity. (Modified from Gray RA, Pertsov AM, Jalife J,[23] with permission from the American Heart Association, Inc.)

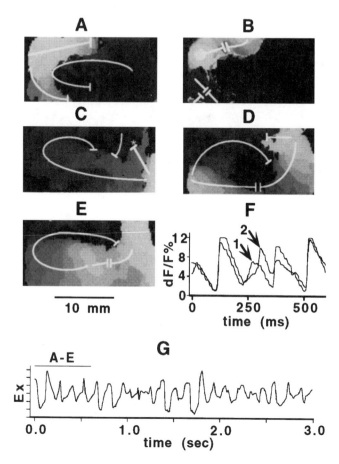

Figure 5. Video imaging of AF. **A-E** sequentially obtained 4-ms isochrone maps during a 600 msec interval of AF; white, arbitrarily selected initial site of activation; black, complete block. T-crossed curves indicate trajectories of epicardial waves moving in complex patterns. Overall, AF was characterized by incomplete reentrant waves, breakthrough patterns, and collisions of waves. **F**: Tracings of change in fluorescence (i.e., membrane potential) obtained by two camera pixels from sites located ~500 μm apart (see asterisk in panel C) demonstrate discordant repolarization that leads to asynchronous activation. **G**: Pseudo electrogram showing that the pattern corresponds to AF. Horizontal bar indicates segment that corresponds to panels A-E. (Modified from Gray RA, Pertsov AM, Jalife J,[23] with permission from the American Heart Association, Inc.)

in panel G, with a horizontal bar indicating the time interval used to create the respective isochrone maps. In panel A, a wave propagated at t = 29 ms (white) from the sulcus terminalis on the upper left side of the preparation and blocked in the middle; then the wave propagated at the top and bottom but later blocked as a result of late activation in the previous sequence. At t = 117 ms a breakthrough (light gray) occurred at the right side; the wave front propagated to the left and then curled down and back to the right but blocked at t = 158 ms (dark gray). In panel B, a new wave entered the field of view at t = 175 ms (light gray), it collided with another wave entering from the top right and was then blocked because of refractoriness in a large area of the right atrial free wall (black). Immediately thereafter, three new waves entered at the bottom left at 192, 204, and 208 ms but were also unable to activate the rest of the atrium. In panel C, a wave entered from the right atrial appendage (RAA) at t = 246 ms (white), activated the lower margin of the right atrial fee wall and then curled upward and then to the right to block at t = 313 ms and result in an incomplete reentrant pattern. This wave collided from another incoming wave (dark gray) that moved downward from the top right at t = 292 ms. In panel D, two waves (white) appeared during the next beat; one emerged at t = 371 ms from the RAA (top right), then conducted downward, and subsequently curled toward the left and collided with another wave that emerged from the lower left at t = 375 ms. The wave that came from the lower left propagated upward and then to the right to block at t = 463 ms. In panel E, a wave (white) conducted from the upper right at t = 521 ms; it fused with a large breakthrough site near the center of the right atrial free wall (t = 525 ms) and then curled upward and back, to the right.

In panel F, we show the signals from two neighboring sites (separated by 2.8 mm) near the region of block shown in panel C (the asterisk in panel C indicates the location of these sites). The sites exhibited similar patterns of activity from the beginning of the recording (panel A) and both sites activated at t = 125 ms. When the next wave propagated into this region (panel C), it activated site 1 at t = 271 ms, but was blocked at site 2. The wave then circumvented a line of block, propagating to the left then curling upward and back to the right, activating site 2 at t = 304 ms. Therefore, the wave propagated through site 1, 154 ms after the previous activation, but blocked at site 2. The reason why conduction block occurred in this region is probably because of transient heterogeneity in refractoriness as a result of different times to full repolarization at the two sites during the previous beat. Such heterogeneities were probably the result of the complex sequence of activation resulting from multiple breakthrough sites, wave collisions, and apparently incomplete reentrant activity on the epicardial surface of the right atrium, which provides strong support for the idea that propagation through the complex structure of the subendocardial layers of the atrial free wall plays a major role in determining the highly unstable patterns of epicardial activation.

Breakthrough sites were identified as the center of regions where activation initiated and propagated in all directions, as in panel E of Figure 5. These breakthrough patterns were very frequent and occurred every 215 ms on average. They were not randomly distributed but were located approximately along the horizontal direction in the middle of the right atrium and the right atrial appendage. On the other hand, the length of the lines of block around which incomplete reentry occurred ranged from 0.92 cm to 3.4 cm (2.1 ± 0.7 cm). These lines of block were concentrated in the middle to lower right atrium and right atrial appendage where there is a dense endocardial network of pectinate muscles. Furthermore, these lines of block qualitatively corresponded to the breakthrough sites.

A histological study of the right atrium supported the idea that the breakthrough sites and lines of block shown in Figure 6 during AF correspond to the subendocardial structure. Thin sections (5 μm) of the entire right atrial free wall at 100 μm intervals were prepared as described elsewhere.[23-25] The sections were cut transversely to the main axis of the right atrium as shown in the top panel. Examples of sections taken at distances of 5 mm from each other and approximately at the locations of the gray vertical bars are shown in the bottom panel. The crista terminalis (CT) separated the smooth portion of the excitable tissue near the right atrium from the pectinate muscle structure of the right atrial subendocardium. The right atrium was comprised of a thin sheet attached to a network of pectinate muscle bundles. Computer reconstruction (not shown) of the right atrial free wall confirmed that three main muscle bundles as well as the CT are oriented horizontally in the right atrial free wall. The direction of these bundles corresponded to the lines of block and the location of the breakthrough sites in AF experiments.

Role of Three-Dimensional Atrial Structure

(1) *Frequency-dependent block at branch sites and discordant endocardial-to-epicardial activation in the right atrium:* To further establish the role of the multidimensional atrial structure in establishing com-

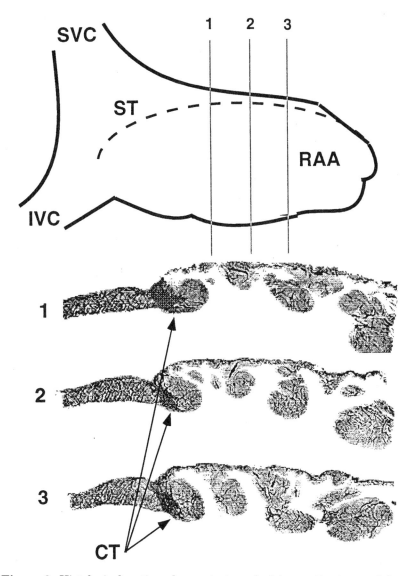

Figure 6. Histological sections demonstrate underlying pectinate muscle bundles orientated along the horizontal axis of the right atrial free wall. **Top**: Diagram of the right atrial free wall illustrating the sites from which 5 μm transverse slices were obtained. **Bottom**: Individual slices show a complex organization of muscle bundles in the endocardium. SVC = superior vena cava; IVC = inferior vena cava; ST = sulcus terminalis; RAA = right atrial appendage; CT = crista terminalis. (Reprinted from Gray RA, Pertsov AM, Jalife J,[23] with permission from the American Heart Association, Inc.)

plex activation patterns, we have carried out pacing experiments in which we simultaneously recorded from the endocardium and the epicardium in a different preparation consisting of the open, superfused right atrial free wall. A diagram of the experimental arrangement is shown in Figure 7. The two cameras were synchronized and set up to face both the epi- and endocardial surfaces. Only one light source, located on the epicardial side, was used to illuminate (excite the fluorescent dye). Thus, the camera focused on the epicardial side of the preparation recorded epifluorescence, whereas the camera facing the endocardial surface recorded transillumination. Since the transillumination signal is the integrated signal throughout the wall, and the pectinate muscles are much thicker than the epicardial sheet, the signal obtained was dominated by the pectinate muscles. Therefore, we could record from the epicardial sheet using epifluorescence and simultaneously record the activity within the pectinate muscles using transillumination.

We determined the frequency-dependence of propagation from a pectinate muscle to the underlying atrial free wall. The tissue was paced by an electrode placed on the crista terminalis (CT). In Figure 8, panel A shows results obtained at a BCL of 500 ms; temperature was somewhat low (32° C). The endocardial signal is shown on the left and the epicardial signal is shown on the right; depolarized tissue is shown as white. Activation is first seen 16 ms after the stimulus and the wave front propagated along the CT initially. After ~32 ms, the wave front began to invade other major pectinate muscle bands (left)

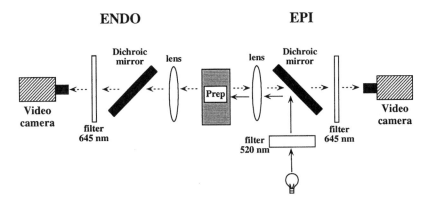

Figure 7. Diagram of dual camera system used to record simultaneously from endocardium (ENDO) and epicardium (EPI) of isolated right atrial free wall. See text for further details.

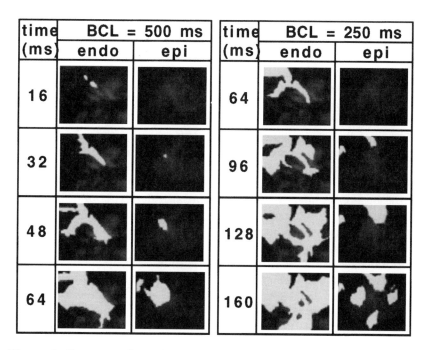

Figure 8. Frequency dependence of discordant endocardial versus epicardial activation in the isolated superfused right atrial free wall. **Left**: Endocardial stimulation at a basic cycle length (BCL) of 500 ms. **Right**: Endocardial stimulation at a BCL of 250 ms. Temperature 32° C. Fluorescence is shown in white superimposed on the real video image of the tissue.

and also appeared as a breakthrough on the epicardial surface. The wave front continued to propagate preferentially along the major bundles on the endocardium (left). In addition, the initial epicardial breakthrough site expanded and collided with another breakthrough pattern that emerged at 83 ms. The entire atrial surface was activated within 120 ms. The latter activation time is similar to that observed by Spach et al.[13] in their superfused preparations.

The activation sequence in this preparation was also studied at BCL = 250 ms (panel B). Propagation was much slower than at BCL = 500 ms. Endocardial activation occurred 24 ms after the stimulus. By 64 ms, the wave front had propagated along the CT and along another major muscle bundle perpendicular to the CT. The wave front then blocked at the junction with an intermediate-sized bundle (left). The first epicardial breakthrough occurred after 90 ms and propagated along the sinoatrial node (SAN) region. Later, two more breakthrough sites were observed leading to a complex sequence of activation with multiple collisions of wave fronts. These data indicate that wave fronts propagate preferentially along major pectinate muscle bundles and that, at rapid pacing, discordant epi- and endocardial activation sequences can be observed. It is important to note, however, that the preparation used for these experiments was superfused at relatively low temperature. This suggests the possibility that somewhat ischemic conditions prevailed, which together with the hypothermia would explain the exceedingly long activation times. Indeed, such activation times are comparable to those measured by Spach et al.[13] in similarly superfused atrial preparations. In addition, the results are consistent with those of Schuessler et al.,[12] who also demonstrated discordant activation between endocardium and epicardium. Our high resolution optical mapping experiments provide a detailed account of how such discordant activation occurs and the role of pectinate muscle activation in the mechanism of epicardial breakthroughs.

(2) *Computer model predictions:* (The "pectinate-muscle bridge" simulation). As demonstrated by the AF isochrone maps, the spatiotemporal complexity during AF is so high that it is usually not possible to observe well-organized reentrant activity on the epicardial surface of the right atrium for more than one beat. On the other hand, the data presented in Figure 8 show that there may be significant discordance in the activation sequences between subendocardial and subepicardial tissues, with major delays in epicardial activation when the frequency of endocardial stimulation is changed. Such discordance usually results in epicardial breakthrough wave fronts that shift from one site to another as a function of the activation cycle length. Taken together, the above data suggest that propagation through a pectinate muscle into the underlying atrial free wall may act to destabilize functional reentry by the interaction of such wave fronts with any reentrant activation front which may form in the atrial free wall. We tested this hypothesis in computer simulations using an oversimplified model in which a single pectinate muscle bundle was attached to a two-dimensional epicardial sheet. These simulations demonstrate that even a simple bridge connecting two sites on a sheet acts to destabilize reentrant vortices. We first utilized a two-dimensional sheet (80 × 80 matrix) incorporating simple Fitzhugh-Nagumo kinetics.[21] We initiated a spiral wave with S1-S2 cross field stimulation generating two perpendicular waves. This induced a spiral wave that rotated around a circular core and whose location was determined by the timing of the premature S2 wave.[20] For these parameters the spiral wave was stationary and gave rise to repetitive activation sequences.

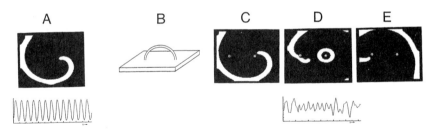

Figure 9. Computer simulations predict that a single pectinate muscle can destabilize reentry. **A**: A two-dimensional sheet of 6400 FitzHugh-Nagumo "cells"[21] underwent self-sustained and stable spiral wave activity during 13 rotations. **B**: Diagram illustrating the connection of a "pectinate muscle" to the two-dimensional sheet. **C-E**: Individual snapshots illustrating dynamics of reentry in the presence of pectinate muscle activation. Note drifting of spiral wave induced by the appearance of breakthrough (target) patterns from the pectinate muscle junctions, which results in fibrillatory activity throughout the sheet (**bottom tracing**). (Reprinted from Gray RA, Pertsov AM, Jalife J,[23] with permission from the American Heart Association, Inc.)

A snapshot of activity is shown in panel A of Figure 9 and the horizontal pseudo-ECG (shown below) exhibits a stable monomorphic pattern. After 13 rotations, the geometry of the matrix was changed by connecting a thin handle (6 cells wide, 3 cells thick) to the top of the two-dimensional grid as shown in panel B. Only the ends of the handle were attached to the grid. The conduction velocity in the handle was slightly greater than in the sheet. The right end of the handle was placed within the core region of the stationary spiral. The length of the handle was varied and therefore it was placed at various horizontal locations at the same vertical location (row) as the right end. The right end of the handle is shown in panels C-E as an asterisk and the left end is labeled as a circle. These data correspond to a simulation for a handle length of 36 cells. Panel C shows the initial position of the rotor. Since the right end of the handle was located within the silent core region, initially no activity propagated through this end. As the spiral wave rotated, however, a wave front entered the handle from its left end and then invaded the core region as a breakthrough (panel D). This acted to push the spiral wave core toward the left. This pattern of activity continued with breakthrough patterns emerging from the right end of the handle and forcing the spiral to move toward the other end. After 9 rotations, the core reached the left end and interrupted the left to right sequence of propagation in the handle (panel E). This resulted in a transient pause in activity along the handle. After one period, however, the spiral wave front activated the right end causing waves to propagate along the handle from right to left. The horizontal pseudo-ECG shown in the bottom panel exhibits a complex pattern not unlike AF. Therefore, the addition of the handle resulted in destabilization of spiral wave activity. The handle resulted in breakthrough patterns of activity that interacted with the spiral wave core and caused it to move. This movement resulted in aperiodic activity and complex spatial patterns. These results show that even a single pectinate muscle bundle can have profound effects on the dynamics of reentry. This suggests that during AF preferential propagation through the complicated pectinate muscle bundles can greatly destabilize activation sequences in the epicardium.

Summary and Conclusions

Our results can be summarized as follows:

(1) During the initiation of AF, reentrant waves often propagate around thin lines of functional block. The waves rotate completely around these lines of block. However, epicardial activation may be absent for a significant time during the rotation period, which suggests that transmural and endocardial pathways make up part of the circuit. The length of the incomplete reentrant circuits calculated from isochrone maps (3.7 cm) was shorter than the calculated wavelength (conduction velocity × action potential duration at BCL = 160 msec) in the horizontal direction (~5 cm), but slightly longer than the wavelength in the vertical direction (~3.5 cm; for coordinates see Fig. 2). Depending on the orientation of the line of block, the length of the reentrant pathway for continuous propagation to occur would range from 3.4 cm to 4.9 cm (vertical and horizontal wavelengths at BCL = 160 ms). If the head of a reentrant wave followed a path length less than this wavelength, the wave would block because the wave front would collide with tissue that was refractory. The lines of block appeared to be oriented preferentially along the pectinate muscles (Fig. 4A and B, and Fig. 6B). Therefore, the reentrant pathway was shorter than the wavelength. Furthermore, we never observed a reentrant wave propagating continuously on the epicardial surface for more than one rotation. When this wave front blocked, however, the activity did not terminate, indicating that transmural activation occurred. Rensma et al.[26] estimated the atrial wavelength of the 30 kg dog to be approximately 6–7 cm. Our value of 4 to 5 cm for the 20 kg sheep compares favorably.

(2) During AF, epicardial activation patterns were characterized

by a combination of incomplete reentry, breakthrough patterns, and collisions of waves (Fig. 5). Our recordings of AF in the sheep heart are consistent with those observed in both intact canine and human atria.[8,27] The sequences of activation on the endocardial surface of the RA free wall during AF in canines and humans show incomplete reentry similar to our recordings.[8,27] In fact, in Allessie's study,[8] only exceptional cases showed that an impulse follows the same circular route more than once.

(3) The lifetime of the individual AF wavelets recorded on the epicardium was short, and rotating waves rarely survived for more than a few hundred milliseconds. In addition, the location of breakthrough sites and the lines of block during incomplete reentry were not randomly distributed but appeared to be related to preferential propagation in the underlying subendocardial structures. Our experiments and computer simulations provide insight into these phenomena. Indeed, the experiments demonstrate that pectinate muscles provide preferential pathways for endocardial wave propagation (Fig. 8). On the other hand, the simulations suggest that breakthrough patterns in the atrial free wall are the result of pectinate muscle activation, and are responsible for destabilization of reentry (Fig. 9). Thus, it seems likely that the observation by us and others of apparently short-lived and often incomplete vortices of reentrant activity during AF is the result of the complex highly-dimensional structure of the atria, which enables discordant epicardial and endocardial activation and the appearance of multiple sites of block and breakthrough sites.

In conclusion, taken together, our experimental and modeling results provide strong support to the idea that the complicated atrial structure, particularly in regard to the highly heterogeneous network of pectinate muscles, may be responsible for destabilization of reentry and, possibly, AF. Hence, our results support the idea that traditional concepts that view the mechanisms AF in the light of two-dimensional multiple wavelet propagation need to be revisited.

References

1. Murgatroyd MA, Camm AJ. Atrial fibrillation for the clinician. In: Camm AJ, ed. Clinical Approaches to Tachyarrhythmias. Armonk, NY: Futura, 1995; Vol 4.
2. Kannel WB, Abbot RD, Savage DD, et al. Epidemiologic features of chronic atrial fibrillation: the Framingham study. N Eng J Med 1982;306: 1018–1022.
3. Pritchett EL. Management of atrial fibrillation. N Eng J Med 1992;326: 1264–1271.

4. Stroke Prevention in Atrial Fibrillation Investigators. Predictors of thromboembolism in atrial fibrillation. I. Clinical features of patients at risk. Ann Int Med 1992;116:1–5.

5. Moe GK, Abildskov JA. Atrial fibrillation as a self-sustaining arrhythmia independent of focal discharge. Am Heart J 1959;58:59–70.

6. Moe GK, Rheinboldt WC, Abildskov JA. A computer model of atrial fibrillation. Am Heart J 1964;67:200–220.

7. Moe GK. Computer simulation of cardiac arrhythmias. In: Manning GW, Ahuja SP, eds. Electrical Activity of the Heart. Springfield, IL: Charles C. Thomas; 1969.

8. Allessie MA, Lammers WEJEP, Bonke FIM, et al. Experimental evaluation of Moe's multiple wavelet hypothesis of atrial fibrillation. In: Zipes DP, Jalife J, eds. Cardiac Electrophysiology and Arrhythmias. Orlando, FL: Grune & Stratton; 1985:265–275.

9. Mines GR. On circulating excitations in heart muscle and their possible relation to tachycardia and fibrillation. Trans Roy Soc Can 1914;8:43–52.

10. Lewis T. The Mechanism and Graphic Registration of the Heart Beat. 3rd ed. London: Shaw & Sons; 1925:319–374.

11. Rosenblueth A, Garcia Ramos J. Studies on flutter and fibrillation. II. The influence of artificial obstacles on experimental auricular flutter. Am Heart J 1947;33:677–684.

12. Schuessler RB, Kawamoto T, Hand DE, et al. Simultaneous epicardial and endocardial activation sequence mapping in the isolated canine right atrium. Circulation 1993;88:250–263.

13. Spach MS, Miller WT III, Dolber PC, et al. The functional role of structural complexities in the propagation of depolarization in the atrium of the dog: cardiac conduction disturbances due to discontinuities of effective axial resistivity. Circ Res 1982;50:175–191.

14. Spach MS, Dolber PC, Anderson PAW. Multiple regional differences in cellular properties that regulate repolarization and contraction in the right atrium of adult and newborn dogs. Circ Res 1989;65:1594–1611.

15. Spach MS, Dolber PC, Heidlage JF. Interaction of inhomogeneities of repolarization with anisotropic propagation in dog atria: a mechanism for both preventing and initiating reentry. Circ Res 1989;65:1612–1631.

16. Schuessler RB, Grayson TM, Bromberg BI, et al. Cholinergically mediated tachyarrhythmias induced by a single extrastimulus in the isolated canine right atrium. Circ Res 1992;71:1254–1267.

17. Pastelin G, Mendez R, Moe GK. Participation of atrial specialized conduction pathways in atrial flutter. Circ Res 1978;42:386–393.

18. Olgin JE, Kalman JM, Fitzpatrick AP, et al. Role of right atrial endocardial structures as barriers to conduction during human type I atrial flutter: activation and entrainment guided by intracardiac echocardiography. Circulation 1995;92:1839–1848.

19. Liu Y, Cabo C, Salomonsz R, et al. Effects of diacetyl monoxime on the electrical properties of sheep and guinea pig ventricular muscle. Cardiovasc Res 1993;27:1991–1997.

20. Gray RA, Jalife J, Panfilov A, et al. Nonstationary vortexlike reentrant activity as a mechanism of polymorphic ventricular tachycardia in the isolated rabbit heart. Circulation 1995;91:2454–2469.

21. Pertsov AM, Davidenko JM, Salomonsz R, et al. Spiral waves of excitation

underlie reentrant activity in isolated cardiac muscle. Circ Res 1993;72: 631–650.

22. Davidenko JM, Pertsov AM, Salomonsz R, et al. Stationary and drifting spiral waves of excitation in isolated cardiac muscle. Nature 1991;355: 349–351.
23. Gray RA, Pertsov AM, Jalife J. Incomplete reentry and epicardial breakthrough patterns during atrial fibrillation in the sheep heart. Circulation 1996;94:2649–2661.
24. Luna LG. Manual of Histologic Staining Methods of the Armed Forces Institute of Pathology. 3rd ed. New York: McGraw-Hill; 1968:94–95.
25. Masson P. Trichrome stainings and their preliminary technique. J Tech Meth 1929;12:75–90.
26. Rensma PL, Allessie MA, Lammers WJEB, et al. The length of the excitation wave as an index for the susceptibility to reentrant atrial arrhythmias. Circ Res 1988;62:395–410.
27. Cox JL, Canavan TE, Schuessler RB, et al. The surgical treatment of atrial fibrillation. II. Intraoperative electrophysiologic mapping and description of the electrophysiologic basis of atrial flutter and atrial fibrillation. J Thorac Cardiovasc Surg 1991;101:406–426.

CHAPTER 25

Drug Cardioversion of Atrial Fibrillation

Ronald W.F. Campbell

Introduction

Atrial fibrillation (AF), while not a fatal arrhythmia, causes significant morbidity and, through its complications, death may occasionally occur. Restoration of sinus rhythm is an important clinical goal. In *paroxysmal* AF, spontaneous reversion to sinus rhythm is by definition the norm, although a variety of measures may be applied to hasten this outcome. In some patients, AF is *permanent*. For them, there is no prospect of restoring sinus rhythm and the management strategy is to control the ventricular response rate. This chapter concerns neither of these patient groups, but rather, patients with *persistent* AF. In a sizeable proportion of this group, sinus rhythm may be restored. During the last 20 years, direct current (DC) cardioversion has been the technique most used, but there is growing interest in drug cardioversion.

The Concept

Human AF is most probably based on multiple interlacing wavelets of reentry. Mapping studies[1a,b] suggest that a minimum of five or six circuits must be present to maintain the arrhythmia. Each circuit behaves as functional reentry and the circuits are not anatomically static. The principle of quenching AF by drug therapy is to reduce the number of reentrant wavelets of activity. Each wavelet has its own wavelength which is the product of the conduction velocity and the refractory period. Drugs that prolong refractoriness should increase the wavelength

Supported by the British Heart Foundation
From *Nonpharmacological Management of Atrial Fibrillation*, edited by F.D. Murgatroyd and A.J. Camm. © 1997, Futura Publishing Co., Inc., Armonk, NY.

and ake it more difficult to fit all the interlacing circuits into the avai able atrial mass. As a consequence, the number of circuits gradually decreases and sinus rhythm is restored. Drugs that have this action include sotolol and amiodarone; they have a proven track record for terminating AF. An alternative approach, in theory, is to increase conduction velocity. This, like increasing refractoriness, would enlarge the size of the reentrant circuit. In clinical practice, drugs that increase conduction velocity may be hazardous. These drugs include catecholamines which through their other effects may create a more problematic arrhythmogenic situation than the one they are being used to treat.

Drugs that slow conduction, principally the class Ic drugs, propafenone and flecainide, would not at first sight seem appropriate for cardioverting AF to sinus rhythm. In practice, however, they have been found to be among the most powerful agents for this purpose. They probably operate by dramatically increasing, or perhaps even blocking, anisotropic slow conduction as the reentrant loop crosses the cell alignment axis of the atrial myocardium. This is a particularly vulnerable part of the arrhythmia circuit. Direct mapping studies in AF, when class Ic drugs have been administered, have revealed that these drugs do indeed reduce the number of reentrant circuits.[1c] Recent evidence has shown that propafenone may also prolong refractoriness in atrial myocardium although this effect is not seen in ventricular myocardium.

An increase in refractoriness or the complete block of conduction are two pharmacological mechanisms by which AF may be terminated. In a very few patients AF may be maintained by adrenergic drive, in which case acute beta blockade may terminate the arrhythmia.

The Clinical Evidence

Many antiarrhythmic agents have been tested for the acute termination of AF (Table 1).[1-27] In general, the studies have been small, the drug dose variable, and the patients have been heterogenous. Nonetheless, some conclusions can be drawn. First, there is no evidence that either digoxin[6,9] or verapamil[12,14] can terminate AF. Second, there are few data for beta-blockers, but the data that exist suggest only a modest efficacy for sotalol.[25,26] Third, there is evidence of moderate efficacy for class Ia drugs (quinidine,[1,15,26] procainamide,[2,4]) a substantial efficacy for class Ic drugs (propafenone,[11,16,24] flecainide[5,8,10,12,23]) and a moderate utility for the class III drug, amiodarone.[6,21,22] Finally, in some studies, important arrhythmogenic reactions have occurred including torsade de pointes.[1,4,25-27]

Table 1
Success Rates for Drug Conversion of Atrial Fibrillation

Study	Year	Drug	n	% SR	% Arrhythmogenic Reaction	Comment
Sokolow	1950	quinidine	30	82	3	VT
Halpern	1980	IV procainamide	21	45	0	
Faniel	1983	IV amiodarone	26	81	0	
Fenster	1983	IV procainamide	26	58	8	nonsustained VT
Borgeat	1986	flecainide	30	67	7	conduction defects
		quinidine	30	60	0	
Cowan	1986	IV amiodarone				
		IV digoxin				
Tiovonen	1987	pirmenol	20	60	0	
		placebo	20	15	0	
Crijns	1988	IV flecainide	14	71	0	
		oral flecainide	13	77	0	
Falk	1987	digoxin	18	50	0	
		placebo	18	44	0	
Goy	1988	flexainide	69	71	0	
Bianconi	1989	propafenone	83	57	0	
Suttorp	1989	flecainide	17	82	0	
		verapamil	17	6	0	
Bertini	1990	amiodarone				
		propafenone				
Kondili	1990	IV verapamil	29	14	0	
		IV flecainide	20	50	0	
		IV propafenone	20	25	0	
McAlister	1990	IV amiodarone	40	41	—	
		oral quinidine	40	64	—	
Negrini	1990	amiodarone	78			
		propafenone	89			
Suttorp	1990	IV propafenone	20	55	0	
		IV flexcainide	20	90	0	
Carr	1991	flecainide	28	68	0	
Donovan	1991	flecainide/dig	51	57	—	
		placebo/dig	51	14	—	
Capucci	1992	flecainide	22	91	4	sinus pause
		amiodarone	19	37	0	
		placebo	21	48	0	
Horner	1992	oral amino		29	—	
		IV amino	86	64	—	
		(DC shock)		42	—	
Zehender	1992	quinidine		25	—	
		quinidine/	40	55	—	
		verapamil				
		amiodarone		60	—	
Madrid	1993	flexcainide	40	92	—	
		procainamide	40	65	—	
Capucci	1994	propafenone		62	4pts	Atrial flutter
		digoxin/quinidine		38	1pt	
		placebo		17	4pts	
Halinen	1995	sotalol	33	52	13	broad QRS tachy
		quinidine/digoxin	28	86	27	broad QRS tachy
Hohnloser	1995	sotalol	25	20	0	
		quinidine	25	60	16	3 torsade 1 VT
Sedgwick	1995	dofetilide		27	1	torsade de pointes
		placebo	16	0	—	

n = number of patients; % SR = percentage of patients restored to sinus rhythm; VT = ventricular tachycardia; pts = patients.

Quinidine

One of the earliest reports of drug conversion of AF was that of Sokolow and Edgar,[1] which described 30 patients who were given between 0.4 and 0.6 grams of quinidine every 2 hours for 10 hours. There was an 82% success rate in converting AF to sinus rhythm with quinidine levels in the range of 4–9 mg/L. This study was also interesting because a 10% adverse reaction rate was reported. Two patients had persistent vomiting and in one, ventricular tachycardia was provoked. This may be the earliest documented instance of drug arrhythmogenesis. Since then, quinidine has been used widely in clinical practice. Its role in research studies has been as a comparative agent against which new therapies have been tested. There has always been concern with quinidine syncope, but the overall safety of quinidine was not questioned until the quinidine meta-analysis of Coplen et al.[28] This study showed that on long-term quinidine therapy there was an excess mortality associated with quinidine treatment, although more quinidine-treated patients were in sinus rhythm than their placebo-treated counterparts. This work has attracted considerable attention and controversy. Quinidine is still widely used in some parts of the world for the management of AF, but there is real and growing concern about its safety.

In comparison with flecainide,[5] quinidine achieved a 60% success rate for restoring sinus rhythm versus 87% for flecainide. Twenty-seven percent of quinidine-treated patients reported adverse effects compared to only 7% treated with flecainide.

In a study comparing amiodarone and quinidine, McAlister et al.[15] recruited 80 patients with sustained atrial flutter or fibrillation post-cardiac surgery. They were treated either with amiodarone 5 mg/kg over 20 minutes intravenously or two 400 mg doses of quinidine separated by 4 hours. Sinus rhythm was restored to 64% of the quinidine-treated group versus 41% of those given amiodarone. Forty-six percent of quinidine-treated patients suffered adverse effects versus 12% of those receiving amiodarone.

In a study reported by Zehender et al.,[22] three managements were tested in 40 patients who had AF for between 4 and 200 weeks. Sinus rhythm was restored in 25% of patients who were given quinidine alone, in 55% given a combination of quinidine and verapamil, and in 60% given amiodarone.

Amiodarone

Amiodarone has been investigated widely with respect to its effects on fibrillation. In an intravenous comparison with digoxin,[6] sinus rhythm was restored more quickly in postinfarct patients suffering AF who were given amiodarone than those given a standard regimen of digoxin. By the end of 24 hours, a similar number of patients in each group were in sinus rhythm.

In another study comparing digoxin and amiodarone for managing AF postcardiac surgery, no differences in antiarrhythmic success were found, leading the authors to conclude that "amiodarone is safe and at least as effective as digoxin".[29] By 24 hours, almost all patients had returned to sinus rhythm, possibly indicating the natural history of AF that occurs following cardiac surgery.

In an observational study,[30] seven patients with AF were treated with amiodarone in a dose of 5 mg/kg over 5 minutes. None reverted to sinus rhythm but the ventricular response rate fell. In a comparison against propafenone,[16] amiodarone achieved a 78% conversion rate in a mean time of 10 hours compared to propafenone's 89% rate in a mean time of 1.7 hours.

Class Ic Drugs

Propafenone and flecainide have emerged as powerful agents for managing AF. They have an important role for drug conversion. Bertini et al.[13] compared amiodarone with propafenone in the field treatment of AF. Eighty-eight percent of patients who were given propafenone returned to sinus rhythm versus 40% given amiodarone. Restoration of sinus rhythm with propafenone was achieved in a remarkably short time (mean, 10 minutes for propafenone; 60 minutes for amiodarone).

The rapid antifibrillatory effects of propafenone were also seen in a study by Bianconi et al.[11] Eighty-three consecutive patients were given 2 mg/kg propafenone intravenously. There was a 57% success rate for conversion to sinus rhythm within a mean time of only 29 minutes. Those converting to sinus rhythm had a shorter duration of AF and tended to have smaller left atria.

In a comparison of propafenone and flecainide, Suttorp et al.[17] reported a 55% success for propafenone versus 90% for flecainide, with unwanted effects occurring in 8% and 40%, respectively. It is likely that these figures reflect the use of nonequivalent doses of the two class Ic drugs.

In another comparative study,[23] flecainide achieved conversion to sinus rhythm in 93% of patients, versus 38% for patients given procainamide. Unwanted effects occurred in 9% of those given flecainide and 2% receiving procainamide.

Flecainide was compared to placebo for drug conversion of AF by Donovan et al.[19] At 1 hour, 57% of flecainide-treated patients were in sinus rhythm compared to only 14% of placebo-treated patients. Adverse effects occurred in 22% of flecainide-treated patients and in 6% of those given placebo.

Interpretation of the Data

There can be no doubt that antiarrhythmic therapies can restore sinus rhythm for at least some patients in AF. There is evidence to support a useful clinical effect of quinidine procainamide, propafenone, flecainide, sotalol, and amiodarone. It is very difficult to establish which, if any, is the best of these agents but in terms of success and rapidity, the most impressive results have been with the class Ic agents. Most of the studies that have been performed to date have been relatively small. Many have included patients with atrial flutter as well as with AF, yet atrial flutter is a fundamentally different arrhythmia. The doses of the agents that were used and the route of administration may not have been ideal, particularly given that in many of the test situations, a relatively high rate of spontaneous conversion to sinus rhythm might have been expected. At this relatively late stage it is unlikely that definitive comparative studies will be undertaken. Clinical practice must be based on an interpretation of current evidence. With growing concerns about the toxicity of quinidine and to a lesser extent, procainamide, the optimal agents would appear to be the class Ic drugs propafenone and flecainide, the beta-blocker sotalol, and the class 3 antiarrhythmic drug, amiodarone. The specific identification of sotalol owes much to its use in clinical research. Ordinary beta-blockers have not been tested in the same way. Thus, it remains uncertain whether sotalol has any special antiarrhythmic advantage over a conventional beta-blocker.

The Benefits of Medical Cardioversion

Medical cardioversion is not uncommon but is often not a planned outcome. Many patients receive antiarrhythmic drugs while they are being treated with anticoagulants pending their later admission for DC cardioversion. A proportion, on returning to the hospital for the DC shock, are found to have "spontaneously" or drug-converted to sinus rhythm. It would be reasonable to have the same concerns about thromboembolism with medical cardioversion as with DC cardioversion but the anticoagulant strategy is by necessity different. When a patient presents in sustained AF and has been in the arrhythmia for some time, immediate management is necessary. It would seem perverse to consider prescribing drugs that only control the ventricular response rate and maintain AF. Such treatment would perhaps allay fear of thromboembolism before warfarin has had its time to act and, in fact, this may be what is achieved by the prescription of digoxin to these patients. When rate control is offered by the Ic drugs, by sotalol or amiodarone, medical conversion is a distinct possibility and this may occur at a relatively early point in the anticoagulation strategy.

There is no evidence to suggest that thromboembolism is less common with medical cardioversion than with DC cardioversion yet the literature is full of reports of this complication associated with DC shocks, while there are relatively few reported instances of thromboembolism with medical conversion. It is biologically plausible that medical cardioversion might be the safer option. If this was proved to be true, it would have considerable importance and would change current medical practice. The evidence supporting this possibility would be gained from registries rather than from randomized controlled studies.

Another advantage of drug cardioversion is that successful drug intervention identifies an agent that is likely to be of value in the future, and which could be used by the patients themselves in the event of an occurrence. This may be an attractive prescribing strategy for those whose events are relatively infrequent.

A final consideration for medical therapy is the speed with which sinus rhythm can be restored, particularly if the patient has ready access to therapy. Allessie et al.[31] have suggested that "atrial fibrillation begets atrial fibrillation". The longer the atrial myocardium fibrillates, the more it undergoes electrophysiological change, which maintains the arrhythmia. Atrial refractory periods shorten quite rapidly. Early medical restoration of sinus rhythm could prevent the deleterious electrophysiological remodeling that occurs with AF.

Conclusions

Medical conversion of AF is a real and reliable prospect with currently available antiarrhythmic drugs. As yet, comprehensive management plans employing this strategy have not been developed, but there are many reasons for this to happen.

References

1. Sokolow M, Edgar AL. Blood quinidine concentrations as a guide in the treatment of cardiac arrhythmias. Circulation 1950;1:576–592.
1a. Smeets JLRM, Allessie MA, Lammers WJEP, et al. The wavelength of the cardiac impulse and reentrant arrhythmias in isolate rabbit atrium. Circ Res 1986;58:96–108.
1b. Cox JL, Schuessler RB, Cain ME, et al. Surgery for atrial fibrillation. In: Cox JL, ed. Seminars in Thoracic and Cardiovascular Surgery. Philadelphia: Harcourt Brace Jovanovitch, Inc; 1989:67–73.
1c. Wang Z, Pagé P, Nattel S. Mechanism of flecainide's antiarrhythmic action in experimental atrial fibrillation. Circ Res 1991;71:271–287.
2. Halpern SW, Ellrodt G, Singh BN, Mandel WJ. Efficacy of intravenous procainamide infusion in converting atrial fibrillation to sinus rhythm: relation to left atrial size. Br Heart J 1980;44(5):589–595.
3. Faniel R, Schoenfeld P. Efficacy of IV amiodarone in converting rapid atrial fibrillation and flutter to sinus rhythm in intensive care patients. Eur Heart J 1983;4(3):180–185.
4. Fenster PE, Comess KA, Marsh R, et al. Conversion of atrial fibrillation to sinus rhythm by acute intravenous procainamide infusion. Am Heart J 1983;106(3):501–504.
5. Borgeat A, Goy JJ, Maendly R, et al. Flecainide versus quinidine for conversion of atrial fibrillation to sinus rhythm. Am J Cardiol 1986;58:496–498.
6. Cowan C, Gardiner P, Reid DS, et al. A comparison of amiodarone and digoxin in the treatment of atrial fibrillation complicating suspected acute myocardial infarction. J Cardiovasc Pharmacol 1986;8(2):252–256.
7. Toivonen LK, Nieminen MS, Manninen V, Frick H. Conversion of paroxysmal atrial fibrillation to sinus rhythm by intravenous pirmenol. Am J Cardiol 1987;59(16):39H-42H.
8. Crijns HJ, van Wijk LM, van Gilst WH, et al. Acute conversion of atrial fibrillation to sinus rhythm: clinical efficacy of flecainide acetate. Comparison of two regimens. Eur Heart J 1988;9(6):634–638.
9. Falk RH, Knowlton AA, Bernard SA, et al. Digoxin for converting recent onset atrial fibrillation to sinus rhythm: a randomized, double-blinded trial. Ann Int Med 1987;106(4):503–506.
10. Goy JJ, Kaufmann U, Kappenberger L, Sigwart U. Restoration of sinus rhythm with flecainide in patients with atrial fibrillation. Am J Cardiol 1988;62(6):38D-40D.
11. Bianconi L, Boccadamo R, Pappalardo A, et al. Effectiveness of intravenous propafenone for conversion of atrial fibrillation and flutter of recent onset. Am J Cardiol 1989;64:335–338.
12. Suttorp MJ, Kingma JH, Lie AHL, Mast EG. Intravenous flecainide versus verapamil for acute conversion of paroxysmal atrial fibrillation or flutter to sinus rhythm. Am J Cardiol 1989;63(11):693–696.
13. Bertini G, Conti A, Fradella G, et al. Propafenone versus amiodarone in

field treatment of primary atrial tachydysrhythmias. J Emerg Med 1990; 8(1):15–20.

14. Kondili A, Kastrati A, Popa Y. Comparative evaluation of verapamil, flecainide and propafenone for the acute conversion of atrial fibrillation to sinus rhythm. Weiner Klinische Wochenschrift 1990;102(17):510–513.

15. McAlister HF, Luke RA, Whitlock RM, Smith WM. Intravenous amiodarone bolus versus oral quinidine for atrial flutter and fibrillation after cardiac operations. J Thorac Cardiovasc Surg 1990;99(5):911–918.

16. Negrini M, Gibelli G, De Ponti C. Comparison of amiodarone and quinidine in the conversion to sinus rhythm of atrial fibrillation of recent onset. Giornale Italiano di Cardiologia 1990;20(3):207–214.

17. Suttorp MJ, Kingma JH, Jessurun ER, et al. The value of class Ic antiarrhythmic drugs for acute conversion of paroxysmal atrial fibrillation or flutter to sinus rhythm. J Am Coll Cardiol 1990;16:1722–1727.

18. Carr B, Hawley K, Channer KS. Cardioversion of atrial fibrillation of recent onset with flecainide. Postgrad Med J 1991;67(789):659–662.

19. Donovan KD, Dobb GJ, Coombs LJ, et al. Reversion of recent onset atrial fibrillation to sinus rhythm by intravenous flecainide. Am J Cardiol 1991; 67(2):137–141.

20. Capucci A, Lenzi T, Boriani G, et al. Effectiveness of loading oral flecainide for converting recent onset atrial fibrillation to sinus rhythm in patients without organic heart disease or with only systemic hypertension. Am J Cardiol 1992;70(1):69–72.

21. Homer SM. A comparison of cardioversion of atrial fibrillation using oral amiodarone intravenous amiodarone and DC cardioversion. Acta Cardiologica 1992;47(5):473–480.

22. Zehender M, Hohnloser S, Muller B, et al. Effects of amiodarone versus quinidine and verapamil in patients with chronic atrial fibrillation: results of a comparative study and a 2-year follow up. J Am Coll Cardiol 1992; 19(5):1054–1059.

23. Madrid AH, Moro C, Marin-Huerta E, et al. Comparison of flecainide and procainamide in cardioversion of atrial fibrillation. Eur Heart J 1993;14(8): 1127–1131.

24. Capucci A, Boriani G, Rubino I, et al. A controlled study on oral propafenone versus digoxin plus quinidine in converting recent onset atrial fibrillation to sinus rhythm. Int J Cardiol 1994;43(3):305–313.

25. Halinen MO, Huttunen M, Paakkinen S, Tarssanen L. Comparison of sotalol with digoxin-quinidine for conversion of acute atrial fibrillation to sinus rhythm (the Sotalol-Digoxin-Quinidine Trial). Am J Cardiol 1995;76(7): 495–498.

26. Hohnloser SH, van de Loo A, Baedeker F. Efficacy and proarrhythmic hazards of pharmacologic cardioversion of atrial fibrillation: prospective comparison of sotalol versus quinidine. J Am Coll Cardiol 1995;26(4):852–858.

27. Sedgwick ML, Lip G, Rae AP, Cobbe SM. Chemical cardioversion of atrial fibrillation with intravenous dofetilide. Int J Cardiol 1995;49(2):159–166.

28. Coplen SE, Antmann EM, Berlin JA, et al. Efficacy and safety of quinidine therapy for maintenance of sinus rhythm after cardioversion: a meta-analysis of randomized control trials. Circulation 1990;82:1106–1116.

29. Cochrane Ad, Siddins M, Rosenfeldt FL, et al. A comparison of amiodarone

and digoxin for treatment of supraventricular arrhythmias after cardiac surgery. Eur J Cardio Thorac Surg 1994;8(4):194–198.

30. Holt P, Crick JC, Davies DW, Curry P. Intravenous amiodarone in the acute termination of supraventricular arrhythmias. Int J Cardiol 1985; 8(1):67–79.

31. Allessie MA, Janse MJ. Atrial fibrillation: is our electrophysiological understanding on the right wavelength? In: Campbell RWF, Janse MJ, eds. Cardiac Arrhythmias: The Management of Atrial Fibrillation. Berlin: Springer-Verlag; 1992:17–26.

CHAPTER 26

Cardioversion and the Risk of Thromboembolism:

Is Cardioversion Thrombogenic?

Richard A. Grimm

Introduction

The risk of thromboembolism following the cardioversion of atrial fibrillation (AF) has been well documented in the literature ever since the initial report by Goldman in 1960 in a large series of patients undergoing chemical cardioversion.[1] However, the presumed mechanistic etiology of cardioversion-related thromboembolism has been speculative at best and poorly investigated. Renewed interest in this subject has been prompted by several factors. These include a widespread resurgence of interest in AF, and a realization that an investigation of fundamental mechanistic data on cardiac chamber thrombogenesis can significantly impact on the advancement of anticoagulation strategies, as well as the development of nonconventional therapeutic approaches to AF such as catheter ablative techniques, implantable defibrillators, and surgical techniques (i.e., the Maze procedure). The presumed cause of stroke following cardioversion was traditionally believed to be the dislodgement of preexisting thrombus with the return of a more forceful atrial contraction following conversion to sinus rhythm.[1] However, this mechanism has never been formally investigated. Recent investigation has unveiled an alternative mechanism which is independent of the presence of preexisting thrombus and suggests that thrombogenesis can occur early following cardioversion and is secondary to left atrial appendage stunning.[2] These observations, along with further advancements in our understanding of thrombogen-

From *Nonpharmacological Management of Atrial Fibrillation*, edited by F.D. Murgatroyd and A.J. Camm. © 1997, Futura Publishing Co., Inc., Armonk, NY.

esis and embolism associated with cardioversion of AF, will have a profound impact on anticoagulation recommendations as well as new technological advances for the treatment and prevention of AF. This chapter will briefly review the historical literature that pertains to the phenomenon of cardioversion-related thrombogenesis and embolism. It will also focus on the rapidly growing scientific literature of recent years which has provided significant, and sometimes surprising, insights into the mechanisms responsible for cardioversion-related embolism as well as their implications for therapy.

Historical Perspective

The literature is replete with studies that highlight the embolic risk following the cardioversion of AF; this risk has ranged from a low of 0.6% to a high of 5.6%.[3] In 1960, Goldman reported the first large series of patients undergoing cardioversion with a 1.5% incidence of thromboembolic events in 400 chemical cardioversions without prior anticoagulation.[1] Subsequently, Lown et al. reported a 1.7% incidence in 50 electrical cardioversions with patients who had mitral stenosis and were receiving anticoagulation.[4] Lown[5] later reported the results of the largest series to date undergoing electrical cardioversion of AF (n = 350) and found a 0.9% incidence of embolism in a patient population in which only 29% were on anticoagulants. Embolic events occurred only in those not receiving warfarin. In 1969, Bjerkelund and Orning[6] reported the results of a prospective study comparing chronic anticoagulant prophylaxis with no prophylaxis in 437 patients undergoing electrical cardioversion for atrial arrhythmias. The incidence of systemic embolization in the chronically anticoagulated group was only 0.8%, whereas the incidence in the nonanticoagulated group was 5.3% despite the greater number of patients at increased embolic risk (congestive heart failure, cardiomegaly, prior embolism) in the anticoagulated group. In a recent study, which retrospectively analyzed 454 elective electrical cardioversions performed for AF or flutter, Arnold et al.[7] reported an incidence of embolic complications of 1.3%. All six embolic events that were described occurred in patients with AF and none of the six were on anticoagulants at the time of the cardioversion. Interestingly, two of the cases of embolism occurred among a group of 115 patients whose AF developed postoperatively.

Recommendations for anticoagulation management in patients undergoing cardioversion of AF have been based largely upon the findings of these studies and many others which have demonstrated the apparent risk of cardioversion-related stroke.[8] This recommendation, as published by the American College of Chest Physicians, states that all patients with AF of greater than 2 days' duration should be placed on warfarin for 3 weeks prior to cardioversion, and 4 weeks following cardioversion, until sinus rhythm has been maintained.

Clearly, these studies, as well as others, have confirmed the association between systemic embolization and cardioversion. However, aside from the suggestion by Goldman that preexisting thrombus was responsible for these rarely occurring thromboembolic events, no investigation of this hypothesis has ever been performed and several observations from the plethora of clinical studies makes one suspicious of the validity of this hypothesis. Historical evidence that is inconsistent with the hypothesis of preexisting thrombi becoming dislodged following conversion to sinus rhythm includes: the occurrence of systemic embolic events in patients with AF of short duration,[9] the occurrence of events within hours or days of the procedure,[6,9,10] and the strong likelihood that it is a freshly formed thrombus that breaks off and embolizes with resultant stroke, peripheral ischemia, or pulmonary embolus.[11] Additionally, Petersen and colleagues have reported that patients with paroxysmal AF had half the incidence of thromboembolic events than those with chronic AF, suggesting that the repeated conversion back and forth from AF to sinus rhythm is not particularly ominous.[12] Finally, echocardiographic studies in patients with AF would imply that most atrial thrombi that exist in these patients do not embolize. The incidence of left atrial thrombi in patients with AF is approximately 10%[13–15] with an incidence of systemic embolization in patients undergoing cardioversion of 1.5–2.0%; therefore, based upon these numbers, 80–85% of thrombi do not result in embolization, or are clinically silent.

Mechanisms of Thromboembolism in Atrial Fibrillation

Our present understanding of the mechanisms involved in thrombogenesis and thromboembolism in AF is rather limited, yet significant strides toward a better understanding of the pathogenesis have been made.[16] Thrombus formation in cardiac chambers during AF is thought to result from Virchows' triad of endocardial injury, stasis of flow, and a hypercoagulable state. Blood stasis and reduced flow intuitively seem to be of utmost importance in the development of thrombus in patients with AF due to impaired atrial activity, as has been proposed by Shrestha and colleagues.[17] Low shear rates in the atrial cavity may lead to increased erythrocyte aggregation and blood viscosity with resultant activation of the coagulation factors and fibrin formation.[18] Erythrocyte aggregation may manifest as spontaneous contrast detectable by echocardiography.[19] Evidence for a hypercoagulable state being present in patients with AF has been scant; however, several investigations have suggested that increased fibrinogen, D-Dimer, and fibrinopeptide-A levels are present along with lower antithrombin III levels.[20-22] Endocardial injury in AF may arise in the form of stretch in the atrial wall with resultant separation of endothelial cells from their basal lamina. Subsequent exposure of subendothelial tissue to intracavitary blood may then serve as a nidus for thrombosis, as is thought to occur in myocardial infarction, with leukocyte infiltration as opposed to myocardial stretch being the triggering event.[23] This mechanism however, has not been demonstrated in AF.

The mechanism of systemic embolization in AF is even less well understood than the process of thrombogenesis. Insight into this problem may be gained by comparing the sequelae of left ventricular thrombi in patients with ventricular aneurysms versus those with thrombi associated with a dilated cardiomyopathy. Fuster et al.[24] suggested that because the thrombus is isolated from the dynamic factors of the circulation in patients with ventricular aneurysms, these thrombi are less likely to embolize than those associated with a dilated cardiomyopathy and this may account for the lower embolic risk observed in these patients. Furthermore, it has been proposed that left atrial appendage thrombi may be analogous to thrombi within ventricular aneurysms (as far as being isolated from the dynamic forces of the circulation) since only a relatively small proportion of atrial appendage thrombi embolize.[17,24] The difference between the two conditions however, is that the left atrial appendage is a contractile structure even in AF,[25] whereas the aneurysm, of course, is not. Therefore, in the case of the left atrial appendage, thrombi may or may not be exposed to the dynamic forces of the circulation. Clearly, further investigation is needed to clarify these issues.

Mechanisms of Cardioversion-Related Stroke

Earlier in this decade, efforts to unravel the etiology of cardioversion-associated thromboembolism began with the recognition that the left atrial appendage was the primary determinant in atrial thrombogenesis. Most atrial thrombi reside within this structure,[17] and the

advent of transesophageal echocardiography (TEE) allowed high resolution interrogation of the left atrial appendage. In an attempt to gain
insights into the etiology for cardioversion-related stroke, we chose to
investigate the pericardioversion period by interrogating atrial structure and function with transesophageal echocardiography.[3] Twenty patients were studied who were successfully cardioverted electrically and
underwent TEE immediately prior to, as well as immediately following,
cardioversion. Left atrial appendage function was evaluated by pulsed
Doppler echo and the presence or absence of spontaneous echo contrast
and thrombus was assessed. This study revealed three main observations. First, organized left atrial appendage function returned in 80% of
patients immediately following cardioversion. Second, peak left atrial
appendage fibrillatory emptying velocities precardioversion were significantly greater than peak left atrial appendage late diastolic emptying velocities postcardioversion (Fig. 1). Third, left atrial and left atrial
appendage spontaneous echo contrast was found to develop or intensify
immediately postcardioversion in 35% of patients (Fig. 2). None of the
patients suffered an embolic event; however, most were anticoagulated

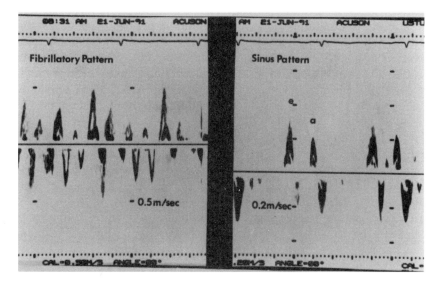

Figure 1. Pulsed Doppler echo of the left atrial appendage immediately before
(**left**) and after (**right**) successful electrical cardioversion, demonstrating that
peak emptying velocities precardioversion while in AF are significantly greater
than peak emptying velocities postcardioversion while in sinus rhythm. (Reproduced with permission from Grimm et al.[16])

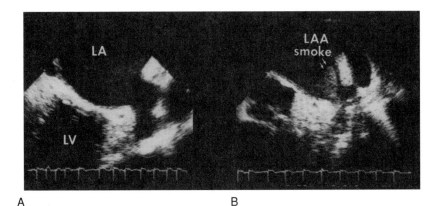

Figure 2. Left atrial appendage pre- (**A**) and postcardioversion (**B**) showing a very mild degree of smoke in the left atrium (LA) and left atrial appendage (LAA) precardioversion, with an increase in the intensity of smoke in the left atrial appendage postcardioversion. (Reproduced with permission from Grimm et al.[3])

at the time of the procedure. Therefore, left atrial appendage function was found to be stunned or impaired and spontaneous echo contrast intensified immediately postcardioversion, as compared to precardioversion, suggesting that a thrombogenic milieu was created. These data implied that postcardioversion thrombogenesis may occur without preexisting thrombus (precardioversion while in AF), thus providing an alternative theory to that of Goldman[1] for the pathogenesis of thromboembolism after cardioversion.

Subsequent to this initial observation of left atrial appendage stunning, other investigators[26] reported similar findings of increased spontaneous echo contrast following electrical cardioversion of 16 patients in whom TEE was also performed before and after the procedure. Left atrial cavity fractional shortening was measured (as opposed to left atrial appendage function) and found to be reduced when compared to normal subjects. Hence, the increase in spontaneous echo contrast that was reported was an indirect indication of the phenomenon of atrial stunning following cardioversion as left atrial cavity fractional shortening was not measured prior to cardioversion, and therefore only the spontaneous contrast assessment provides a before and after comparison. Nonetheless this study confirmed our initial observations in an independent study group. Although historical clinical observations were consistent with the hypothesis of left atrial appendage stunning resulting in thrombogenesis, the fact that all of our patients were on anticoagulants at the time of the procedure precluded thromboembolic events and, therefore, precluded a cause and effect relationship as well. Coincidentally, however, isolated cases of thromboembolic events despite a negative TEE for thrombus began appearing in the literature.

Black et al.[27] compiled a series of 17 such cases of thromboembolic events following a negative TEE examination for thrombus and questioned the utility of TEE for obviating the need for anticoagulation after cardioversion. Importantly, all of these patients suffered events relatively early following cardioversion and all were subtherapeutically anticoagulated. At the time of the embolic event, three patients had AF of <7 days duration. This series, therefore, dispelled many conventional beliefs including: (1) that TEE can preclude the need for anticoagulation; (2) that events occur in patients with long duration AF; and 3) that events occur secondarily to preexisting thrombus. More importantly, however, this report provided support for the theory of thrombogenesis and embolism following cardioversion secondary to left atrial appendage stunning.

The observation of left atrial appendage stunning in patients undergoing direct current countershock raises several intriguing issues relative to its clinical implications. These include: the role of atrial appendage stunning in patients with atrial flutter; the role of electrical energy in the stunning phenomenon; the effect of antiarrhythmic agents on left atrial appendage function pre- and postcardioversion; and finally, the question of duration of the atrial appendage stunning phenomenon. Although definitive studies designed to answer many of these questions are ongoing, recent observations and investigations may provide insights into several of these issues.

Left Atrial Appendage Stunning in Atrial Flutter

Once the phenomenon of left atrial appendage stunning was identified as a potential cause of thromboembolic events, a logical extension of the study was to investigate patients with atrial flutter. It is widely believed that patients with atrial flutter are less susceptible to embolic complications of cardioversion than those with AF. Yet, despite the low event rate, thromboembolic events have been reported.[28] A longstanding weakness of previous studies on atrial flutter has been small sample size. However, this limitation in our understanding of this population is being rectified by a renewed interest in atrial flutter, which is unveiling rather unexpected results. A report from Bikkina and colleagues[29] found a surprisingly high incidence of thrombus in 24 consecutive hospitalized patients with atrial flutter. Intra-atrial thrombus was detected by transesophageal echocardiography in 21% (5/24) of patients with atrial flutter versus 3% (6/184) in a control group. Therefore, it would appear from this isolated report that the potential for thrombogenesis in atrial flutter may have been underestimated in the past.

The key to a better understanding of embolic risk in patients with atrial flutter is an understanding of the mechanisms involved in thromboembolism. Some investigators have suggested that this is the result of a more synchronous atrial activity while in atrial flutter;[8] however, the mechanism of this reduced embolic risk has not been explored. A similar mechanism for thromboembolic events, as has previously been described in patients with AF,[3,26] seems likely in patients with atrial flutter. In an effort to test this hypothesis, we studied left atrial appendage function before and after cardioversion in a group of patients with atrial flutter and compared the results to those with AF using transesophageal Doppler echocardiography.[30] This investigation demonstrated that, following cardioversion, left atrial appendage flow velocities decreased in comparison to precardioversion velocities in patients with AF as well as in those with atrial flutter (Fig. 3). This decrease in flow velocity from pre- to postcardioversion occurred in 82% of patients with AF and 74% of patients in atrial flutter. These results provide the first mechanistic support for historical data that suggests that patients with atrial flutter are less likely (yet still prone) to experience

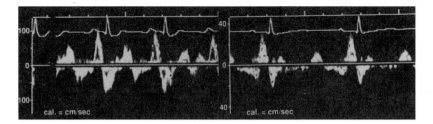

Figure 3. Representative left atrial appendage pulsed Doppler flows illustrating the "stunning" phenomenon following electrical cardioversion in a patient with atrial flutter. Left atrial appendage flow in atrial flutter before cardioversion (**left**) with "flutter waves" on the ECG tracing preceding each forward and reverse Doppler flow, and left atrial appendage flow in sinus rhythm following cardioversion (**right**) with a p-wave preceding the late diastolic forward and reverse flow. (Reproduced with permission from Grimm et al.[30])

thromboembolic complications following cardioversion than those in AF. These data suggest that the potential for the development of a thrombogenic milieu does exist in patients with atrial flutter as a result of left atrial appendage stunning and, therefore, these patients should not be considered risk free for thromboembolic events following cardioversion. Furthermore, anticoagulation for even a short duration around the time of cardioversion would seem prudent for all patients with atrial flutter in view of these results, or until further data are available for better risk stratification of patients, either by clinical or echocardiographic parameters or by detailed interrogation of left atrial function relative to its thromboembolic potential.

Is Electrical Energy Causing Atrial Stunning?

The debate over whether electrical cardioversion has any untoward myocardial effects has loomed in the literature for many years[31,32] with little significance or clinical effect ever having been proven. However, the recent reports of left atrial appendage stunning have fueled the controversy. Despite the views of some investigators suggesting that this stunning effect is due to the electrical energy applied, most of the data argue otherwise. Fatkin and co-workers[26] found an association between the number of electrical shocks applied, as well as a higher mean energy shock level, and the development of new or increased spontaneous echo contrast. In our original study of 20 patients with AF, who underwent complete echocardiographic assessment for the presence of spontaneous echo contrast as well as an evaluation of left atrial appendage function before and following cardioversion, a relationship was not observed between the presence of increased spontaneous echo contrast after cardioversion and the amount of electrical energy or number of shocks applied. Additionally, we did not demonstrate a correlation between decreased left atrial appendage flow velocity postcardioversion and electrical energy. Furthermore, this lack of correlation between electrical energy and/or number of shocks with atrial appendage stunning held up when the original analysis on a sample size of 20 was extended to 63 patients in a follow up study.[30] More recently, investigators examined left atrial appendage function before and after several ineffective attempts at electrical cardioversion. Sixteen patients were studied with TEE, seven of which were successfully converted to sinus rhythm, while nine patients were unsuccessfully cardioverted. These investigators reported no decrease in left atrial appendage emptying velocity or increase in spontaneous echo contrast following ineffective electrical shocks. A decrease in left atrial appendage emptying velocity was observed, however, when patients were successfully converted to sinus rhythm, which was consistent with left atrial appendage stunning.[33]

Additional evidence from the observations reported during two independent cases of spontaneous conversion from AF and atrial flutter to normal sinus rhythm during a transesophageal echocardiographic procedure appears to exonerate electrical energy as the culprit responsible for the atrial appendage stunning phenomenon.[34] One patient with AF of 2 weeks duration spontaneously converted to sinus rhythm during the TEE procedure performed prior to an intended cardioversion (Fig. 4). Left atrial appendage flow velocities prior to spontaneous conversion measured 0.56 m/sec while emptying velocities following the conversion to sinus rhythm measured 0.25 m/sec. Of note, an increase in the intensity of left atrial spontaneous echo contrast was also observed

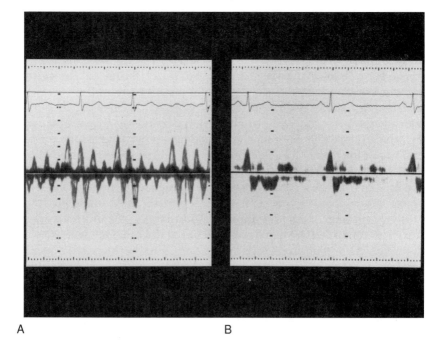

A   B

Figure 4. Pulsed Doppler flow profiles from a patient while in AF (**A**) and in sinus rhythm (**B**) immediately following spontaneous conversion. Peak emptying flow velocities were greater in AF than in sinus rhythm (Reproduced with permission from Grimm et al.[34])

following cardioversion. In a subsequent case of a 68-year-old male with atrial flutter of 4 days duration following open heart surgery, flow velocities in the left atrial appendage averaged 0.67 m/sec before, and 0.4 m/sec after, spontaneous conversion. The results of these two case studies demonstrate that worsening left atrial appendage function occurs following *spontaneous* conversion from AF and flutter to sinus rhythm, independent of electrical or chemical therapeutic interventions. Moreover, spontaneous echo contrast can intensify following spontaneous conversion from AF to sinus rhythm, again without the interference of electrical or chemical intervention. Therefore, it appears as though the mere conversion to sinus rhythm may be sufficient to predispose the left atrial appendage to thrombogenesis and embolism. The precise etiologic mechanism underlying this impaired atrial appendage function following spontaneous conversion to sinus rhythm, however, is unclear.

The clinical implications of these isolated case studies are pertinent to the embolic risk associated with cardioversion of AF as well as the embolic risk attributed to acute, chronic, and paroxysmal AF. Electrical cardioversion should not be rejected due to a concern for potentially "causing" left atrial appendage stunning which may in turn place the patient at increased risk for stroke following the procedure. Additionally, it is unlikely that pharmacological cardioversion has any more or less of an effect on left atrial appendage function than electrical cardioversion. Therefore, all patients undergoing cardioversion of atrial arrhythmias (whether chemical or electrical) should be considered at equivalent risk for the development of postcardioversion thromboembolism, and similar anticoagulation strategies should be employed regardless of the modality of cardioversion. Clinical studies support this contention as a similar incidence of thromboembolic complications has been reported following chemical as well as electrical cardioversion.[2]

Chemical Versus Electrical Cardioversion

Historical data clearly implicate chemical as well as electrical cardioversion as equal triggers for thromboembolic events in patients undergoing cardioversion.[1,2] However, the mechanism involved in the provocation of events by antiarrhythmic drugs is less clear. Currently, few reports exist in the literature that compare the relative effects of chemical cardioversion with electrical cardioversion, and those that have been reported either exhibit significant limitations or have studied too few patients to draw definitive conclusions. Manning and colleagues[35] compared chemically cardioverted patients with those electrically cardioverted by examining atrial function as assessed via Doppler interrogation of mitral inflow in 33 patients at 2 hours, 24 hours, and 7 days following cardioversion. They concluded that recovery of atrial mechanical function is related to the mode of cardioversion, as a more prompt return of atrial function was seen in the group that was chemically converted. Because of the lack of randomization to treatment arms as well as the design of the study, which first employed an attempt at conversion with procainamide or quinidine followed by electrical cardioversion if chemical conversion failed, this study is seriously flawed. This study simply demonstrated that patients successfully cardioverted with antiarrhythmic agents had "healthier atria" and, therefore, less severe dysfunction following the conversion. Hence, inherent in the study design was a bias against direct current cardioversion, as electrically cardioverted patients were more likely to have sicker atria and, therefore, a more prolonged recovery of function compared to chemically cardioverted patients. In fact, those in the electrically cardioverted group had significanly larger atria, were older, and had a longer duration of AF.

A small series, recently reported in abstract form, evaluated left atrial appendage function before and after chemical cardioversion with procainamide, and compared atrial appendage flow velocities as a parameter of atrial function.[36] In this series, the authors found that a decrease in left atrial appendage flow velocities occurred in three patients converted chemically, as well as in the comparison group of five patients converted by electrical countershock. This study (although limited by a small number of observations) would appear more in line with the data from our laboratory,[34] which suggests that the mere conversion to sinus rhythm is sufficient to result in left atrial appendage stunning, independent of the mode of cardioversion selected. Additional, and more scientifically rigorous, investigation will be required to definitively answer this important question.

Recovery of Atrial Function Following Cardioversion

Clearly, left atrial appendage stunning can result in the immediate aftermath of conversion to sinus rhythm and, therefore, the potential for thrombogenesis is real. A more important issue, however, may be the duration of this stunning phenomenon, and therefore, the duration of this thrombogenic potential and subsequent need for anticoagulant prophylaxis. Most studies to date have observed and described the stunning phenomenon solely in the immediate postcardioversion period. Unfortunately, there are few data which describe the progression and time period of subsequent return of atrial function to normal levels. Manning and colleagues[37] have demonstrated that *atrial cavity* function as assessed by transthoracic echo Doppler interogation of mitral inflow and mitral A waves returns to normal levels by 3–4 weeks after cardioversion. Hence, the recommendations are for 4 weeks of anticoagulation following the procedure.[8] In a subsequent study, this same group of investigators demonstrated that the extent of impaired left atrial mechanical dysfunction is related to the duration of AF.[38] They found that full atrial mechanical recovery of function is achieved within 24 hours in brief AF, within 1 week in patients with moderate duration AF, and within 1 month in patients with prolonged AF as determined by mitral A wave analysis postcardioversion. *Left atrial cavity* function, however, is not always equivalent to left atrial appendage function (unpublished data) and, therefore, not necessarily representative of the primary factor responsible for thrombogenesis and embolism, as the left atrial appendage is where the majority of thrombi reside. The function of the main left atrial cavity (as opposed to the atrial appendage) has been implicated in playing a role in thrombogenesis postcardioversion, yet the data are less convincing than those described for the left atrial appendage. In addition to the delay in return of normal left *atrial* activity, which occurs in the majority of patients as assessed by Doppler interrogation of mitral inflows, left atrial mechanical asystole occurs in only a small minority of patients immediately after electrical cardioversion of AF.[39-41] Although some investigators have implied that this early absence of atrial mechanical activity may predispose patients to late embolic events postcardioversion[37,39]; O'Neil et al.[42] have reported an embolic event in a patient with immediate and "vigorous" return of atrial contraction following electrical cardioversion as assessed by Doppler evaluation of mitral inflow. In contrast to the atrial cavity, where effective contraction almost always improves from pre- to postcardioversion (going from no effective contraction pre-, to attenuated contraction postcardioverion), effective contraction in the left atrial appendage is usually reduced.

Preliminary data from our laboratory would suggest that a spectrum of functional recovery of the left atrial appendage exists depending on severity of atrial dysfunction, left atrial size, AF duration, and underlying structural heart disease. This hypothesis would be at least partly supported by recently published data in a canine AF model. Louie et al.[43] studied the return of left atrial appendage function after spontaneous reversion to sinus rhythm in 10 dogs with 60 minutes of rapid-pacing induced AF. Sinus rhythm returned within 1–5 minutes of termination of rapid pacing in all cases, and although left atrial appendage velocities were initially depressed by as much as 50 ± 23% compared to pre-AF velocities, left atrial appendage function returned to baseline values within 40 minutes of conversion. These data imply that recovery of left atrial appendage impairment may be a function of the duration of AF. Certainly, further investigation into this area is imperative for the understanding of atrial cavity thrombogenesis and embolism, with significant implications for anticoagulant therapy following cardioversion for patients with paroxysmal AF, and for future developments in this arena, such as internal defibrillator use.

Clinical Implications

The primary implication resulting from an improved understanding of atrial thrombogenesis and embolism following cardioversion is in regard to anticoagulation management. Significant interest in a TEE-guided anticoagulation management strategy has been generated; it is believed that such an approach can enable earlier cardioversion while at the same time allowing a safer procedure to be performed.[3,14,16] The theoretical basis for this strategy addresses both potential thromboembolic mechanisms, including those proposed by Goldman[1] involving preexisting thrombus in the left atrium or atrial appendage, and a second mechanism that involves worsening left atrial appendage function and thrombogenesis postcardioversion.[3] This echo-guided strategy employs TEE to address the preexisting thrombus mechanism and therapeutic anticoagulation at the time of the index procedure and 4 weeks thereafter to address the postcardioversion thromboembolic mechanism (Fig. 5). By identifying patients with left atrial or left atrial appendage thrombus prior to cardioversion, the procedure can be postponed so as to allow at least 6 weeks of anticoagulation for stabilization of the thrombus. In addition, antithrombotic therapy at the time of the TEE and for 4 weeks following the cardioversion is an integral part of this anticoagulation management strategy, as the potential for thrombogenesis early postcardioversion should be eliminated. It is important to recognize, however, that although the TEE-guided anticoagulation management strategy is thought to be more efficacious, more convenient, and enables earlier cardioversion, the conventional strategy of 3 weeks of warfarin precardioversion, followed by 4 weeks postcardioversion, remains a very viable and effective anticoagulation management strategy. The Assessment of Cardioversion Using Transesophageal

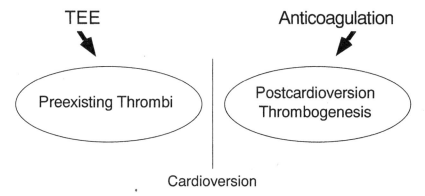

Figure 5. The rationale for a TEE-guided anticoagulation management strategy for patients with atrial fibrillation undergoing cardioversion.

Echocardiography Trial (ACUTE) is a multicenter clinical trial, currently in progress, which is randomizing patients with AF and flutter to either a TEE-guided approach or conventional anticoagulation management, with the stated purpose of clarifying the relative benefits of both strategies.[44] Other clinical implications emerging from a greater insight into mechanisms of atrial thrombogenesis and embolism will involve improved risk stratification and further anticoagulation management modifications for patients in AF and flutter, as well as for those undergoing therapeutic procedures such as external and internal electrical cardioversion, chemical cardioversion, catheter ablation, and surgical procedures (e.g., the MAZE procedure).

Conclusion

The theory on the mechanism underlying cardioversion-related thromboembolism, as first proposed by Goldman approximately 30 years ago, has been challenged in recent years. It now appears that at least two mechanisms exist, one based on the theory of preexisting thrombus, and a second mechanism suggesting that thrombogenesis can occur in the immediate postcardioversion period. Despite the recent flurry in investigation into this important area of stroke research, many key questions are unsolved such as the management and treatment of AF; its incumbent need for anticoagulant prophylaxis continues to be one of the most troublesome and ill-defined areas of cardiac care for practitioners. A more comprehensive understanding of the mechanisms involved in cardiac chamber thrombogenesis and embolism will lead to significantly improved risk stratification of patients, which will direct anticoagulation therapy toward those patients at greatest risk for thromboembolism and, potentially, away from those who are at negligible or absent risk of thromboembolism. The potential for reducing the embolic event rate following cardioversion to near zero is eminently feasible given current technology. The tools required for this risk stratification will undoubtedly include clinical and echocardiographic parameters and, possibly (but not necessarily), an assessment of left atrial and left atrial appendage mechanics via transesophageal echocardiography.

References

1. Goldman MJ. The management of chronic atrial fibrillation. Prog Cardiovasc Dis 1960;2:465–479.
2. Stein B, Halperin JL, Fuster V. Should patients with atrial fibrillation be anticoagulated prior to and chronically following cardioversion? In: Cheitlin MD, ed. Dilemmas in Clinical Cardiology. Philadelphia: F.A. Davis Co; 1990:231–249.
3. Grimm RA, Stewart WJ, Maloney JD, et al. Impact of electrical cardioversion of atrial fibrillation on left atrial appendage function and spontaneous echo contrast: characterization by simultaneous transesophageal echocardiography. J Am Coll Cardiol 1993;22:1359–1366.
4. Lown B, Perlroth MG, Kaidbey S, et al. "Cardioversion" of atrial fibrillation: a report on the treatment of 65 episodes in 50 patients. N Engl J Med 1963;269:325.
5. Lown B. Electrical reversion of cardiac arrhythmias. Br Heart J 1967;29: 469–489.
6. Bjerkelund CJ, Orning OM. The efficacy of anticoagulant therapy in preventing embolism related to DC electrical conversion of atrial fibrillation. Am J Cardiol 1969;23:208–216.
7. Arnold AZ, Mick MJ, Mazurek RP, et al. Role of prophylactic anticoagulation for direct current cardioversion in patients with atrial fibrillation or atrial flutter. J Am Coll Cardiol 1992;19:851–855.
8. Laupacis A, Albers G, Dunn M, Feinberg W. Antithrombotic therapy in atrial fibrillation. 3rd ACCP Conference on Antithrombotic Therapy. Chest 1992;102(suppl):426S-433S.
9. Rokseth R, Storstein D. Quinidine therapy of chronic auricular fibrillation: the occurrence and mechanism of syncope. Arch Intern Med 1963;111:184.
10. Weinberg DM, Mancini GBJ. Anticoagulation for cardioversion of atrial fibrillation. Am J Cardiol 1989;63:745–746.
11. Belcher JR, Sommervill W. Systemic embolism and left auricular thrombosis in relation to mitral valvotomy. Brit Med J 1955;2:1000.
12. Petersen P, Gottfredsen J. Embolic complications in paroxysmal atrial fibrillation. Stroke 1986;17:622–626.

13. Manning WJ, Silverman DI, Gordon SPF, et al. Cardioversion from atrial fibrillation without prolonged anticoagulation with use of transesophageal echocardiography to exclude the presence of atrial thrombi. N Engl J Med 1993;328:750–755.
14. Black IW, Grimm RA, Walsh WF, et al. Risk factors for atrial thrombus and stroke in 156 patients undergoing electrical cardioversion: a multicenter transesophageal echocardiographic study. J Am Coll Cardiol 1993;21(suppl A):28A. Abstract.
15. Black IW, Hopkins AP, Lee LCL, Walsh WF. Evaluation of transesophageal echocardiography prior to cardioversion of atrial fibrillation and flutter in non-anticoagulated patients. Am Heart J 1993;126:375–381.
16. Grimm RA, Stewart WJ, Black IW, et al. Should all patients undergo transesophageal echocardiography prior to electrical cardioversion of atrial fibrillation? J Am Coll Cardiol 1994;23:533–541.
17. Shrestha NK, Moreno FL, Narcisco FV, et al. Two dimensional echo diagnosis of left atrial appendage thrombus in rheumatic heart disease: a clinicopathologic study. Circulation 1983;67:341–346.
18. Stein B, Fuster V, Halperin JL, Chesebro JH. Antithrombotic therapy in cardiac disease: an emerging approach based on pathogenesis and risk. Circulation 1989;80:1501–1513.
19. Beppu S, Nimura Y, Sakakibara H, et al. Smoke-like echo in the left atrial cavity in mitral valve disease: its features and significance. J Am Coll Cardiol 1985;6:744–749.
20. Uno M, Tsuji H, Sawada S, et al. Fibrinopeptide A (FPA) levels in atrial fibrillation and the effects of heparin administration. Jpn Circ 1988;52: 9–12.
21. Gustafsson C, Blomback M, Britton M, et al. Coagulation factors and the increased risk of stroke in nonvalvular atrial fibrillation. Stroke 1990;21: 47–51.
22. Kumagi K, Fukunami M, Ohmori M, et al. Increased intracardiovascular clotting in patients with nonvalvular atrial fibrillation. J Am Coll Cardiol 1990;16:377–380.
23. Hochman JS, Platia EB, Bulkley BH. Endocardial abnormalities in left ventricular aneurysms: a clinicopathologic study. Ann Intern Med 1984; 100:29–35.
24. Fuster V, Halperin JL. Left ventricular thrombi and cerebral embolism: an emerging approach. N Engl J Med 1989;320:392–394.
25. Pollick C, Taylor D. Assessment of left atrial appendage function by transesophageal echocardiography: implications for the development of thrombus. Circulation 1991;84:223–231.
26. Fatkin D, Kuchar DL, Thorburn CW, Feneley MP. Transesophageal echocardiography before and during direct current cardioversion of atrial fibrillation: evidence for "atrial stunning" as a mechanism of thromboembolic complications. J Am Coll Cardiol 1994;23:307–316.
27. Black IW, Fatkin D, Sagar KB, et al. Exclusion of atrial thrombus by transesophageal echocardiopgraphy does not preclude embolism after cardioversion of atrial fibrillation: a multicenter study. Circulation 1994; 89: 2509–2513.
28. Roy D, Marchand E, Gagne P, et al. Usefulness of anticoangulant therapy

in the prevention of embolic complications of atrial fibrillation. Am Heart J.1986;112:1039–1043.

29. Bikkina M, Alpert MA, Mulekar M, et al. Prevalence of intraatrial thrombus in patients with atrial flutter. Am J Cardiol 1995;76:186–189.

30. Grimm RA, Stewart WJ, Thomas JD, Klein AL. Left atrial appendage "stunning" following electrical cardioversion of atrial flutter: an attenuated response when compared to atrial fibrillation as a mechanism for lower susceptibility to thromboembolic events. J Am Coll Cardiol 1997;29: 582–589.

31. Ehsanin A, Ewi GA, Sobel BE. Effects of electrical countershock on serum creatinine phosphokinase isoenzyme activity. Am J Cardiol 1976;37:12–18.

32. Metcalfe MJ, Smith F, Jennings K. Does cardioversion of atrial fibrillation result in myocardial damage? Br Med J 1988;296:1364.

33. Falcone R, Morady F, Armstrong WF. Continuous transesophageal echocardiography during sequential electrical cardioversion attempts for atrial fibrillation: effect on left atrial appendage function and spontaneous echo contrast. J Am Coll Cardiol 1995;(suppl):231A. Abstract.

34. Grimm RA, Leung DY, Black IW, et al. Left atrial appendage "stunning" after spontaneous conversion of atrial fibrillation demonstrated by transesophageal Doppler echocardiography. Am Heart J 1995;130:174–176.

35. Manning WJ, Silverman DI, Katz SE, et al. Temporal dependence of the return of atrial mechanical function on the mode of cardioversion of atrial fibrillation to sinus rhythm. Am J Cardiol 1995;75:624–626.

36. Falcone R, Morady F, Armstrong WF. Effect of chemical vs electrical cardioversion of atrial fibrillation on left atrial appendage function and spontaneous contrast formation assessed by transesophageal echocardiography. J Am Coll Cardiol 1995;(suppl):65A. Abstract.

37. Manning WJ, Leeman DE, Gotch PJ, Come PC. Pulsed Doppler evaluation of atrial mechanical function after electrical cardioversion of atrial fibrillation. J Am Coll Cardiol 1989;13:617–623.

38. Manning WJ, Silverman DI, Katz SE, et al. Impaired left atrial mechanical function after cardioversion: relation to the duration of atrial fibrillation. J Am Coll Cardiol 1994;23:1535–1540.

39. Ikram H, Nixon P, Arcan T. Left atrial function after electrical cardioversion to sinus rhythm. Br Heart J 1968;30:80–83.

40. DeMaria A, Lies J, King J, et al. Echocardiographic assessment of atrial transport, mitral movement and ventricular performance following electroversion of supraventricular arrythmias. Circulation 1975;51:273–282.

41. Shapiro E, Effron M, Lima S, et al. Transient atrial dysfunction after conversion of chronic atrial fibrillation to sinus rhythm. Am J Cardiol 1988; 62:1202–1207.

42. O'Neil P, Puleo P, Bolli R, Rokey R. Return of mechanical function following electrical conversion of atrial dysrhythmias. Am Heart J 1990;120: 353–359.

43. Louie EK, Liu D, Reynertson SI, et al. Time course of recovery of left atrial appendage function after reversion to sinus rhythm from atrial fibrillation. Circulation 1995;92(suppl):I-141. Abstract.

44. Klein AL, Grimm RA, Black IW, et al. Cardioversion guided by transesophageal echocardiography: the ACUTE pilot study. Ann Internal Med 1997; 126:200–209.

PART VIII

Termination of Atrial Fibrillation Without Drugs

CHAPTER 27

Can Pacemakers Terminate Atrial Fibrillation?

Mårten Rosenqvist

Introduction

A prerequisite for pace termination of an arrhythmia is that it is a reentrant tachycardia and that cardiac pacing can interfere with the reentrant circuit. In contrast to supraventricular reentrant arrhythmias, atrial fibrillation (AF) has traditionally been considered a chaotic rhythm disturbance, and thus not suitable for antitachycardia pacing. In the early 1960s, Moe[1] suggested that AF was based on the continuous propagation of multiple wavelets in the atria, the so-called multiple wavelet hypothesis. Later work by Allessie's group[2] provided experimental evidence that supported this hypothesis.

These observations have recently created an interest in the feasibility of cardiac pacing to interfere with AF. This chapter will focus on studies that evaluate artificial cardiac pacing in the context of AF, and discuss mechanisms and future possibilities.

Prerequisites for Antitachycardia Pacing

In order for a tachycardia to be terminated by pacing, it has to originate from a reentrant circuit. Such a circuit usually consists of an area in the myocardium with electrophysiological properties that differ from those of the normal conduction system. These areas usually consist of a myocardial scar or an accessory pathway. In contrast, in patients with AF, an area of abnormal tissue does not appear to be a

This work was supported by the Swedish Heart and Lung Foundation.
From *Nonpharmacological Management of Atrial Fibrillation*, edited by F.D. Murgatroyd and A.J. Camm. © 1997, Futura Publishing Co., Inc., Armonk, NY.

prerequisite, as AF can be induced in patients with an apparently normal heart.

A reentrant tachycardia is characterized by its ability to be induced and terminated by programmed electric stimulation. Termination of a tachycardia is dependent on the critical timing of the stimulated wave front arriving early enough to cause conduction block before refractoriness expires. El-Sherif[3] has suggested three factors that determine whether the wave front can reach into the critical part of the circuit in time to cause block: (1) the cycle length of stimulation; (2) the number of stimulated beats; and (3) the site of stimulation.

In order for the tachycardia to be susceptible to termination, it is necessary that the refractory period within the circuit be shorter than the time taken by the wave front to complete the cycle. If the refractory period approaches the revolution time, the circuit will be refractory to external stimuli. An excitable gap will thus exist only if the refractory period is shorter than the cycle length. Pacemaker therapy for termination of tachycardia aims to insert a stimulus into this gap in such a way that conduction is no longer possible, owing to the refractoriness. Retrograde conduction in the circuit will thus collide with the oncoming wave front already in the circuit, thereby extinguishing it.

Despite these critical prerequisites, more than 90% of both supraventricular and ventricular reentrant tachycardias can usually be terminated by antitachycardia pacing.

Is Atrial Fibrillation a Reentrant Arrhythmia?

In 1915, Hewlett et al.[4] observed that, using the surface electrocardiogram, AF could have different morphologies, i.e., "coarse" and "fine" fibrillation. Later, Wells et al.[5] identified four different types of AF based on the recordings from bipolar atrial electrograms in postoperative patients. In type I, the atrial electrogram showed distinct complexes of slightly variable morphology separated by a discrete isoelectric line. Type II was also characterized by the same type of distinct complexes as in type I, but differed from type I in that the baseline showed continuous perturbation. Type III was characterized by highly fragmented atrial electrograms showing no discrete complexes and with no isoelectric interval. Wells also noted that the same patient could alternate between different types of AF—a phenomenon that was classified as type IV.

In 1985, Allessie et al. performed mapping studies in isolated canine hearts showing the first experimental evidence confirming Moe's multiple wavelet hypothesis.[2] They also observed that a critical number of an average of at least three wavelets was required for perpetuation. Wang et al.[6] contributed additional support to this observation by demonstrating that termination of AF by flecainide, sotalol, procainamide, and propafenone was preceded by a decrease in the number of wavelets.

Cox et al.[7] studied 13 patients with Wolff-Parkinson-White (WPW) syndrome during surgery for interruption of the accessory pathway. Atrial fibrillation was induced with burst pacing, and the atria were mapped with an interelectrode distance of about 1 cm on average. In six out of the 13 patients, an atrial activation pattern during AF was suggestive of reentry in the right atrium.

Konings et al.[8] performed atrial mapping during AF in 25 patients undergoing WPW surgery, using high resolution mapping with a spoon-shaped electrode with 244 unipolar electrodes. Using the complete pattern of activation, they classified AF into three different categories based on the number and complexity of wavelets in the mapped area. With this classification, 40% of the patients had only one wave front which propagated without significant conduction delay (type I). Thirty-two percent of the patients had either two wavelets or a single wavelet that was associated with conduction block or slow propagation (type II). The remaining 28% of patients exhibited three or more wavelets in combination with conduction block and areas of slow conduction (type III). Interestingly, there was no correlation between the type of fibrillation and various clinical variables such as age, sex, or previously reported AF. However, there was a correlation between the type of fibrillation and the fibrillation intervals and intra-atrial conduction. Thus, the more wavelets and lines of conduction block that were observed, the shorter the fibrillation intervals. In accordance with the observation by Wells,[5] various types of fibrillation could be seen in the same patient. Although there is no clear substrate for a reentrant arrhythmia in AF it can be speculated that degenerative microscopic changes seen with increasing age[9] can promote development of AF.

In conclusion, the available data strongly suggest that AF can be classified as a reentrant arrhythmia which, however, consists of multiple circuits with varying propagation properties.

Can the Fibrillating Atrium Be Captured by Pacing?

The second prerequisite for terminating fibrillation with pacing is that the excitable gap of the reentrant circuit can be reached by the electrical stimulus. In order to terminate the arrhythmia, the stimulus has to be inserted in a way such that retrograde conduction collides with the oncoming wave front and thus extinguishes it. Allessie et al.[10] and Kirchhof et al.[11] recently published data exploring these concepts in animal studies. Using both a closed-chest and an open-chest model, these studies evaluated the possibility of achieving local capture of the left atrium during induced and sustained AF. The activation pattern of the atrium was analyzed using a spoon-shaped mapping electrode consisting of 248 unipolar electrodes with an interelectrode distance of 2.5 mm.

The main observation from these studies was that it was possible to achieve local capture of the left atrium over an average distance from the pacing site of 3.1 ± 0.8 cm. Mapping analysis before and during capture showed that, before pacing, the area of interest was characterized by multiple wavelets from various directions. When capture occurred, this pattern changed and the entire mapping area was activated by a single wave front. Another important observation was that the window for capture was quite narrow, approximately 10–12 ms. However, termination of AF was never observed, which the authors attribute to the fact that the area of capture was too small and the remaining uncaptured area was large enough to sustain the fibrillation.

Is it Possible to Terminate Atrial Fibrillation by Pacing?

The macroscopically chaotic nature of AF is probably the reason why few studies have been published that attempt to evaluate the efficacy of pacing for termination of AF. Although the studies previously discussed have claimed that AF is in fact a reentrant arrhythmia with multiple circuits, studies on pacing to capture the atrium have shown that this is possible only very locally.

Recently, however, some preliminary reports have evaluated the possibility of termination of AF in patients. Haffajee et al.[12] studied 25 patients with AF; 17 had had fibrillation for more than 3 weeks, and the remaining eight for less than 48 hours. Prior to elective cardioversion, high frequency burst pacing was delivered in a randomized fashion during various time intervals up to 5 seconds. Among the eight patients with AF of short duration, three converted to sinus rhythm, whereas none of the patients with long-lasting fibrillation converted. Giorgberidze et al.,[13] in a similar study, studied 10 patients with either paroxysmal type II flutter or fibrillation. During 11 episodes of flutter or fibrillation, 143 trains of high frequency pacing at a cycle length of 20 ms were delivered for a duration of up to 250–4,000 ms. In no patient was fibrillation terminated, but four patients with type II flutter had the arrhythmia stopped. In eight patients, a transient change in the atrial electrogram was also seen during pacing. The authors conclude that high frequency atrial pacing can alter local atrial activation during atypical flutter and thus destabilize the flutter and terminate the arrhythmia.

It is difficult to draw any reliable conclusions from these observations for several reasons. Firstly, it cannot be ruled out that the arrhythmia terminations actually occurred spontaneously since neither study had a control group. It is well known that induced AF can be difficult to sustain and often converts spontaneously. Secondly, the observation by Allessie et al.[10] and Kirchhof et al.[11] makes it difficult to see how atrial burst pacing at a random rate could maintain capture in an atrial area large enough and for a long enough time to terminate the tachycardia. These observations will thus have to be confirmed in future controlled studies. In addition, electrodes probably need to cover a larger area of the atrium either by increasing the size of the site, or by using multiple sites, or a combination of both to capture an area large enough to reliably convert fibrillation.

Can Pacing Facilitate Termination of Atrial Fibrillation?

Although at present it seems unlikely that termination of AF is possible using high frequency pacing, one could speculate that pacing might facilitate the termination of AF by other means. The previously discussed studies by Allessie et al.[10] and Kirchhof et al.[11] clearly show that atrial pacing changed the activation pattern to become more organized. A similar type of transformation of the atrial activity was observed by Wang et al.[6] just before conversion to sinus rhythm, during administration of antiarrhythmic drugs. It would thus be interesting to study whether the combination of antiarrhythmic drugs and high frequency pacing could facilitate conversion to sinus rhythm.

Another hypothetical application of these findings is that rapid pacing prior to internal cardioversion of AF might decrease the atrial defibrillation threshold. A study to evaluate this concept has recently begun in two centers in Sweden.

Conclusions

• Atrial fibrillation fulfills several criteria for consideration as a reentrant arrhythmia. However, it consists of several (4–6) coexistent circuits and can alternate between various degrees of organized rhythm.

• It is possible to capture the atrium locally with rapid atrial pacing. The area of capture is, however, limited ($\approx$3 cm), and the window of cycle lengths for achieving capture is narrow ($\approx$10–12 ms).

• Rapid atrial overdrive pacing, using standard techniques and electrodes, can probably organize the atrial electrogram but rarely converts AF to sinus rhythm.

• As rapid atrial pacing may transform AF to a more organized rhythm, it can be speculated that pacing might facilitate conversion to sinus rhythm by other methods.

• Electrode configuration and pacing techniques probably need to be improved in order to reliably achieve sustained capture during AF.

References

1. Moe GK. On the multiple wavelet hypothesis of atrial fibrillation. Arch Int Parmacodyn Ther 1962;140:183–188.
2. Allessie MA, Lammers WJEP, Bonke FIM, et al. Experimental evaluation of Moe's multiple wavelet hypothesis of atrial fibrillation. In: Zipes D, Jalife J, eds. Cardiac Arrhythmias. New York: Grune and Stratton; 1985: 265–276.
3. El-Sherif N. Electrophysiologic mechanisms in electrical therapy of ventricular tachycardia. In: Saksena S, Goldschlager N, eds. Electrical Therapy for Cardiac Arrhythmias. Philadelphia: WB Saunders Co; 1990:395–410.
4. Hewlett AW, Wilson FN. Coarse auricular fibrillation in man. Arch Int Med 1915;15:786–793.
5. Wells JL, Karp RB, Kouchoukos NT, et al. Characterization of atrial fibrillation in man: studies following open heart surgery. PACE 1978;1:426–438.
6. Wang Z, Pagé P, Nattel S. Mechanism of flecainide antiarrhythmic action in experimental atrial fibrillation. Circ Res 1992;71:271–287.
7. Cox JL, Canavan TE, Scheussler RB, et al. The surgical treatment of atrial fibrillation. II. Intraoperative electrophysiologic mapping and description of the electrophysiologic basis of atrial flutter and fibrillation. J Thorac Cardiovasc Surg 1991;101:406–426.
8. Konings KTS, Kirchhof CJHJ, Smeets JRLM, et al. High density mapping of electrically induced atrial fibrillation in man. Circulation 1994;89: 1665–1680.
9. Spach MS, Dolber P. Relating extracellular potentials and their derivatives to anisotropic propagation at a microscopic level in human cardiac muscle:

evidence for electrical uncoupling of side to side fiber connections with increasing age. Circ Res 1987;60:206–219.

10. Allessie MA, Kirchhof CJHJ, Scheffer GJ, et al. Regional control of atrial fibrillation by rapid pacing in conscious dogs. Circulation 1991;84: 1689–1697.

11. Kirchhof CJHJ, Chorro FJ, Scheffer GJ, et al. Regional entrainment of atrial fibrillation studied by high-resolution mapping in open-chest dogs. Circulation 1993;88:736–749.

12. Haffajee C, Stevens S, Mongeon L, et al. High frequency pacing atrial burst pacing for termination of atrial fibrillation. PACE 1995;18:804. Abstract.

13. Giorgberidze I, Saksena S, Ryszard BK, et al. Clinical efficacy and electrophysiologic effects of high frequency atrial pacing for type II atrial flutter and atrial fibrillation. PACE 1995;18:804. Abstract.

CHAPTER 28

Low Energy Atrial Defibrillation:

Experimental Background

David Keane, Jeremy Ruskin

Introduction

Following the recognition of the risk of ventricular fibrillation (VF) induction by alternating current, the technique of direct current "high energy" cardioversion of atrial fibrillation (AF) was introduced by Lown et al. in 1962.[1-3] Thirty-five years later, the routine clinical practice of cardioversion of AF continues to involve the transthoracic administration of 100 to 360 joules (J) under general anesthesia. Although the use of large surface area cutaneous electrodes would be expected to result in a homogenous distribution of potential gradient within the atria, the principal factors leading to such a high energy requirement are, foremost, the low transcardiac current fraction (approximately 4%[4]) of transthoracic shocks and, secondly, the high impedance of the skin, chest wall, and lungs. The third element of inefficacy associated with conventional external defibrillator units is the persistent use of a damped sinusoidal waveform. Despite these shortcomings, conventional high energy cardioversion has been found to be effective in approximately 80% of patients with AF (depending on patient selection) and to be associated with minimal risks. The technique of high energy cardioversion is most satisfactory in the setting of recent onset AF where precipitating factors may be partly controlled or reversible. For the patient with recurrent AF, however, particularly those in whom AF may result in hemodynamic embarrassment, the concept of repeated hospital visits for semielective cardioversion under general anesthesia is eminently unsatisfactory. The need to explore more efficient "low energy" cardioversion of AF arises from (a) the prospect of introducing

From *Nonpharmacological Management of Atrial Fibrillation*, edited by F.D. Murgatroyd and A.J. Camm. © 1997, Futura Publishing Co., Inc., Armonk, NY.

Table 1
Experimental Steps Taken over the Last 27 Years Towards Lower
Energy Cardioversion

A single right atrial electrode combined with an external electrode
↓
Biatrial electrodes-right atrium combined with a coronary sinus (or epicardial)
electrode)
↓
Up-sizing of electrodes to customized large surface area defibrillation electrodes
↓
Application of biphasic waveforms

an implantable atrial defibrillator for patients with recurrent AF, and (b) the elective cardioversion of patients in whom conventional transthoracic cardioversion is unsuccessful.

To this end, the last 27 years of atrial defibrillation research has witnessed the introduction of the following steps towards lower energy cardioversion (Table 1): (1) the placement of an intra-atrial electrode—initially as a single right atrial electrode combined with an external electrode; (2) the use of exclusively biatrial electrodes whereby a right atrial electrode is combined with a left atrial electrode as provided by a coronary sinus location or a left atrial epicardial electrode; (3) up-sizing of conventional catheter electrodes to customized large surface area defibrillation electrodes; and (4) the application to atrial defibrillation of biphasic waveforms. Of these steps, the most effective measure has undoubtedly been the elimination of noncardiac electrode locations.

The primary limitation of the present exclusively intracardiac right atrial-coronary sinus electrode configuration, is that the potential gradient is likely to be lowest in the high left atrium, thus requiring suprathreshold potential gradients to generated in the left atrioventricular groove (coronary sinus) with subsequent energy wastage. To this aim the use of the left pectoral active can configuration may improve the uniformity of the potential gradient in the left atrium and thus improve efficiency.[66] With ventricular defibrillation, however, the use of the exclusively cardiac (pericardial) configuration of right and left ventricular patches continues to be significantly more efficient than the active can configuration. Given that patient tolerance will be a crucial factor in determining the success of the implantable atrial defibrillator, the use of an epicardial left atrial electrode (introduced minimally invasively by the use of a pericardioscope) or the use of a microcatheter in the oblique vein of the left atrium should not be excluded at this early stage.

Implications from Studies of Ventricular Defibrillation

With the advent of the implantable ventricular defibrillator, extensive experimental and clinical research has been carried out on subcutaneous, epicardial, and endocardial electrode configurations for ventricular defibrillation. While it is unknown if the mechanism of atrial defibrillation is identical to that of ventricular defibrillation, it is likely that the atria and ventricles share some of the more basic principles of defibrillation. One such principle is that extracellular current density and potential gradient correlate most closely with changes in transmembrane potentials caused by shocks and, hence, the ability to defibrillate.[5] Furthermore, it appears that a certain minimum potential gradient throughout most of the myocardium is required for defibrillation.[6] In what proportion of the atria the minimal gradient is required will depend on the atrial critical mass that remains undetermined. Tang et al. studied potential gradients generated by shocks delivered between a right ventricular endocardial electrode (V), a right atrial endocardial electrode (A), and a left lateral cutaneous patch (P) using a 128 electrode three-dimensional recording system in the ventricles and atria.[7] The mean ratio of the highest to the lowest gradient was used as an index of the unevenness of the potential gradient distribution. This ratio ranged from 16.5 : 1 for the V + A→P electrode configuration to 26.5:1 for the V→A electrode configuration. This unevenness of the gradient field contributes to the inefficiency of ventricular defibrillation. Excessively high potential gradients (seen in the immediate proximity to intracardiac electrodes) may have a deleterious effect on the myocardium and may induce conduction block and arrhythmias, while areas containing potential gradient below the "threshold gradient" may result in persistent fibrillation. Defibrillation could probably be improved by electrode configurations that produce a more even gradient field in which the minimum gradient is higher for a given shock strength. The minimum threshold gradient required for atrial defibrillation has yet to be determined and studies are needed to investigate the distribution of potential gradients for exclusively atrial electrode configurations. The principles of more efficient electric waveforms such as the biphasic waveform had already been extensively studied in ventricular defibrillation prior to their application to atrial defibrillation. As a result of their previously demonstrated limited advantages over biphasic waveforms in ventricular defibrillation, triphasic waveforms and dual pathway sequential waveforms have not been adequately addressed in atrial defibrillation research. Our investigative strategies should remain wide and open until such time as we can devise the optimal system which can achieve atrial defibrillation with shocks of adequately low energy so as to be acceptable to the conscious patient.

Mechanism of Atrial Defibrillation

In order to study the mechanism of atrial defibrillation Gray et al. recently performed optical mapping studies of perithreshold shocks in a Langendorff-perfused sheep heart preparation.[60] Four distinct outcomes of perithreshold shocks were documented—two of which resulted in early defibrillation, one in delayed defibrillation, and one in failure—as follows: (1) immediate cessation of epicardial activity; (2) a single postshock activation followed by sinus rhythm; (3) organized activation for 0.8 to 1.5 seconds followed by termination; and (4) organized activity followed by degeneration back to AF. The repolarization time after a shock was significantly longer for successful (99 ± 14 ms) compared with unsuccessful (83 ± 15ms) shocks. Although the dispersion in activation on the anterior right atrial wall was significantly reduced during type (2), (3), and (4) outcomes compared to the preshock AF, the degree of synchronization achieved by the shock was not related to outcome. The results of this study suggest that auxiliary measures that can augment postshock refractory period extension may lower defibrillation energy requirements. Furthermore, the finding that atrial shocks organized the epicardial pattern of activation regardless of whether the attempted defibrillation was successful or not raises the question as to whether additional therapies delivered in the immediate postshock phase may increase the proportion of perithreshold shocks that results in sinus rhythm, i.e. to convert type (4) outcomes to type (3) outcomes. Such adjuvant therapies may be an additional very low energy shock delivered more than 100 ms after the initial shock or, alternatively, multisite pacing. The results of this study do not provide evidence against either the critical mass hypothesis of defibrillation or the upper limit of vulnerability hypothesis and further studies of high-density mapping will be required before we can have a comprehensive understanding of the nature of atrial defibrillation. In particular, we need to perform high-density mapping studies of the smooth wall of the atria such as the posterior left atrium in the region of the pulmonary veins in addition to the more accessible trabeculated (pectinate) free walls of the right and left atrial epicardium. Moreover, we need to perform high-density mapping studies of the atrial endocardium with particular interest in the interatrial septum—this might be achieved either by using a down-sized internal optical mapping system or, alternatively, indirectly achieved using a noncontact multielectrode catheter utilizing boundary element inverse solution mathematics in conjunction with a roving locator catheter.[63]

Electrode Configurations or Atrial Defibrillation

Details of the historical development of atrial defibrillation and the results of the seminal experimental studies leading to low energy internal atrial defibrillation have previously been reviewed in detail.[25,29,61–62] For the purpose of reviewing their cumulative clinical implications, the earlier experimental studies can be grouped according to the electrode configuration deployed.

Partially Internal Electrode Configurations for Atrial Defibrillation

In view of the immediate proximity of the esophagus to the posterior wall of the left atrium, this location has not only been used for atrial pacing but has also been evaluated for atrial defibrillation. In 1966, McNally et al. reported the deployment of an esophageal electrode in combination with a precordial electrode in the cardioversion of thirteen patients with chronic AF.[8] Eleven of the patients cardioverted with 40 joules (J) or less, while the other two patients required 60 J. Five of the patients were cardioverted by both the esophageal and, subsequently, the conventional antero-posterior external technique; the energy requirement for the esophageal configuration averaged less than one third that of the conventional technique. Of particular interest, five patients in this study were unanesthetized during the administration of esophageal shocks, although they did receive a sedative 1 hour prior to the procedure; no patient experienced severe pain and all said they would not mind having the procedure repeated.

Subsequently, in 1969, Jain and colleagues reported combining a single right atrial lead with an external electrode on the chest wall.[9] Ten shocks of 200 J were given in quick succession to six anesthetized dogs. Examination of the hearts was performed immediately after the shocks in three of the dogs and after 72 hours in the other three. No functional or anatomical effect was discernible. The same electrode configuration was then applied, with a 6 French electrode of 10 mm length, in the right atrium in seven patients. Shock strengths of 10, 30, 50, 75, and 100 J were administered until cardioversion of AF occurred. The mean energy requirement for the right atrial electrode configuration was 65 ± 23 J. No changes were noted on subsequent serial EKG or S.G.O.T. monitoring.

A similar approach of combining one right atrial electrode with an external electrode was described by Levy et al. who adapted the electrode configuration of conventional high energy direct current (DC) His bundle ablation for atrial defibrillation.[10] High energy (200 and 300 J) transcatheter cardioversion was performed by pulling back the atrioventricular junctional catheter just inferior to the site of the His bundle recording and delivering the shock between a proximal electrode (intended not to be in contact with the endocardium) and a backplate (anode). Sinus rhythm was restored by this technique in nine of the 10 patients with chronic AF resistant to external cardioversion of 400 J. In a second evaluation of this high energy technique, when Kumagai et al. studied 10 patients with chronic lone AF, cardioversion with 200 J or 300 J was successful in all patients, although one patient developed transient AV block requiring temporary pacing for 9 minutes.[11] A subsequent randomized comparison of this technique with conventional external cardioversion in 112 patients confirmed the greater efficacy of this partly internal technique of cardioversion which achieved a 91% success rate compared to the 67% rate of conventional external cardioversion.[12]

This partly internal electrode configuration was also used by Cotoi and colleagues who combined a right atrial electrode with a precordial paddle placed on the left anterior thoracic wall (anode).[13] This configuration was assessed in the cardioversion of four patients; two had AF and sick sinus syndrome and two had new onset AF induced by electrical stimulation of atrial flutter. Shocks of 20 J were administered without anesthesia but under sedation. Sinus rhythm was achieved in both patients with pace-induced AF (previously atrial flutter) and transient sinus rhythm was recorded in one of the patients with chronic AF and sick sinus syndrome. Of note, in the cases in which cardioversion was successful, the right atrial electrode lay in contact with the endocardium as evidenced by the recording of monophasic action potentials. While this study involving a precordial external paddle used one tenth of the energy administered in the studies by Levy et al.,[10,12] it is unlikely to have been a more efficacious configuration, as the success rate was poor, and the study population was small and it did not contain patients with chronic AF that had been previously resistant to conventional external cardioversion attempts. Furthermore, only the anterior wall of the right atrium lay in the high-density electrical field between the two electrodes (albeit accepting that current does not flow directly within the thorax between two electrodes due to heterogenous tissue impedances).

The right atrial catheter electrode-cutaneous patch configuration was further studied by Powell and colleagues[14] in a pace-induced AF model in sheep weighing 25 kg to 45 kg. Atrial defibrillation was achieved with low energies in this study by the use an endocardial electrode of large stimulating surface area (a spring coil of 655 mm^2) and a biphasic waveform. Cardioversion occurred at a success rate of 50% (E50) at 1.5 J and 80% (E80) at 2.5 J. Eighteen (2.4%) of 768 shocks induced VF, all due to T-wave sensing from the surface ECG, while in a further study of 45 shocks synchronized to a right ventricular bipolar electrogram, VF did not occur. Of note, there was no association between the level of delivered energy and induction of VF.

While configurations deploying one internal (esophageal or endocardial) electrode in combination with an external electrode (precordial or posterior patch or paddle)—equivalent to a subcutaneous patch—may achieve a higher intracardiac current density than an entirely external transthoracic system, they still involve a considerable amount of extracardiac tissue in their pathway. Thus, it is unlikely that such electrode configurations would ever be either adequately efficient or tolerable to a conscious patient. Intracardiac or epicardial electrode configurations, on the other hand, might be expected to achieve higher atrial current densities.

Intracardiac Configurations Limited to the Right Atrium

Several investigators have assessed bipolar endocardial defibrillation with both electrodes positioned on a single catheter within the right atrium. In 1974, Mirowski, Mower, and Langer studied the transvenous cardioversion of atrial tachyarrhythmias in the dog.[15] Atrial tachyarrhythmias were induced by topical acetylcholine and gentle trauma to the left atrial appendage.[15] A bipolar defibrillating catheter was positioned in the right atrium and truncated exponential shocks were administered between a proximal electrode in the superior vena cava and a distal electrode in the right atrium. In 125 episodes of atrial tachyarrhythmia, shocks of 0.05 J to 0.5 J were usually effective and only occasionally were 1 J to 3 J required, while conversion of these tachyarrhythmias with transthoracic paddles required 40 J to 100 J.

In another study of bipolar endocardial cardioversion of pace-induced atrial tachyarrhythmias in the dog, Benditt et al. assessed electrode catheters positioned in the right atrial appendage.[16] Shocks of 0.16 J to 1 J (rapidly decaying truncated exponential waveform) that were delivered through electrodes with a stimulating area of 20 mm^2 and 26 mm^2 were universally unsuccessful, while shocks administered through electrodes with a stimulating area of 53 mm^2 and 85 mm^2 did succeed intermittently, particularly when the shocks were delivered within 40 msec to 60 msec of the preceding atrial electrogram. The overall success rate of cardioversion was 23% and, in the majority of cases, termination of the atrial tachyarrhythmia was achieved by acceleration or deceleration of atrial activity for 5 to 14 cycles, while abrupt termination with restoration of sinus rhythm occurred in the minority of successful cardioversions. In a further study by the same group, a cathodal electrode was maintained in the right atrial appendage, while three different anodal positions were compared within the right atrium; the superior vena cava, the mid-right atrium, and the inferior vena cava.[17] Successful cardioversion was achieved at each of the three anode positions with delivered energies of ≤0.75 J, and the position of the anodal electrode within the right atrium had no consistent effect on energy requirements when the results were combined. In this latter study, success of cardioversion was not significantly influenced by the timing of energy delivery with respect to the atrial or ventricular electrocardiogram. Timing of atrial shocks was intended to be synchronized with the atrial electrocardiogram and VF was induced in nine (2.4%) of 372 cardioversion attempts. The incidence of VF induction increased with higher delivered energies: 0% at 0.01 J to 0.1 J; 3.1% at 0.25 J to 0.75 J; and 6.5% at energies of 1 J to 5 J.

Three alternative electrode configurations in the cardioversion of atrial flutter and AF in dogs of 9 kg to 20 kg with talc-induced pericarditis were compared by Kumagai et al:[18] A = conventional external paddles; B = combination of a right atrial catheter electrode (cathode) and an external backplate (anode); C = combination of a proximal and a distal electrode on a right atrial catheter. Shocks of ≤1 J resulted in successful cardioversion in 12% in configuration A, 70% in configuration B, and 74% in configuration C. Mean minimal effective energy for cardioversion was 4.0 ± 3.52 J for configuration A, 0.62 ± 0.67 J for configuration B, and 0.58 ± 0.71 J for configuration C.

A bipolar right atrial configuration was assessed in humans in a study of low energy endocardial cardioversion of a variety of arrhythmias by Nathan and colleagues.[19] In this study of five patients with AF, a catheter electrode of 250 mm^2 surface area was placed in the right atrium in two patients and in the right ventricle in three patients. Low energy shocks (either truncated exponential or damped sinusoidal) were administered with a mean energy of 0.7 J. None of the patients with AF were converted to sinus rhythm, and one asynchronous atrial shock of 5 J resulted in VF. General anesthesia was used in only one patient and sedation was given in two; some patients complained of severe pain with shocks of less than 5 J, and it was felt that shocks delivered in the right atrium induced more pain than shocks delivered in the ventricle.

While the comparative study in dogs by Kumagai et al. demonstrated the greater efficacy of transcatheter cardioversion over conventional external cardioversion,[18] it is unlikely that the confinement of both electrodes to the right atrium would incorporate a sufficient amount of the left atrium to be highly effective. This exclusively right atrial configuration, however, is at least as effective as the combination of a right atrial electrode with an external electrode. These studies indicated that alternative cardiac configurations (preferably with greater proximity to the left atrium) should be investigated.

Intracardiac Configurations Involving More than the Right Atrium

Scott et al. evaluated two lead configurations using a right atrial J lead (RA) (7.4cm^2), a right ventricular apical lead (RV) (5cm^2), and two subcutaneous catheter electrodes (SQ) (6cm^2) inserted in the 5th and 7th intercostal spaces, in a study on defibrillation of the atria and ventricles in the dog.[20] The defibrillation threshold with a 10 msec biphasic waveform for the RV (cathode)—RA (anode) configuration was 180 ± 63 V, and 187 ± 48 V for the RV (cathode)—RA and SQ (anode) configuration. Of interest, the defibrillation threshold of the ventricles for the latter lead configuration was 370 ± 130 V.

In a comprehensive investigation of multiple waveforms and lead configurations for atrial defibrillation in sheep (50 to 65 kg), Cooper and colleagues positioned spring coil electrodes (2.95cm^2) in the right atrium (RA) and left pulmonary artery (LPA), a hexapolar catheter in the coronary sinus (CS), and a subcutaneous patch ($133cm^2$) in the left upper chest wall (P).[21] The optimal waveform tested was a 3/3 msec biphasic waveform with which the energies associated with 50% success for the four electrode configurations were: RA→P 6.9 ± 1.5 J; RA→LPA 3.3 ± 1.8 J; RA→CS + LPA 2.0 ± .9 J; and RA→CS 1.3 ±.4 J. In a substudy by the same group, endocardial configurations in the sheep were evaluated further.[21] Electrode configurations limited to the right atrium (right→right) were compared with electrode configurations involving the right atrium and coronary sinus (right→left). All right→left configurations were more efficient than right→right configurations and the lowest 50% successful energy requirement (1.1 ± 0.3 J) was associated with a right atrial appendage and coronary sinus combination. A study of endocardial cardioversion in the same sheep model by Ayers et al.[22] suggests that further reduction in energy requirements may be possible when electrodes are placed in various locations within the great cardiac vein in combination with a right atrial appendage electrode. The results of epicardial and endocardial atrial defibrillation in patients are concordant with the results of Cooper et al., indicating that the atria can be defibrillated more effectively with a biphasic waveform than with a monophasic waveform,[23-25] and that endocardial cardioversion using a right atrial and coronary sinus lead configuration offers an effective system for internal atrial defibrillation.[26-30]

Effect of Electrode Location on Conduction Block

In a study of eight different electrode configurations for atrial defibrillation in the sheep, Cooper et al. found that sinoatrial block only occurred during shocks administered between the superior vena cava → right atrial appendage leads, while atrioventricular block only occurred with either the low right atrium → coronary sinus or the middle right atrium → coronary sinus electrode system.[21] Thus, not surprisingly, it appears that electrode configurations that generate high potential gradients near the sinoatrial and atrioventricular nodes are more prone to result in postshock conduction disturbances.

Effect of Electrode Location on Ventricular Arrhythmia Induction

The risk of provoking VF by an asynchronous discharge is less than 5%.[31] The induction of VF from poorly synchronized atrial shocks was reported in several of the studies on internal cardioversion described above.[14,17,19] These studies, however, used a surface ECG for R-wave synchronization and all shocks of VF resulted from failure of R-wave synchronization and the consequent delivery of T-wave shocks; furthermore, no shock was reported to induce VF when a local bipolar ventricular electrocardiogram was used for synchronization.[14] A right ventricular endocardial signal, in addition to providing a reliable signal of stable amplitude, would not be prone to synchronization with high-voltage repolarization waves after bandpass filtering. The intensity of electrical gradients within the ventricles resulting from low energy shocks in the atria would be expected to fall far below the upper limit of vulnerability of the ventricles. Of note, in the study by Dunbar et al. in which both the cathodal and anodal electrodes were within the dog's right atrium, the incidence of VF induction increased with the administration of shocks of higher energy,[17] while in the study by Powell and colleagues, when one electrode was positioned in the sheep's right atrium and the other electrode was a lateral cutaneous patch, no association was found between delivered energy and induction of VF.[14]

Cooper et al. reported that although no sustained ventricular arrhythmias occurred during the administration of atrial shocks that were synchronized with the R wave, episodes of nonsustained ventricular tachycardia were occasionally observed.[21] During testing of VF induction by the administration of atrial shocks on the T wave, no difference was found between the different atrial electrode configurations and the minimum energy required to induce VF (0.07 ± 0.01 J). It is unclear if the placement of electrodes distant to the ventricles would necessarily further reduce the likelihood of VF induction.

To study the influence of the preceding ventricular cycle length and likelihood of VF induction by atrial defibrillation shocks, Ayers et al. undertook a study in a rapid pace-induced (assisted by topical methacholine as required) model of AF in the healthy ovine heart.[22] A right ventricular sensing catheter was used for synchronization of all atrial shocks which were delivered between the right atrial appendage and the great cardiac vein. In a total of four protocols (three with programmed ventricular stimulation during sinus rhythm) involving the delivery of 1,870 synchronized shocks in 16 sheep, 11 episodes of VF were induced. All shocks resulting in VF were preceded by a ventricular cycle of ≤300 ms, whereas no episodes of VF were seen when the preceding cycle length was >300 ms. As outlined by Ayers et al., three possible mechanisms exist to account for the induction of VF by internally delivered cardioversions shocks.[22] One is a lack of synchronization of the cardioversion shock with respect to intrinsic ventricular depolarization, resulting in the shock being delivered on the T wave. The second is the delivery of a synchronized shock that occurs prior to complete repolarization of the previous beat, which from a surface electrogram may appear as an R on T. The third mechanism pertains to the delay of shock delivery from the sensed ventricular depolarization and the effect of irregular and rapid cycle lengths on the refractory period of the ventricle and, therefore, the time from depolarization to the end of the vulnerable period. Short and irregular preceding cycle lengths give rise to dispersion of ventricular refractoriness, and it was assumed that if sufficient time had elapsed since the last beat for all ventricular cells to fully repolarize, none of the ventricular myocytes should be vulnerable. This hypothesis was supported by the work of Elharrar and Surawicz[67] who showed in canine myocardium that ventricular action potential durations approached a maximum of 330 ms at long preceding cycle lengths. No correlation was found by Ayers et al. between shock strength or the characteristics of the preceding rhythm (other than cycle length) and the occurrence of VF.

In a recent study by Osswald et al.[32] in a canine model of ischemic cardiomyopathy, the effect of synchronization and sensing lead configuration was investigated using a transvenous tripolar lead (Endotak 0062, CPI, St. Paul, MN, USA) with defibrillation coils in the superior vena cava and right ventricle. Ventricular fibrillation developed immediately after 7/160 (4.38%) shocks which were deliberately delivered in an asynchronous mode, compared to 3/2179 (0.14%) synchronized shocks. In the synchronized mode, VF was induced by 3/1062 (0.28%) shocks with "integrated bipolar" sensing (right ventricular coil-electrode tip) compared to 0/1117 shocks when a separate true bipolar right ventricular sensing electrode was used for synchronization. The results of this study emphasize the importance of incorporating a bipolar ventricular sensing electrode in an implantable atrial defibrillator, particularly if a single chamber defibrillator is deployed, and underscore the need for reliable default programming in the event of a sensing lead fracture.

Electrode Polarity

In most studies on atrial defibrillation, the right atrial electrode was assigned to be cathodal for the delivery of shocks. The rationale for consistently administering cathodal shocks to the right atrium with the external electrode as an anode appears to have been based primarily on tradition. The only support for such an approach stems from the results of ventricular pacing studies which examined strength-interval curves for cathodal and anodal stimuli during diastole. Given, however, that during fibrillation most of the myocytes may be in a state of depolarization or incomplete repolarization,[33] and that during the relative refractory period anodal stimuli may be more effective than cathodal stimuli,[34-39] it is conceivable that lower defibrillation energy requirements may have been achieved by reversing the polarity in many of the above studies.

A number of studies have evaluated the role of right and left ventricular electrode polarity on defibrillation energy requirements during the delivery of monophasic shocks for VF. Most of the reported studies found a tendency (albeit inconsistent) towards a polarity effect for either the right or left ventricle in both experimental animal models (right ventricle anodal)[40] and in individual patients at the time of device implantation (left ventricle anodal).[34,35] Following the introduction of biphasic shocks, most of which were symmetrical dual capacitor shocks in the early studies,[41] it may have been felt that a polarity effect for the first phase would be less significant. Presently, however, several implantable ventricular defibrillators are designed to deliver single capacitor (or single capacitor emulated) biphasic shocks with a greater amount of energy delivered during the first phase.[42] This again raises the issue of whether the polarity of the first phase of single capacitor biphasic shocks could influence defibrillation energy requirements. A recent study by Kalman et al.[43] reported a polarity effect during atrial defibrillation in a canine model in which a right atrial anode/right ventricle cathode polarity during the first phase of single 150 μF capacitor 3 ms:3 ms biphasic shocks was found to be more efficacious than right atrial cathode/right ventricle anode biphasic shocks. Studies are required to confirm whether an "anodal dip"[34,39] occurs on atrial pacing during the relative refractory period of the atria, and to determine whether any lowering of energy requirements can be achieved by testing right and left (coronary sinus) atrial polarity during the delivery of interatrial single capacitor biphasic shocks in individual patients. While the left ventricle contains substantially greater muscle mass than the right ventricle, the possible effects of the ratio of muscle mass between the left atrium (3 mm thick) and right atrium (2 mm thick but larger volume[44]) and the presence of the sinus node in the right atrium on interatrial shock polarity remain to be determined.

Hybrid Therapies

It has been hypothesized that the creation of linear lesions in the atria might organize AF and thereby facilitate defibrillation. This hypothesis was recently tested by Kalman et al. who created four linear lesions in the right atrium by radiofrequency catheter ablation in a chronic rapid pacing model of AF in dogs.[64] Following ablation, fibrillation in both the left as well as the right atrium was found to be more organized and the atrial defibrillation threshold was significantly reduced from 1.3 ± 0.3 J to 0.6 ± 0.2 J. These interesting results raise the prospect that a proportion of patients previously found to be unsuitable for an implantable atrial defibrillator due to high defibrillation energy requirements or shock intolerance, may be rendered amenable to such therapy by right atrial catheter ablation. Such a limited right atrial catheter ablation should avoid the systemic thromboembolic risks of left atrial ablation, yet hopefully result in a significant improvement in the organization of atrial fibrillary activity.

Another approach towards the facilitation of low energy atrial defibrillation may be the use of regional entrainment of the atria by rapid pacing. Kirchhof et al. have shown that a local area of the atria can be entrained by rapid pacing during AF.[52] Preliminary attempts to achieve pan-atrial entrainment by simultaneous multisite pacing have so far been disappointing due to difficulties in merging the entrained regions. If two or more remote regions of the atria were entrained immediately prior to shock delivery, then overall improvement in atrial organization might be expected to lower atrial defibrillation energy requirements. Regional entrainment of the atria should be enhanced by compartmentalization of the atria by catheter ablation. The interaction of hybrid therapies is likely to be a focus of intense research efforts over the coming years with implications for the multiple functionality of the implantable atrial defibrillator.

Timing of Atrial Shock Delivery

Conventionally, the timing of atrial shocks has been exclusively synchronized with ventricular depolarization and the information from atrial electrograms has not been utilized. Based on earlier research in a finite element model, Karch et al. were able to demonstrate that the timing of delivery of low energy atrial shocks significantly effected the energy required to cardiovert atrial flutter.[65] This finding might be expected for any single macroreentrant arrhythmia including that of ventricular tachycardia when the activation wave front is in the zone of slow conduction. It is unknown whether such a 'defibrillation window' might exist for AF. Upon initial consideration, the number of coexistent wavelets and their random pattern of reentry in stable AF would suggest that, if such a window did exist, it would convey only a marginal reduction in energy requirements and its critical timing would be difficult to determine. Of interest, Gerstenfeld et al. recently demonstrated transient linking of atrial excitation during stable AF by the use of an orthogonal catheter in patients undergoing cardiac catheterization thereby providing evidence that AF in humans may not be entirely random.[59] Botteron and Smith subsequently provided further evidence for spatial organization by the placement of five equally spaced catheters in the right atrium in patients.[58] They they found that patients with chronic AF had the lowest level of organization (as determined by the mean activation space constant) and that patients with induced AF but no history of clinical AF had the highest level of organization, while patients with paroxysmal AF had an intermediate level of organization. These studies indicate that AF, particularly when of recent onset, may have an element of organization. Whether such partial organization provides a potential 'defibrillation window' will depend on the presence of zones of slow conduction and the ability of integrated electrograms to detect such a point in time.

Experimental Models of Atrial Fibrillation

The ideal experimental animal model for AF remains to be determined. Thus far, AF has been studied in the sheep, goat, dog, rabbit, and baboon. A variety of methods for the induction and maintenance of fibrillation have been reported including vagal stimulation, gentle trauma with the topical application of acetyl choline, or rapid pacing in acute animal studies, and talc pericarditis, disruption of the atrioventricular valve apparatus, and chronic rapid pacing in studies of chronic AF.

The degree of organization of atrial electrical activity in acute dog models of AF appears to be high and its mechanism and energy requirements for termination may not be directly comparable to true AF.[16,45] Furthermore, even in a study of the talc pericarditis dog model, 32 of 38 episodes of atrial tachyarrhythmias were found to be regular and reproducible with standard deviations in mean atrial cycle length within each dog of 0.6 ms to 6.6 ms.[17] The level of electrophysiological organization in this model may, however, be suitable for the study of atrial flutter.[46] Although the absolute values for energy requirement for cardioversion in such studies may not be directly applicable to atrial defibrillation in humans, they may provide valuable data on the relative energy requirements for different lead configurations under comparision within the same model.

A model of AF in a canine heart failure model has recently been described, whereby the circumflex artery is repeatedly instilled with microspheres resulting in progressive left ventricular dysfunction with subsequent left atrial distension and inducibility of sustained AF.[32,47,48] This model may be of particular interest to the study of a predominantly left atrial spectrum of AF as may be seen in patients with cardiomyopathy of coronary artery disease. It remains to be determined to what extent microembolization and possible ischemia of the left atrium occurs with this current model, and to what extent further manipulation of this model might be achieved with microembolization of right atrial and sinus node arterial branches. One limitation of this model is the intensive animal care required after coronary artery embolization.

The use of continuous rapid atrial pacing or repeated AF induction by bursts of rapid pacing over a prolonged period has recently been described to shorten atrial refractory periods and, to a lesser extent (and inconsistently), lengthen conduction velocity in the atria in order to achieve sustained AF.[49,50] Serial echocardiographic examination demonstrated marked biatrial dilatation following 6 weeks of continuous rapid atrial pacing in the dog, and an increase in atrial area of more than 40% was strongly correlated with the inducibility of AF.[49] This technique generates a reliable model of AF which provides a number of useful endpoints for the study of interventional and pharmacological therapies.[49–51]

A human model of AF has also been examined on cardiopulmonary bypass.[23] The inducibility of AF in this model may arise from the right atriotomy, from reduced conduction velocity during the systemic hypothermia of 31°, and from an ischemic component associated with intermittent aortic cross clamping. The model lends itself to epicardial as well as endocardial mapping and open access to left atrial defibrillation electrode sites without the anatomical restrictions (coronary sinus) associated with transvenous access. In addition to comparative defibrillation studies, this model also lends itself to the study of biatrial multisite antitachycardia pacing[52] for the termination of AF in humans.

Atrial Fibrillation Begets Atrial Fibrillation and Sinus Rhythm Begets Sinus Rhythm: Implications for Early Defibrillation

In an elegant study of electrical remodeling in a pace-induced caprine model of AF, Wijffels et al.[50] demonstrated that repeated induction of AF was associated with a progressive shortening of the atrial effective refractory period, a decrease in the median fibrillation interval, and increased inducibility of AF from a single premature stimulus.[50] These changes were not marked until after the first 6 hours of repeatedly induced AF and it took up to 2 weeks before AF became self-sustained (>24 hours). Of particular relevance to the introduction of an implantable atrial defibrillator was a substudy in five of the goats where the reversibility of electrical remodeling was examined after 19 days of chronic AF. Six hours after cessation of AF the median duration of electrically induced paroxysms of AF was already back to normal and lasted only 7 ± 2 seconds.[50] Additionally, following 6 hours of sinus rhythm, the AF interval had significantly prolonged again from 105 ± 10 ms to 139 ± 7 ms. These results of slow onset remodeling during AF and the more rapid reversibility of these changes following termination of AF suggest that if an implantable defibrillator prevents AF from becoming sustained, AF should be more easily terminated, and subsequent sinus rhythm should be more easily sustained. The proportion of the atrial milieu favoring fibrillation in patients that is due to reversible altered cellular metabolism[53] compared to fixed or reversible anatomical changes will greatly determine the clinical implications of these experimental results.

Future Directions and Limitations of Experimental Studies

The experimental studies outlined above have provided clear directions for the optimization of internal atrial defibrillation. Coronary sinus lead placement, in addition to improving left atrial defibrillation, provides the opportunity for dual or multiple site atrial pacing in the prophylaxis of atrial pacing.[54–56] This may serve to decrease the heterogeneity of atrial repolarization in patients with marked intra-atrial conduction delay. The provision of atrial pacing may also be of benefit in a very limited number of patients who consistently demonstrate sinus bradycardia prior to the onset of AF.[57] Furthermore, the value of decremental pacing for the first few minutes immediately following cardioversion of AF in the prophylaxis of very early recurrence needs to be explored (particularly in the presence of early sinus node disease). Validation of such prophylactic pacing may ultimately allow the implantable atrial defibrillator to provide both a preventive and a therapeutic role for patients with paroxysmal AF. The lack of spontaneous and frequently recurrent AF in our current animal models of AF will limit the potential of these models to provide such validation. In addition to this limitation of our current animal models, an inherent unsuitability for the prediction of tolerance of atrial shocks in conscious patients should also be acknowledged. Ultimately, large multicenter clinical trials will be required before the true benefit and general applicability of the implantable atrial defibrillator becomes established.

References

1. Lown B, Amarasingham R, Neuman J. New method for terminating cardiac arrhythmias: use of synchronised capacitor discharge. JAMA 1962;182: 548–555.
2. Lown B, Kleiger R, Williams J. The technique of cardioversion. Am Heart J 1964;67:282.
3. Lown B. Electrical reversion of cardiac arrhythmias. Br Heart J 1967;29: 469–489.
4. Lerman B, Deale OC. Relation between transcardiac and transthoracic current during defibrillation in humans. Circula tion Research 1990;67: 1420–1426.
5. Lepeschkin E, Jones JL, Rush S, Jones RE. Local potential gradients as a unifying measure for thresholds of stimulation, standstill, tachyarrhythmia and fibrillation appearing after strong capacitor discharges. Adv Cardiol 1978;268–278.
6. Ideker RE, Tang ASL, Frazier DW, et al. Ventricular defibrillation: basic concepts. In: El-Sherif N, Samet P, eds. Cardiac Pacing and Electrophysiology. Philadelphia: WB Saunders Co; 1991:713–726.
7. Tang AS, Wolf PW, Afework Y, et al. Three-dimensional potential gradient fields generated by intracardiac catheter and cutaneous patch electrodes. Circulation 1992;85:1857–1864.
8. McNally EM, Meyer EC, Langendorf R. Elective countershock in unanesthetized patients with use of an oesophageal electrode. Circulation 1966; 33:124–127.
9. Jain SC, Bhatnagar VM, Azami RU, Awasthey P. Elective countershock in atrial fibrillation with an intracardiac electrode: a preliminary report. Proceedings of the Association of Physicians of India and Cardiology Society of India. 1970:8214.
10. Levy S, Lacombe P, Cointe R, Bru P. High energy transcatheter cardioversion of chronic atrial fibrillation. J Am Coll Cardiol 1988;12:514–518.
11. Kumagai K, Yamanouchi Y, Hiroki T, Arakawa K. Effects of transcatheter cardioversion on chronic lone atrial fibrillation. PACE 1991;14:1571–1575.
12. Levy S, Lauribe P, Dolla E, et al. A randomised comparison of external and internal cardioversion of chronic atrial fibrillation. Circulation 1992; 86:1415–1420.
13. Cotoi S, Carasca E, Incze A, Podoleanu D. Intracardiac electrical discharge in terminating atrial fibrillation. Rev Roum Physiol 1990;27:21–24.

14. Powell A, Garan H, McGovern B, et al. Low energy conversion of atrial fibrillation in the sheep. J Am Coll Cardiol 1992;20:707–711.

15. Mirowski M, Mower M, Langer A. Low-energy catheter cardioversion of atrial tachyarrhythmias. Clin Res 1974;22:290A. Abstract.

16. Benditt D, Kriett J, Tobler H, et al. Cardioversion of atrial tachyarrhythmias by low energy transvenous technique. In: Steinbach K, ed. Cardiac Pacing: Proceedings of the VII World Symposium on Cardiac Pacing. Darmstadt: Steinkopff; 1982:845–851.

17. Dunbar D, Tobler G, Fetter J, et al. Intracavitary electrode catheter cardioversion of atrial tachyarrhythmias in the dog. J Am Coll Cardiol 1986;7: 1015–1027.

18. Kumagai K, Yamanouchi Y, Tashiro N, et al. Low energy synchronous transcatheter cardioversion of atrial flutter/fibrillation in the dog. J Am Coll Cardiol 1990;16:497–501.

19. Nathan A, Bexton R, Spurrell R, Camm AJ. Internal transvenous low energy cardioversion for the treatment of cardiac arrhythmias. Br Heart J 1984;52;377–384.

20. Scott S, Accorti P, Callaghan F, et al. Ventricular and atrial defibrillation using new transvenous tripolar and bipolar leads with 5 French electrodes and 8 French subcutaneous catheters. PACE 1991;14(II):1893–1898.

21. Cooper R, Alferness C, Smith W, Ideker R. Internal cardioversion of atrial fibrillation in sheep. Circulation 1993;87:1673–1686.

22. Ayers GM, Alferness CA, Ilina M, et al. Ventricular proarrhythmic effects of ventricular cycle length and shock strength in a sheep model of transvenous atrial defibrillation. Circulation 1994;89:413–422.

23. Keane D, Boyd E, Anderson D, et al. Comparison of biphasic versus monophasic waveforms in epicardial atrial defibrillation. J Am Coll Cardiol 1994;24:171–176.

24. Johnson EE, Yarger MD, Wharton JM. Monophasic and biphasic waveforms for low energy internal cardioversion of atrial fibrillation in humans. Circulation 1993;88:I-592. Abstract.

25. Keane D. Impact of pulse characteristics on atrial defibrillation energy requirements. PACE 1994; 17II:1048–1057.

26. Keane D, Sulke N, Cooke R, et al. Endocardial cardioversion of atrial flutter and fibrillation. PACE 1993;16:928. Abstract.

27. Alt E, Schmitt C, Ammer R, et al. Initial experience with intracardiac atrial defibrillation in patients with chronic atrial fibrillation. PACE 1994; 17(Part II):1067–1078.

28. Murgatroyd FD, Slade AK, Sopher SM, et al. Efficacy and tolerability of transvenous low energy cardioversion of paroxysmal atrial fibrillation in man. J Am Coll Cardiol 1995;25:1347–1353.

29. Keane D. Internal cardioversion of atrial arrhythmias: a review of experimental and clinical studies with implications for the design of an implantable atrial defibrillator. Eur J Cardiac Pacing Electrophysiol 1993: 4:308–314.

30. Keane D. Electrode configurations for internal atrial defibrillation. In: Camm AJ, Lindemans FW, eds. Transvenous Defibrillation and Radiofrequency Ablation. Armonk, NY: Futura Publishing Co; 1995;31–42.

31. DeSilva RA, Graboys T, Podrid PJ, Lown B. Cardioversion and defibrillation. Am Heart J 1980;100:881–895.
32. Osswald S, Trouton T, Roelke M, et al. Transvenous single lead atrial defibrillation: efficacy and risk of ventricular fibrillation in an ischemic canine model. Circulation 1996. In press.
33. Leim LB, Clay DA, Swerdlow CD, Franz MR. Distinct differences in human action potential characteristics during induction of ventricular fibrillation and ventricular tachycardia. Circulation 1986;(suppl)74:II-483. Abstract.
34. Bardy GH, Ivey TD, Allen MD, et al. Evaluation of electrode polarity on defibrillation efficacy. Am J Cardiol 1989;63:433–437.
35. O'Neill P, Boahene KA, Lawrie G, et al. The automatic implantable cardioverter-defibrillator: effect of patch polarity on defibrillation threshold. J Am Coll Cardiol 1991;17:707–711.
36. Mehra R, Furman S. Comparison of cathodal, anodal and bipolar strength-interval curves with temporary and permanent pacing electrodes. Br Heart J 1979;41:468–476.
37. Mehra R, McMullen M, Furman S. Time dependence of unipolar cathodal and anodal strength-interval curves. PACE 1980;3:526–530.
38. van Dam RT, Durrer D, Strackee J, van der Tweel LH. The excitability cycle of the dog's left ventricle determined by anodal, cathodal and bipolar stimulation. Circ Res 1956;IV:196–204.
39. Cranefield PF, Hoffman BF, Siebens AA. Anodal excitation of cardiac muscle. Am J Physiol 1957;190:383–390.
40. Schuder JC, Stoeckle H, McDaniel WC, Dbeis M. Is the effectiveness of cardiac ventricular defibrillation dependent upon polarity? Med Instrun 1987;21:262–265.
41. Jones JL, Jones RE, Balasky G. Improved cardiac cell excitation with symmetrical biphasic defibrillator waveforms. Am J Physiol 1987;253. Heart Circ Physiol 22:H1418-H1424.
42. Chapman PD, Vetter JW, Souza JJ, et al. Biphasic nonthoracotomy internal defibrillation: can it be done with a single capacitor? PACE 1988;11: 499. Abstract.
43. Kalman JM, Power JM, Chen JM, et al. Importance of electrode design, lead configuration and impedance for successful low energy transcatheter atrial defibrillation in dogs. J Am Coll Cardiol 1993;22:1199–1206.
44. Guiraudon GM, Guiraudon CM. Atrial functional anatomy. In: Kingma JH, van Hemel NM, Lie KI, eds. Atrial Fibrillation: A Treatable Disease? Boston: Kluwer Academic Publishers; 1992;23–40.
45. Strackee J, Hoelen AJ, Zimmerman AN, Meijler FL. Artificial atrial fibrillation in the dog: an artefact? Circ Res 1971;28:441–445.
46. Pagé PL, Plumb VJ, Okumura K, Waldo AL. A new animal model of atrial flutter. J Am Coll Cardiol 1986;8:872–879.
47. Sabbah HN, Stein PD, Kono T, et al. A canine model of chronic heart failure produced by multiple sequential coronary microembolizations. Am J Physiol 1991;260:H1379–84.
48. Sabbah HN, Goldberg AD, Schoels W, et al. Spontaneous and inducible ventricular arrhythmias in a canine model of chronic heart failure: relation

to hemodynamics and sympathoadrenergic activation. Eur Heart J 1992; 13:1562–1572.

49. Morillo CA, Klein GJ, Jones DL, Guiraudon CM. Chronic rapid atrial pacing: structural, functional and electrophysiological characteristics of a new model of sustained atrial fibrillation. Circulation 1995;91:1588–1595.

50. Wijffels M, Kirchhof C, Frederiks J, et al. Atrial fibrillation begets atrial fibrillation. Circulation 1993;88:I-18. Abstract.

51. Allessie MA, Wijffels M, Kirchhof C. Experimental models of arrhythmias: toys or truths? Eur Heart J 1994;15(suppl A):2–8.

52. Kirchhof C, Chorro F, Scheffer GJ, et al. Regional entrainment of atrial fibrillation studied by high-resolution mapping in open-chest dogs. Circulation 1993;88:736–749.

53. Katz AM. T wave "memory": possible causal relationship to stress-induced changes in cardiac ion channels? J Cardiovasc Electrophysiol 1992;3: 150–159.

54. Daubert JC, Gras D, Leclerq C, et al. Biatrial synchronous pacing: a new therapeutic approach to prevent refractory atrial arrhythmias. J Am Coll Cardiol 1995;25:230A. Abstract.

55. Prakash A, Saksena S, Hill M, et al. Outcome of patients with drug refractory atrial fibrillation/flutter and bradyarrhythmias using long-term dual site atrial pacing. PACE 1995;18(Part II):809. Abstract.

56. Prakash A, Saksena S, Hill M, et al. Electrophysiology of acute prevention of atrial fibrillation and flutter with dual site atrial pacing. PACE 1995; 18(Part II):803. Abstract.

57. Attuel P, Pellerin D, Mugica J, Coumel PH. DDD pacing: an effective treatment modality for recurrent atrial arrhythmias. PACE 1988;11: 1647–1654.

58. Botteron G, Smith JM. Quantitative assessment of the spatial organization of atrial fibrillation in the intact human heart. Circulation 1996;93: 513–518.

59. Gerstenfeld E, Sahakian A, Swiryn S. Evidence for transient linking of atrial excitation during atrial fibrillation in humans. Circulation 1992;86: 375–382.

60. Gray R, Ayers G, Jalife J. Video imaging of atrial defibrillation in the sheep heart. Circulation 1997;95:1038–1047.

61. Griffen JC, Ayers GM, Adams J, et al. Is the automatic atrial defibrillator a promising approach? J Cardiovasc Electrophysiol 1996;7:1217–1224.

62. Hillsley R, Wharton M. Implantable atrial defibrillators. J Cardiovasc Electrophysiol 1995;6:634–638.

63. Kadish A, Hauck J, Beatty G, et al. Mapping of atrial activation and tachyarrhythmias using a non-contact right atrial catheter. J Am Coll Cardiol 1997;29:331A. Abstract.

64. Kalman JM, Olgin J, Karch M, et al. Effect of right atrial linear lesions on atrial defibrillation threshold: implications for "hybrid therapy". PACE 1996;19(Part II):625. Abstract.

65. Karch M, Ellis W, Roithinger F, Lesh MD. Timing of shock during atrial flutter cycle predicts outcome of internal cardioversion. J Am Coll Cardiol 1997;29(suppl A):473A. Abstract.

66. Min X, Mongeon L, Mehra R. An electrode system Can + CS-RA with low atrial defibrillation threshold by finite element human thorax model and comparisons with clinical data. Circulation 1996;94(suppl):I-67. Abstract.
67. Elharrar V, Atarashi H, Surawicz B. Cycle length-dependent action potential duration in canine cardiac Purkinje fibers. Am J Physiol 1984;247: H936–945.

CHAPTER 29

Implantable Dual Chamber Defibrillators for Atrial Defibrillation

Rasmakota K. Reddy, Gust H. Bardy

Introduction

The frustration and difficulty of suppressing atrial fibrillation (AF) with antiarrhythmic drugs has given rise to a host of alternative non-pharmacological approaches to the problem. The implantable atrial defibrillator is one such therapy, but its potential benefit for patients with AF, most notably those with paroxysmal AF, is unknown. Where implantable atrial defibrillators fit into our therapeutic strategies, along with AV node interruption and catheter and surgical Maze procedures, remains to be defined. Fortunately, because AF is usually a non-lethal rhythm, a thoughtful assessment of the potential advantages and dangers of implantable atrial defibrillators can be made *prior* to wholesale adoption of this expensive and potentially dangerous therapy.

Potential Value of Atrial Defibrillators

Although the mortality benefit from aggressive maintenance of sinus rhythm over providing only rate control and anticoagulation in patients with AF has yet to be proven in a randomized clinical trial, the symptomatic benefit of normal sinus rhythm in individual patients is undeniable. Clearly, aggressive therapy can be warranted in such symptomatic patients on the basis of quality of life, regardless of mortality issues.

From *Nonpharmacological Management of Atrial Fibrillation*, edited by F.D. Murgatroyd and A.J. Camm. © 1997, Futura Publishing Co., Inc., Armonk, NY.

The potential value of an implantable atrial defibrillator lies not only in the immediate alleviation of symptoms for the arrhythmia itself; preliminary work suggests that prompt termination of AF will also decrease the likelihood of recurrence.[1] The longer AF persists, the more difficult it is to restore normal sinus rhythm. To the extent that many of the adverse consequences of AF, most notably stroke, are probabilistic in nature, even postponing the onset of chronic AF may be of benefit by decreasing the total life-years spent in AF.

Possible Dangers of Implanted Atrial Defibrillators

Despite the potential value of an implantable atrial defibrillator, there are two pressing concerns with this type of therapy: shock-related pain and shock-induced ventricular fibrillation.[2,3] As will be discussed later, these limitations strongly argue for the use of dual chamber defibrillators instead of stand-alone atrial defibrillators.

Shock-Induced Pain

The first of these problems, shock-induced pain or discomfort, can result in considerable psychological distress, a phenomenon well described in patients treated with implantable cardioverter defibrillators for ventricular tachycardia (VT) or ventricular fibrillation (VF).[4-8] In these VT/VF patients, the problem of shock-induced pain is considered an unfortunate side effect of a life-saving therapy. However, in the case of patients with AF and not VT/VF, it may be difficult to justify treatment of a less catastrophic arrhythmia with therapy that might prove worse than the disease.

The problem of shock-induced pain is a consequence of the need to use shock energy levels for atrial defibrillation well above the pain threshold. This is the case even when using optimal shock waveforms and the best shock vectors available, as is the case when biphasic coronary sinus (CS) to right atrial defibrillation is used. Almost no conscious patient will undergo successful atrial defibrillation at energies that are imperceptible, and few can be defibrillated at levels deemed acceptable, if shocks occur frequently.[2,9]

The pain associated with shocks does not in and of itself make an implantable atrial defibrillator unviable in the conscious patient. In patients with significant disability or hemodynamic distress associated with drug refractory AF, an implantable atrial defibrillator would be reasonable if the shock-induced distress was infrequent enough to not become more disabling than the arrhythmia itself. Such a candidate might have had infrequent episodes, such as two episodes per year, that sustain for at least 24 hours, with disabling symptoms or hemodynamic compromise. In addition, an implantable atrial defibrillator would be a more reasonable therapy for those patients who are refractory to antiarrhythmic drug therapy, have undergone recurrent transthoracic cardioversions, and are not candidates for other nonpharmacological therapies such as catheter ablation. In such circumstances, an implantable atrial defibrillator should be given serious thought. Otherwise, in our opinion, shock-induced distress is a very serious problem that makes a stand-alone implantable atrial defibrillator an untenable therapy in patients with frequent episodes of AF.

Device Proarrhythmia

The second and more serious concern with a stand-alone atrial defibrillator is inadvertent induction of VF with the delivery of the atrial defibrillation shock. Studies in healthy animals demonstrate a risk of induction of VF, even with R-wave synchronized shocks, at 0.5% per shock.[3] Considerable effort has been expended to find strategies minimizing this risk. It is not clear whether these strategies, usually developed in a sedated healthy animal model, will be applicable to awake humans with chronic heart disease.

Even if a perfect strategy were developed to make synchronized shocks nonproarrhythmic, the everyday reality that pacemakers and defibrillators at least occasionally oversense and undersense makes proarrhythmia an unavoidable concern. Changes in the underlying cardiac substrate, the influence of antiarrhythmic drugs, the occurrence of lead dislodgements, the development of new conduction abnormalities, and the onset of high amplitude T-wave changes all harbor the potential for fooling a device to deliver an atrial defibrillation shock into the vulnerable period of ventricular repolarization, and thus to induce VF. This risk is especially high when shock energy is lower (much lower than the upper limit of ventricular vulnerability) and when the current density across the ventricles is inhomogeneous, as when using an atrial shock vector. Thus, it is our opinion that a stand-alone atrial defibrillator cannot be used safely without protection from the proarrhythmic response that is the inevitable consequence of an atrial defibrillatory shock, no matter how diligent the attempt to synchronize shock delivery.

As a result of the potential for induction of a lethal arrhythmia, an implantable atrial defibrillator has an onus of safety beyond that of a standard ventricular implantable defibrillator that often corrects its own proarrhythmic mistakes. The risk of inadvertent induction of VF makes the use of a stand-alone atrial defibrillator too risky in most cases of AF, except for those rare individuals with refractory AF associated with immediate hemodynamic collapse. Whether by antiarrhythmic drug or antiarrhythmic device, inadvertent induction of unprotected VF and death in the course of treating a noncalamitous arrhythmia is a tragedy that must be avoided. We believe it will be difficult to justify stand-alone atrial defibrillators unless there is substantial additional evidence that these patients are not at risk of more harm from the therapy than from the disease.

Rationale for Dual Chamber Defibrillators

A Solution to the Risk-Benefit Dilemma of Atrial Defibrillators

The conservative perspective on the risk of atrial defibrillation discussed above does not mean that we advocate the abandonment of work on implantable atrial defibrillators. Rather, we propose that such devices are best evaluated in circumstances where the patient can benefit from therapy directed at more that just AF, e.g. VT/VF or bradyarrhythmias. Because dual chamber ICDs offer protection from proarrhythmia, shock-induced pain becomes the major factor that limits this form of therapy for AF. If pain were to surface as a limiting issue, abandonment or curtailment of atrial defibrillation therapy would not leave the patient adrift with an expensive therapy that has become a failed therapeutic exercise.

The possibility that the patient would benefit from ventricular defibrillation or antibradycardia pacing in this context is not trivial. It is known that the presence of AF is itself a marker for arrhythmic death, with a 2.2% to 2.5% risk of arrhythmic death in patients not on antiarrhythmic drug therapy and a 5% risk in patients on specific drug therapy.[10,11] Thus, it may be found that implantation of a dual chamber defibrillator for the primary indication of AF may actually result in reduction of ventricular arrhythmic deaths in this population.

Simple Versus Complex Lead Systems: Is the Coronary Sinus Lead of any Value?

Low-energy defibrillation, unless extremely low, i.e., <0.5 joules (J), will likely result in shock-related psychological distress.[9] Atrial defibrillation, even with optimal shock vectors between the right atria and coronary sinus, requires energies of >1.0 J to defibrillate, and often much more. Even with a CS lead, the pain associated with atrial defibrillation in the conscious patient can not be avoided with shock strengths that ensure effective defibrillation.[9] In addition, the CS lead is subject to lead dislodgement and a host of other problems related to coronary sinus instrumentation.[12] If the managing physician and the patient are willing to incur the psychological distress associated with atrial defibrillation, then one must question the use of a lead system that requires greater skill and adds an extra lead to an already complicated therapy.

Atrial defibrillation with lead systems comparable to a standard dual chamber pacemaker (Fig. 1) using RV, SVC, and CAN electrodes for atrial defibrillation, albeit requiring higher shock strength, offers the significant advantages of simplicity and safety. Simplicity increases safety in two ways. First, the fewer the electrodes and leads, the lower the complication rate. Second, the use of a single lead atrial defibrillator lends itself naturally to a device and lead system that provides ventricular defibrillation.

The ability to perform both atrial and ventricular defibrillation makes research into atrial defibrillation especially viable in its early stage. The problem of proarrhythmia is not the ethical and legal issue it becomes in a stand-alone atrial defibrillator. Moreover, if significant pain occurs as a consequence of atrial defibrillation, one can simply turn off this aspect of the device without the dilemma of abandoning

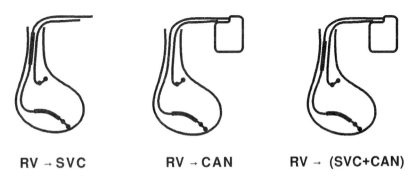

RV → SVC   **RV → CAN**   **RV → (SVC+CAN)**

Figure 1. Two lead AV-ICD systems.

an expensive therapy with significant psychological and financial implications for the patient. The ability to perform both atrial and ventricular defibrillation makes it less likely that the pain problem will have
a negative impact on atrial defibrillation research, by allowing a more
reasonable venue for its careful study.

Potential for Use of Dual Chamber
Defibrillators: Two Lead Systems

There are two types of atrial-ventricular implantable cardioverter
defibrillators (AV-ICDs) to consider: single lead and dual lead systems.
These devices would be comparable in lead system complexity to standard VVI and DDD pacemakers. Illustrations of three practical dual
lead systems that could be considered safe (i.e., able to rescue the patient from an atrial shock-related proarrhythmic outcome) are shown
in Figure 1.

Use of an RV→CAN, RV→SVC, or RV→(SVC + CAN) shock configuration certainly satisfies requirements for ventricular defibrillation
while simultaneously providing atrial defibrillation, albeit at energies
levels that are higher than those of optimal shock vectors. We found
the atrial defibrillation threshold (DFT) utilizing a biphasic waveform
with an RV→CAN configuration to be 9.3 ± 7.1 J (n = 25). The atrial
DFT with RV→SVC configuration was 4.8 ± 3.8 J, and with RV→(SVC
+ CAN) configuration, 4.2 ± 2.5 J (n = 11, unpublished data).

The choice of a single or dual lead AV-ICD would depend upon the
ability of single lead systems to sense AF reliably. Single lead systems,
without a dedicated right atrial sensing electrode, must rely either on
far-field atrial signal detection, which is a difficult prospect, or on inversion of current stability algorithms for detection rather than rejection
of AF. Most physicians would likely not use an AV-ICD without a dedicated atrial sensing electrode. Thus, the simplicity of a single lead AV-
ICD system that uses an indirect means to detect AF at least merits
evaluation in controlled circumstances.

Other Benefits of AV-ICDs

In addition to atrial defibrillation, there are other important benefits of a pace-sense lead in the atrium.

Ventricular and Supraventricular Tachycardia Discrimination

Discrimination of supraventricular tachycardia (SVT) from slow ventricular tachycardia (VT) is a problem in current Icds. In the case of a dual lead system AV-ICD, this arrhythmia discrimination problem would be largely solved. All current SVT-VT discrimination algorithms use some indirect measure derived solely from the ventricular electrogram, and do not directly test for ventriculo-atrial dissociation, the most reliable means to sort SVT from slow monomorphic VT. If an ICD had an atrial electrogram available to incorporate into its detection algorithm, one would expect much greater VT detection specificity than is now available.

Prevention of Atrial Fibrillation

The use of a dual lead system AV-ICD also offers the value of atrial pacing for the prevention of AF. Prevention of bradycardia and coordination of atrial and ventricular activity during minor atrial arrhythmias, with or without rhythm-smoothing algorithms, may have a prophylactic role in AF.

Antitachycardia Pacing to Terminate AF

The use of an atrial pacing electrode will also allow research into the use of rapid overdrive pacing for the termination of AF. Several studies have explored this approach to AF termination but the results so far are disappointing.[10,11,13] Nevertheless, this approach has obvious appeal and merits continued clinical investigation.

Standard Antibradycardia Pacing

Dual lead system AV-ICDs also carry the potential value of dual chamber pacing for standard antibradycardia pacing. Eliminating the use of two devices is a clear benefit for the VT/VF patient who also requires atrial pacing.

How Many Patients Could Conceivably Benefit from Dual Chamber AV-ICDs?

If the use of dual chamber AV-ICDs was predicated upon the need for therapy of VT/VF and one of the other arrhythmia problems men-

Table 1

AV-ICD Indication	Patients
Need for anti-bradycardia pacing	74 (16%)
VT/SVT discrimination	97 (20%)
Atrial fibrillation	166 (35%)
Any one or more of the above	**241 (51%)**

Potential additional benefit from a dual chamber ICD in 477 consecutive patients implanted with an ICD for VT/VF.

tioned above, how often would such a device actually be useful or, at minimum, potentially useful? To answer this question, we reviewed our VT/VF ICD patient population from the last six years for the concomitant occurrence of AF, slow VT (cycle length <360 ms), and/or the need for antibradycardia pacing.

From 1990–1996, 477 patients received an ICD for VT/VF. Of these, 97 could have benefited from a dual chamber AV-ICD for SVT-VT discrimination, 74 for antibradycardia pacing, and/or 166 for the concomitant therapy of AF. A total of 241 of 477 patients (51%) would have benefited from more than just VT/VF therapies if a dual lead AV-ICD were used (Table 1).

As pertains particularly to the problem of AF, it becomes more justifiable to explore these as yet unproven therapies if, paradoxically, we could comfortably abandon the therapy should it prove too painful or psychologically disturbing to the patient. The ICD would still be useful to the patient as a standard ventricular defibrillator and not leave the patient feeling that the therapy was a complete failure.

Conclusion

Combined atrial and ventricular ICDs may serve an increasingly valuable role in the management of patients with cardiac arrhythmias. In the case of AF management, such devices may serve both a prophylactic role as well as offer shock and nonshock therapies for the termination of AF. Concerns over atrial defibrillation-related ventricular proarrhythmia would be fewer in dual chamber devices because of their ability to treat induced ventricular arrhythmias. If the use of an implantable device for the therapy of AF is ever to be a feasable strategy, the proof will almost certainly derive from information gleaned from investigation with dual chamber defibrillators. Dual chamber ICDs would also provide improved arrhythmia discrimination of VT from SVT and limit the need for multiple devices in those patients who could benefit from dual chamber antibradycardia pacemaking. Evolution of implantable defibrillator therapy to include the atria can be practical, but only if we recognize the risks associated with such therapy and prospectively take measures to limit them.

References

1. Wijffels MC, Kirchhof CJ, Dorland R, Allessie MA. Atrial fibrillation begets atrial fibrillation: a study in awake chronically instrumented goats. Circulation 1995;92(7):1954–1968.
2. Nathan AW, Bexton RS, Spurrell RA, Camm AJ. Internal transvenous low energy cardioversion for the treatment of cardiac arrhythmias. Br Heart J 1984;52(4):377–384.
3. Ayers GM, Alferness CA, Ilina M, et al. Ventricular proarrhythmic effects of ventricular cycle length and shock strength in a sheep model of transvenous atrial defibrillation. Circulation 1994;89(1):413–422.
4. Dougherty CM. Longitudinal recovery following sudden cardiac arrest and internal cardioverter defibrillator implantation: survivors and their families. Am J Crit Care 1994;3(2):145–154.
5. Morris PL, Badger J, Chmielewski C, et al. Psychiatric morbidity following implantation of the automatic implantable cardioverter defibrillator. Psychosomatics 1991;32(1):58–64.
6. Pycha C, Gulledge AD, Hutzler J, et al. Psychological responses to the implantable defibrillator: preliminary observations. Psychosomatics 1986; 27(12):841–845.
7. Pycha C, Calabrese JR, Gulledge AD, Maloney JD. Patient and spouse acceptance and adaptation to implantable cardioverter defibrillators. Cleve Clin J Med 1990;57(5):441–444.
8. Sneed NV, Finch N. Experiences of patients and significant others with automatic implantable cardioverter defibrillators after discharge from the hospital. Prog Cardiovasc Nurs 1992;7(3):20–24.
9. Murgatroyd FD, Slade AK, Sopher SM, et al. Efficacy and tolerability of transvenous low energy cardioversion of paroxysmal atrial fibrillation in humans. J Am Coll Cardiol 1995;25(6):1347–1353.
10. Flaker GC, Blackshear JL, McBride R, et al. Antiarrhythmic drug therapy and cardiac mortality in atrial fibrillation. The Stroke Prevention in Atrial Fibrillation Investigators. J Am Coll Cardiol 1992;20(3):527–532.
11. Kannel WB, Abbott RD, Savage DD, McNamara PM. Epidemiologic features of chronic atrial fibrillation: the Framingham study. N Engl J Med 1982;306(17):1018–1022.
12. Jones GK, Swerdlow C, Reichenbach DD, et al. Anatomical findings in patients having had a chronically indwelling coronary sinus defibrillation lead. Pacing Clin Electrophysiol 1995;18(11):2062–2067.
13. Allessie M, Kirchhof C, Scheffer GJ, et al. Regional control of atrial fibrillation by rapid pacing in conscious dogs. Circulation 1991;84(4):1689–1697.

CHAPTER 30

Clinical Experience with Low-Energy Atrial Defibrillation

Francis D. Murgatroyd

Introduction

Direct current capacitor discharge between skin paddle electrodes was described by Lown et al. in 1962,[1] and is now the standard method for cardioverting atrial fibrillation (AF). The technique is successful in 70–95% of cases (depending on clinical variables, especially the duration of AF[2]), but the energy required is usually between 100 J and 300 J, and general anesthesia is therefore necessary. Alternate skin paddle positions do not consistently yield lower defibrillation thresholds.[3] Animal studies have shown that myocardial defibrillation requires shocks to produce a minimum potential gradient in the tissues, and this gradient is greatest near the electrodes.[4,5] It follows that the total energy requirement for defibrillation can be reduced by delivering shocks between high surface area electrodes in a configuration that surrounds the target tissue, at a minimal distance from that tissue.[6] This could be achieved for the atria using an invasive approach of some kind, with esophageal, epicardial, or intracavitary electrodes. Clinical experience with ventricular defibrillation supports this possibility, as energies <20 J are usually sufficient if epicardial or endocardial electrodes are used instead of external paddles. A technique that substantially reduced the atrial defibrillation threshold would enable cardioversion to be achieved without the need for general anesthesia. This would open the door to the development of an implantable atrial defibrillator. For such a device to be feasible, it would have to be demonstrated that a technique can be found to achieve cardioversion with very low energy, that this technique is safe, and that the shocks are tolerable to the patient group concerned. The experimental background to low-energy

From *Nonpharmacological Management of Atrial Fibrillation*, edited by F.D. Murgatroyd and A.J. Camm. © 1997, Futura Publishing Co., Inc., Armonk, NY.

atrial defibrillation has been covered in an earlier chapter of this book; in this and subsequent chapters the issues of efficacy, safety, and tolerability will be discussed from a clinical perspective, along with initial experience with an implantable atrial defibrillator.

The Feasibility of Low-Energy Internal Cardioversion in Humans

Esophageal Shocks

Because of its proximity to the left atrium, the esophagus has been investigated as a temporary cardioversion electrode site. In a canine sterile pericarditis model, Yamanouchi et al. obtained an atrial defibrillation threshold of 1.30 ± 0.46 J for shocks delivered between proximal and distal esophageal electrodes, and 1.29 ± 0.35 J for shocks delivered between the distal esophageal electrode and a chest plate.[7] This was three to four times lower than the energy required for transthoracic cardioversion in the same model. A similar lowering of threshold was obtained by McNally et al. in eight patients using a 7 cm esophageal electrode and a precordial plate.[8] Cardioversion was achieved with energies ≤60 J, compared with ≤215 J for conventional cardioversion in the same patients. McKeown et al. were able to cardiovert 80% of 88 patients with AF using an esophageal electrode, with a mean delivered energy of 63.1 ± 4.2 J; the maximum energy of 200 J was required in four patients.[9]

Endocavitary Right Atrial Shocks

Early attempts to obtain lower atrial defibrillation thresholds using conventional intracavitary electrodes were disappointing. In 1970, Jain et al. successfully cardioverted seven patients using right atrium-precordial shocks, but high energies were required.[10] Hartzler and Kallock found that shocks of up to 5 J delivered between the superior vena cava and the right atrium were unsuccessful in terminating AF or flutter.[11] Nathan et al. delivered bipolar and unipolar (with superior or inferior vena caval electrodes acting as anode) right atrial shocks of up to 10 J in nine patients. One episode of atrial flutter and no episodes of AF were terminated.[12] Unipolar right atrial shocks of 200–300 J (with a skin plate acting as indifferent electrode) have, however, been shown to be more effective than external cardioversion. Lévy et al. and Kumagai et al. each reported success with this technique in ten patients who were resistant to pharmacological or transthoracic cardioversion.[13,14] In a multicenter study, 112 patients resistant to electrical and/or pharmacological cardioversion were loaded orally with amiodarone and randomized to internal or external shocks. Internal shocks of 200–300 J were successful in 91% of patients, whereas conventional shocks of 300–360 J were successful in 67% (*P*<0.002). There was no difference between the techniques in the maintenance of sinus rhythm following successful cardioversion.[15] Concern has been expressed regarding the use of this technique, however, as shocks above 2.5 J using conventional low surface area electrodes cause the formation of a gas bubble. Arcing occurs within this bubble, causing a shock wave and consequent barotrauma.[16] It is even possible that the efficacy of the technique owes as much to this barotrauma as it does to a direct electrical effect on the arrhythmia.

Biatrial Shocks

The most efficient defibrillation electrode configuration induces a high potential gradient in the target tissue, and wastes minimal energy elsewhere. As the entirety of the atrial myocardium is involved in the perpetuation of AF, it would seem likely that a successful shock field must involve at least a significant proportion of both atria. Esophageal and unipolar right atrial techniques are anatomically far from ideal from this respect, and greater efficacy would be expected using an electrode configuration that encompasses both atria, from close quarters. A systematic comparison of transvenous right atrial and biatrial lead configurations and shock waveforms was therefore conducted by Cooper et al. in a series of experiments using a pacing-induced model of AF in sheep.[17] This model examined four right atrial electrode positions (superior vena cava, right atrial appendage, mid- and low right atrium) and three left atrial positions (coronary sinus, left pulmonary artery, and a left axillary subcutaneous patch) (Fig. 1). As expected, the lowest defibrillation thresholds were obtained using left-right atrial configurations, with those using an electrode pair in the right atrium and the coronary sinus somewhat lower than others. Using this configuration and a 3 ms + 3 ms biphasic truncated exponential shock, the mean energy requirement for cardioversion of AF was 1.3 ± 0.4 J.

The remarkably low atrial defibrillation thresholds seen in these animal experiments have prompted several centers to investigate the use of biatrial shocks in patients with clinical AF.

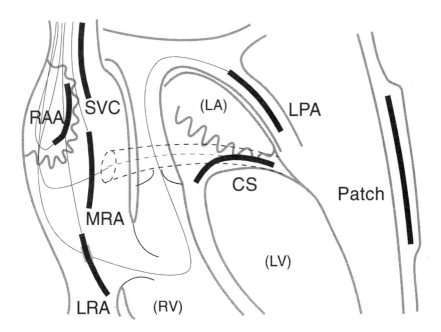

Figure 1. Electrode configurations in the study of Cooper et al.[17] Four right atrial sites were examined: superior vena cava (SVC), right atrial appendage (RAA), mid-right atrium (MRA), and low-right atrium (LRA); and three left atrial sites: coronary sinus (CS), left pulmonary artery (LPA), and subcutaneous patch (Patch). LA = left atrium; LV = left ventricle; RV = right ventricle. (Modified with permission from Cooper et al.[17])

Keane et al. compared 8 ms monophasic shocks and 4 ms + 4 ms biphasic shocks using epicardial paddle electrodes on the surface of each atrium in 21 patients undergoing cardiopulmonary bypass.[18] Fifty percent success was obtained at a mean energy of 1.44 J with monophasic shocks and 0.37 J with biphasic shocks. This study used large surface area paddles in direct contact with the epicardium, and AF was artificially induced and of short duration. For these reasons, the study may not have constituted a realistic model of the clinical application of transvenous systems. However, the study is of considerable theoretical importance for the same reasons, as it probably gives an indication of the lowest defibrillation thresholds that are likely to be achieved, although further improvements may be obtained with different waveforms.

Applying the findings of Cooper et al.[17] to patients with paroxysmal AF, we studied the efficacy of 3 ms + 3 ms biatrial shocks delivered between transvenous electrodes situated in the high right atrium and coronary sinus.[19] Each electrode was of a nine-segment, unipolar design with a total length of 6 cm and surface area of 2.83 cm². Twenty-two patients with acute AF were studied in the context of electrophysiological investigations. Seventeen of the patients had a history of documented, spontaneous AF. The episode of AF studied was induced by catheter manipulation or pacing in 18 patients (duration 0.25–1.25 hours) and spontaneous (duration 18–72 hours) in the other four. The technique was successful (Fig. 2) in the 19 patients who completed the study, with the mean energy requirement for cardioversion, 2.16 ± 1.02 J, somewhat higher than with the epicardial shocks of Keane et al.[18]

Early studies also showed the technique of biatrial transvenous shocks to be effective in persistent and resistant AF. The defibrillation thresholds are somewhat higher than with paroxysmal AF but still remarkably low. Alt et al. delivered shocks between electrodes (similar to the above) in the right atrium and the coronary sinus or left pulmonary artery in 14 patients with established AF.[20] In six of these patients, external cardioversion had previously failed. Shocks of up to 520 V (7,9 J) were delivered, and sinus rhythm was obtained in 10/14 cases. Cardioversion was achieved by Sopher et al. in 8 out of 11 patients with highly resistant AF[21] using the right atrium-coronary sinus configuration and shocks of up to 400 V (≈6 J). All patients had previously failed to cardiovert with repeated external shocks of up to 360 J delivered using both apex-base and anteroposterior paddle configurations—in many cases using adjunctive class III antiarrhythmic medication. Fi-

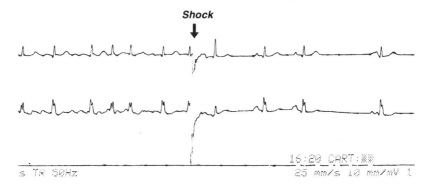

Figure 2. Electrogram of cardioversion using a 1.6 J biphasic shock delivered between transvenous biatrial leads.

nally, Baker et al.[22] reported successful internal cardioversion using transvenous biatrial shocks of ≤10 J in two morbidly obese patients with previously unsuccessful attempts at conventional cardioversion.

Safety

Proarrhythmic Safety

More widespread applicability of transvenous atrial defibrillation will be contingent on the demonstration of the safety of the technique. The most serious potential adverse consequence is that shocks delivered to cardiovert AF may provoke ventricular arrhythmias. This is of particular concern to the concept of a stand-alone implantable atrial defibrillator, whose use is envisaged out-of-hospital without the possibility of delivering immediate therapy for ventricular tachyarrhythmias.

The risk of ventricular proarrhythmia is likely to be determined by three factors. Firstly, the configuration of electrodes determines the energy required for atrial defibrillation and, therefore, both the strength and distribution of the defibrillation field. Experimental and clinical studies, as well as geometrical considerations and computer modeling all indicate that the right atrium-coronary sinus configuration is the most efficient, with minimum ventricular inclusion within the defibrillation field.[23] Other electrode configurations, such as those using the left pulmonary artery or a subcutaneous patch, require greater total field strengths and deliver a higher proportion of shock energy to the ventricles.

Secondly, the risk of proarrhythmia is likely to be affected by the susceptibility of the ventricle at a given time in individual patients. The inducibility of ventricular arrhythmias is determined by functional (ischemia, autonomic tone, electrolyte imbalance, and antiarrhythmic drugs) as well as structural factors, such as infarction and fibrosis.

Lastly, the timing of shocks within the cardiac cycle is critical to their safety. With transthoracic cardioversion, shocks falling on the T wave carry a high risk of inducing ventricular fibrillation (VF), and for this reason shock synchronization to the surface QRS complex or the endocardial R wave is necessary.[24,25] Even with correct synchronization, it is theoretically possible that an atrial shock delivered following a very short RR interval may fall into the relative refractory period of part of the ventricle, and thus initiate VF. Canine studies by Niwano et al. suggest that the possibility of proarrhythmia from shocks is contingent on the refractory status of the ventricle, and that atrial shocks can be delivered safely by avoiding a window around the QT interval.[26] Ayers et al. studied proarrhythmia from synchronized right atrium-coronary sinus shocks.[27] These were delivered: (1) at two strengths—20 V below the atrial defibrillation threshold and twice the threshold; (2) with a delay of 0–100 ms after the R wave onset; and (3) in paced rhythm, after single and double extrastimuli, and in AF. From a total of 1,870 shocks, four episodes of VF ensued at the lower energy settings, and seven at the higher settings. These episodes were all initiated by shocks following RR intervals of 300 ms or less. It was suggested that biatrial shocks would be safe if they are both QRS-synchronous and delivered after a minimum RR interval. To allow a safety margin, a value of 500 ms was suggested. By prolonging the QT interval, the presence of bundle branch block would be expected to increase the window of ventricular vulnerability. This has been confirmed in experimental bundle branch block in dogs by Keelan et al., who found that the risk associated with a short RR interval was lowered if the preceding RR interval was still shorter by at least 30 ms.[28] Shocks might therefore be safely delivered in AF even at high ventricular rates, if there is a critical RR deceleration interval immediately prior to the selected QRS complex. These findings have not been confirmed in humans, and such confirmation might be very difficult to achieve.

Systematic clinical testing of these hypotheses does not exist at present. No individual center has accumulated sufficient experience to test the safety of transvenous atrial defibrillation, nor is any likely to in the immediate future. A cooperative registry of centers that are investigating biatrial shocks delivered in patients has therefore been instituted. The registry reported initially from a thousand shocks.[29] By the end of 1994, this figure had exceeded 3,000 shocks: no proarrhythmia resulted from synchronized shocks delivered between the right atrium and coronary sinus, though unsynchronized shocks have triggered VF. Higher energies delivered between the right atrium and pulmonary artery have given rise to nonsustained runs of broad complex tachycardia. In addition to data in this registry, two cases have been reported of nonsustained ventricular tachycardia caused by synchronous atrioversion shocks delivered between the right atrium and the right ventricle, in patients with structural heart disease and a history of ventricular arrhythmias.[30]

For a stand-alone atrial defibrillator (without the ability to deliver "rescue" ventricular defibrillation), it is critical that the risk of inducing malignant ventricular arrhythmias approaches zero. This risk is substantial with unsynchronized atrial defibrillation shocks, whatever the electrode configuration used, but appears to be remote if correctly synchronized shocks are delivered between the right atrium and coronary sinus. The order of magnitude of the risk can be estimated if the assumption is made that the cumulative probability of a proarrhythmic occurrence follows a binomial distribution. Using this model, the lack of any events following the approximately 3,000 synchronized shocks observed in the multicenter registry gives an estimated risk of 0.0 per shock—more usefully, the upper 95% confidence interval of the risk is 0.1% per shock. In a device delivering one shock per month on average, this upper confidence interval would yield an annual risk comparable to that of antiarrhythmic drugs in a similar group of patients. This upper confidence limit will be revised downward if the encouraging safety experience with biatrial shocks continues.

It can be concluded that an implantable atrial defibrillator using the right atrium-coronary sinus lead configuration: (1) must guarantee correct QRS synchronization; (2) should probably only shock following RR intervals greater than 400–500 ms (shorter intervals may be permissible if they constitute a deceleration, and equally long-short intervals may be dangerous); (3) should avoid delivering shocks on or immediately after aberrantly conducted beats. A ventricular pace-sense electrode will therefore be necessary. Satisfactory technical demonstration of these capabilities would be a prerequisite for a stand-alone atrial defibrillator to be considered safe.

Bradycardia

In the sheep study of Cooper et al., it was noted that transient bradycardia could result from biatrial shocks at the upper energies studied.[17] If the right atrial electrode was situated in the high right atrium/superior vena caval region, shocks appeared to affect sinus node function, while atrioventricular conduction was sometimes temporarily disturbed with a low right atrium/inferior vena cava electrode. These effects have also been noted in humans: in the multicenter clinical registry, transient disturbance of sinoatrial and atrioventricular nodal function was occasionally seen with higher energy (>4 J) shocks, causing slowing of the ventricular rate during AF, and after cardioversion causing significant pauses before the resumption of sinus rhythm.[29] Although the observed bradycardic effects have been transient and limited to patients with sustained arrhythmia, caution dictates that an implantable atrial defibrillator provide, as a minimum, ventricular postshock backup pacing.

Mechanical Damage

It is clear from both animal and clinical data that direct current shocks delivered to the right atrium using conventional (low surface area) electrodes can cause significant damage. With shocks of 0.5 J in dogs, Dunbar et al. found focal subendocardial necrosis at the electrode contact site which, with shocks of 5J, became more widespread and affected half the atrial wall thickness.[31] Kalman et al. observed full thickness hemorrhagic necrosis in the atria of dogs given multiple shocks of 10–40 J, but using high surface area (braided) electrodes, energies of 0.5–10 J were sufficient for defibrillation, and only focal and superficial hemorrhagic change was seen.[32] Similarly, high-energy shocks delivered by low surface area electrodes to the coronary sinus for catheter ablation and attempted defibrillation have caused intramural rupture of the coronary sinus wall in dogs,[33,34] and coronary sinus rupture causing tamponade has been reported with this technique in a patient.[34] These complications have not been observed with high surface area defibrillation electrodes in the right atrium or coronary sinus,[35,36] presumably because the current density is more uniform, and the total energy requirement is lower, so that both arcing/barotrauma and direct electrical damage are avoided.

Thromboembolism

Conventional cardioversion of AF is associated with a risk of systemic thromboembolism of approximately 5%, which is reduced to around 1% in fully anticoagulated patients.[37,38] It is currently recommended (though the subject of debate) that anticoagulation be given to patients with AF of >48 hours' duration, prior to cardioversion.[39] Transesophageal studies have recently shown that thromboembolism can occur in patients without preexisting atrial thrombus, probably because of the phenomenon of atrial "stunning"—the delay between the return of sinus rhythm and that of normal mechanical function in the cardioverted atria.[40] It is not clear whether stunning is a direct effect of defibrillation shocks on the atria or, more likely, of prolonged AF itself. This issue is of great importance related to the potential benefit of an implantable atrial defibrillator, and is discussed in detail elsewhere in this book. It is hoped that an atrial defibrillator would prevent arrhythmic episodes from lasting more than a few hours, and that this would eliminate the thromboembolic risk. However, until more data are obtained to support this, it would be prudent for patients receiving anticoagulants to continue this therapy for a period after device implant.

Tolerability

The third issue that will determine the applicability of low-energy atrial defibrillation is the tolerability of shocks. Reason would suggest that discomfort increases with shock intensity, and that there is a threshold below which shocks are not felt, and a another above which discomfort is intolerable. Unfortunately, published reports that contribute data in this field are few and contradictory, and most relate to different forms of intracardiac shock delivery. Zipes et al. examined internal shocks for the termination of ventricular tachycardia and fibrillation, and found that energies less than 0.5 J were well tolerated without sedation.[41] Nathan et al. gave internal shocks of 0.1 J to 6.7 J for a variety of arrhythmias using low surface area catheters.[12] Twenty-one of 22 patients reported discomfort, which was severe in 14. No correlation was observed between energy and pain perception. Using high surface area electrodes in ventricular defibrillation configurations, Saksena et al. found that 8 of 10 conscious patients were able to tolerate shocks of less than 2 J.[42] These shocks were reported as uncomfortable but not painful.

In our study of low-energy biatrial shocks using high surface area catheters, no sedation was initially given; patients were asked to score the discomfort caused by each shock, and were offered sedation.[19] If the latter was requested, severe discomfort was automatically noted. All shocks were perceptible to patients, even those of 10–20 V (<0.1 J) given for system testing. The perception of discomfort varied greatly between patients, but appeared to increase uniformly with delivered energy for each patient (Fig. 3). In most patients, the atrial defibrillation threshold was somewhat higher than that of tolerability, with the greatest shock delivered without sedation between 100 V and 180 V, equivalent to ~0.5 J to 1.0 J.

Psychological factors are probably a major determinant of tolerability for internal cardioversion. Most of the patients in the above report had experienced a prolonged period of electrophysiological study immediately prior to the investigation. They were given shocks of steadily increasing intensity, for research purposes rather than clinical benefit, and had no knowledge of the number of shocks likely to restore sinus rhythm. The apparent relationship between intensity and discomfort may actually have reflected increasing distress with each successive

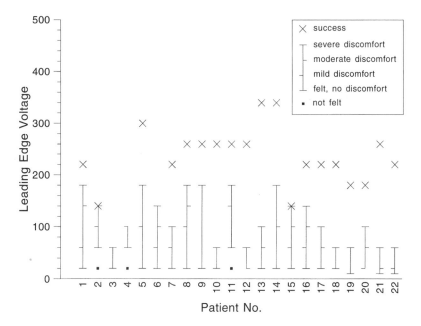

Figure 3. Discomfort in transvenous biatrial defibrillation, from the study of Murgatroyd et al. For each patient, the energy causing each level of discomfort is shown, together with the energy of the first successful shock. (Reproduced with permission from Murgatroyd et al.[19])

(ineffective) shock. This is supported by the experience of Steinhaus et al., who studied the tolerability of synchronized shocks of either 0.4 J or 2.0 J delivered in random order to 18 patients using standard epicardial or nonthoracotomy implantable cardioverter defibrillator systems.[43] Tolerability declined with the number of shocks delivered (100% for the first shock, 89% for the second, 50% for the third, and 33% for the fourth) but no relationship was found between discomfort and the two shock strengths. The anticipation of a clinical benefit from cardioversion seems to improve patient tolerance greatly, as does reducing the number of shocks to a minimum. Thus, patients with severely symptomatic chronic AF are frequently able to tolerate internal cardioversion with one or two shocks, despite the need for higher energies than with paroxysmal AF (Lau CP, Lévy S, personal communications). Baker et al. found that two morbidly obese patients with symptomatic AF refractory to transthoracic shocks were able to tolerate internal cardioversion using biatrial shocks of up to 10 J, with only light sedation.[22]

The recent advent of biphasic, biatrial shocks has enabled investigators to reduce the atrial defibrillation threshold by two orders of magnitude compared with external cardioversion. Nevertheless, this threshold remains well above that of perception, and a little higher than that of discomfort—a further lowering in threshold could enable the technique to become tolerable to the majority of patients. Clinical data regarding the determinants of atrial defibrillation threshold, and of shock-induced discomfort, are the subject of active investigation in several centers. They will be discussed in detail in a later chapter of this book, and are therefore only briefly summarized here.

Determinants of Atrial Defibrillation Threshold

Shock Waveform

The experiments of Cooper et al. in sheep[17] indicated the superiority of biphasic waveforms over monophasic waveforms for atrial defibrillation. This was confirmed in humans by Keane et al., with epicardial shocks.[18] Almost all investigations with transvenous leads have therefore used biphasic shocks exclusively, but the optimum waveform has recently been examined in more detail. Cooper et al. compared equivalent biphasic and monophasic waveforms over a range of total durations.[44] For total shock durations greater than 4 ms, the strength-duration curve for biphasic waveforms was fairly flat and uniformly lower than that for monophasic waveforms. Experiments in both sheep and humans, also by Cooper et al., indicate that asymmetric shocks with the second phase shorter than the first may yield lower defibrillation thresholds.[45,46] The effects of capacitance and the tilt of the biphasic waveform on biatrial defibrillation threshold have been examined in dogs by Mongeon et al.[47] Using 90 μF capacitors in this model, the leading edge voltage threshold varied little over a range of tilts between 15% and 85% (total shock duration 4 ms to 14 ms), but with a larger (180 μF) capacitor, threshold increased markedly with tilt, the optimum being 25% (total shock duration 4 ms to 8 ms). Barold et al. examined tilt in patients with induced AF.[48] A 50% tilt appeared optimal if waveforms with equal tilt in both phases were used, but lower energies were required using asymmetric waveforms with a greater tilt in the second phase than the first. The ideal waveform may therefore have a first phase that is longer and has a greater tilt than the second phase.

Electrode Configuration

Interest in the possible use of conventional ventricular lead systems for atrial defibrillation has led several groups to compare these lead systems with biatrial electrode configurations in small groups of patients; preliminary reports have recently appeared from many studies of optimum electrode position and size. Desai et al. were able to terminate induced AF (6 patients) and chronic AF (3 patients) with mean energies, respectively, of: 1.5 J and 9.3 J using the right atrium-coronary sinus configuration; 4.3 J and 10.4 J, using electrodes in the superior vena cava and right ventricle; and 5.4 J and 12.1 J, using a right atrial electrode and a pectoral can.[49] Saksena et al. compared transvenous ventricular defibrillator lead configurations in 10 patients.[42] The mean energy required was approximately 10 J for a right atrium (or superior vena cava)-right ventricle configuration, and 17.5 J for a right ventricle/patch lead system. Kalman et al. were successful in cardioverting only 1 of 10 patients with refractory AF using right atrium-right ventricle shocks of up to 10 J.[50] The addition of a cutaneous patch did not improve this efficacy. However, Geiger et al. recently reported, in a series of 13 patients, that the addition of a superior vena cava electrode to the right atrial electrode, or of a prepectoral patch to the coronary sinus electrode reduced the atrial defibrillation from approximately 220 V to approximately 150 V—equivalent to a 50% reduction in delivered energy.[51] The precise site and size of electrodes may also affect the defibrillation threshold. Schmitt et al. randomly compared the coronary sinus and left pulmonary artery as the location for a left atrial electrode in 56 patients.[52] Although impedances were similar, the defibrillation threshold was significantly lower for the coronary sinus group (3.9 vs. 6.9 J, $P<0.05$), suggesting that lead location rather than impedance determines the efficacy of biatrial shocks. Lok et al. examined right atrial electrode locations, and found that the mid-right atrium was associated with lower success rates than low or high right atrial sites, although it may have been more tolerable.[53] Hillsley et al. compared electrode lengths of 3 cm and 6 cm in a randomized fashion in seven patients.[54] The 6 cm electrode was associated with both lower impedance and a lower defibrillation threshold. It is not clear whether further electrode lengthening would be advantageous. Thus, while a range of electrode configurations can be used for internal atrial defibrillation, the right atrium-coronary sinus pairing currently offers the lowest threshold, though increased electrode length, the addition of a superior vena electrode, and/or that of a left pectoral patch or active can may lower the threshold further.

Clinical Variables

It is clear from the clinical studies described above that the atrial defibrillation threshold increases with arrhythmia duration. In the only large scale investigation to date, the multicenter study reported by Lévy et al., the mean conversion voltage was 216 V for acutely induced AF, 234 V for paroxysmal AF (≤7 days' duration), 257 V for AF of intermediate (7–30 days) duration, and 313 V for chronic AF (>30 days) (Fig. 4).[15] Apart from AF duration, left atrial size was significantly correlated with atrial defibrillation threshold. It is not clear whether these two factors are independent, or whether age, arrhythmia etiology, and other clinical factors may also affect the defibrillation threshold. However, a small study by Santini et al. suggests that exercise does not affect the threshold.[55]

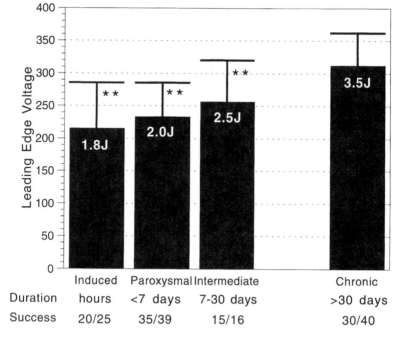

Figure 4. Atrial defibrillation thresholds for different arrhythmia durations, using a right atrium-coronary sinus lead configuration and 3 ms + 3 ms biphasic shocks. (From the multicenter XAD trial.[63])

Drugs and Catheter Ablation

Few data are available regarding the effects of antiarrhythmic drugs on the atrial defibrillation threshold. Amiodarone appears to reduce this threshold when conventional shocks are used[15]; anecdotal and largely retrospective reports from various investigators suggest that this is the case for both amiodarone and sotalol with internal shocks. Baker et al. have prospectively examined the effects of amiodarone, sotalol, and procainamide in a canine model. All three drugs lowered the atrial defibrillation threshold, but this was only significant for procainamide.[56] Similar prospective evaluations of the effects of antiarrhythmic drugs on human atrial defibrillation thresholds are being conducted but have not yet appeared in the published literature. Some of the most interesting effects may be seen with Vaughan Williams class III drugs, because of their capacity to increase the organization of AF and their relative lack of ventricular proarrhythmia. Drug/device hybrid therapy is likely to be commonplace for atrial defibrillators as with ventricular implantable cardioverter defibrillators (ICDs), for the same reason—many patients do not have rare, isolated arrhythmic events, but require drugs to reduce recurrences to a minimum, which can be satisfactorily treated by a device. Another form of hybrid therapy has been proposed by Kalman et al., who found that linear right atrial ablation lesions in a canine model increased the spatiotemporal organization of AF and reduced the atrial defibrillation threshold by approximately 50%.[57]

Applications of Low-Energy Atrial Defibrillation

The above studies have confirmed that cardioversion of AF using biphasic shocks and transvenous biatrial electrodes requires very low energies. General anesthesia is not required, and though shocks remain uncomfortable with current techniques, several modifications may lower the defibrillation threshold sufficiently for this problem to resolve. This technique may be of clinical importance in three types of applications.

Acute AF

Internal cardioversion may be indicated in the acute setting. Atrial fibrillation frequently complicates diagnostic electrophysiological procedures and catheter ablation, and general anesthesia for cardioversion causes delays while the use of antiarrhythmic drugs may make continuation of the procedure difficult. Internal cardioversion is used by several electrophysiology laboratories as a matter of routine in this situation, as it carries none of these disadvantages. The technique could be extended to intensive care settings, such as the management of patients following cardiac surgery and acute myocardial infarction, and to patients in whom general anesthesia may be hazardous, such as the morbidly obese.[22] Similarly, cardiac surgery patients frequently suffer repeated episodes of AF that may be poorly tolerated; temporary biatrial leads could be attached to the pericardium at the time of surgery for the purpose of cardioversion in the postoperative intensive care unit. This method was found to be uniformly effective in the canine sterile pericarditis model, with a mean atrial defibrillation threshold of 0.46 ± 0.07 J.[58] However, cardioversion using epicardial wires has yet to be formally evaluated in patients.

Resistant AF

Internal shocks can be used to terminate AF that has been highly resistant to conventional methods of cardioversion, as described earlier. While the efficacy of the technique in these patients is remarkable, the spontaneous recurrence rate is likely to be high, and there is no reason to believe that the use of a different technique of cardioversion will affect this. Internal cardioversion of resistant AF is therefore likely to be reserved for those cases in whom the benefit of sinus rhythm is particularly important, and those in whom maintenance antiarrhythmic therapy is contemplated.

Atrial Defibrillation by Implantable Devices

The most exciting potential application of low-energy internal cardioversion is undoubtedly its use in implanted devices. Atrial fibrillation occurs frequently in patients with ICDs, and is probably the most common cause of inappropriate therapy.[59] As discussed earlier, existing (ventricular) defibrillation electrode systems can be used for cardioversion, but the energy required is of the order of 5–10 J for paroxysmal AF, and 10–20 J for chronic AF.[42,49] Future ICDs may offer the ability to detect and treat AF using conventional electrodes. However, it is not clear that patients would tolerate automatic shocks of the required intensity for a non-life-threatening arrhythmia, and an additional coronary sinus electrode may be necessary to allow low-energy cardioversion.

The Implantable Atrial Defibrillator

The most radical application of low-energy atrioversion is an implantable device which has the sole purpose of terminating AF. Such a device has been developed and tested extensively in sheep.[60] It uses defibrillation electrodes in the right atrium and coronary sinus—in the former it has a screw for active fixation, in the latter it is held in place by assuming a helical conformation when its stylet is withdrawn after positioning (Fig. 5). A conventional bipolar lead is used for R-wave synchronization and backup pacing. The functioning of the atrial defibrillator is very different to that of ICDs; because AF is rarely a life-threatening emergency, the device does not need to detect and treat each episode immediately. Function in an atrial device must be based on the principle *primum non nocere* (first, do no harm). This applies especially to the arrhythmia diagnosis and shock synchronization algorithms; if an episode of AF is not treated, little harm is likely to ensue, but a shock delivered during another arrhythmia or poorly synchronized to the QRS could cause a life-threatening proarrhythmia. Therefore, in contradistinction to ICDs, atrial defibrillators must be highly specific in arrhythmia diagnosis, and the sensitivity of the detection algorithms is of secondary importance. The design aspects of the device that relate to safety, especially the arrhythmia detection and R-wave synchronization algorithms, will be discussed in more detail in a later chapter of this book.

The implantable atrial defibrillator can be programmed to several modes of functioning: (1) automatic, (2) patient-activated, (3) monitor only, (4) acute testing, (5) VVI pacing, and (6) off. In automatic mode, the device "wakes up" at preprogrammed intervals and records intracardiac electrograms for a number of seconds. Off-line analysis is performed to determine whether AF may be present. If not, the device returns to "sleep". If AF is suspected, highly specific algorithms using data sampled from lead pairs are used to establish a definite diagnosis of AF. If these algorithms are satisfied, the device charges its capacitors, reconfirms the diagnosis, and attempts to find a suitable R wave on which to deliver a synchronized shock. This process, from initial suspicion of AF to shock delivery, can easily take over a minute, and a small programmable warning shock can also be used to alert the

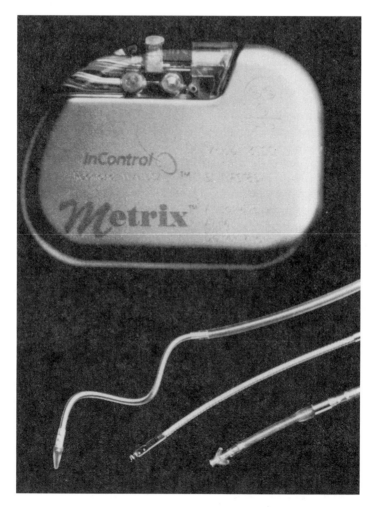

Figure 5. The implantable atrial defibrillator (METRIX™ 3000, InControl, Inc., Redmond, WA, USA). The three leads used are, from above, (1) a coronary sinus defibrillation electrode lead which assumes a helical shape upon withdrawal of its stylet, in order to retain its location; (2) an active fixation right atrial defibrillation electrode; and (3) a conventional bipolar ventricular pace/sense electrode. (Photograph courtesy of InControl, Inc.)

patient to the imminent delivery of a therapeutic shock. In the patient-activated mode, the device is "woken" up by magnet application rather than a timer. Thus, the patient suspecting AF can effectively switch the device on. If it agrees with the diagnosis, and a suitable R wave can be found within a given period of time, a therapy will be delivered; if not, the device will return to sleep. In monitor mode, function is exactly as in automatic mode, except that no therapy is delivered. This mode is used to obtain stored electrogram and other data, to verify correct device functioning. Because of the lack of urgency for therapy delivery, the device remains in "sleep" mode most of the time, and the capacitors need not be charged rapidly. This enables smaller batteries and capacitors to be used than in ICDs, reducing the overall size of the device.

The first human implants of this system (METRIX™ 3000, InControl Inc., Redmond, WA, USA), began in late 1995 (Fig. 6).[61] In this initial

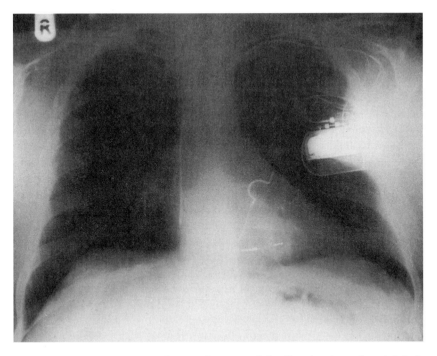

Figure 6. Posteroanterior chest radiogram of the first implanted atrial defibrillator. The right atrial electrode lies vertically above its attachment to the low lateral right atrial wall, and the helical coronary sinus electrode extends to the obtuse margin.

phase of evaluation of the device, automatic and patient-activated therapy is not permitted. All patients are programmed to monitor mode while out-of-hospital, and must return for arrhythmia treatment under medical supervision. By April 1996, six devices had been implanted worldwide. Correct function has been observed in all cases, and defibrillation thresholds have not been found to fluctuate significantly from those observed at time of implant. Data collected in these and future devices in monitor mode will enable the arrhythmia diagnosis algorithms to be validated during thousands of episodes, and the R-wave synchronization algorithms to be observed on tens of thousands of beats. Only then may out-of-hospital use of the device be permitted.

Conclusions

Recent developments, particularly the combination of biphasic shock waveforms, high surface area electrodes, and biatrial lead configurations, have dramatically reduced the voltage and energy required to terminate all types of AF. The atrial defibrillation threshold for internal cardioversion approaches, and has often reached, a level at which patients are able to tolerate the procedure without sedation, though not without some discomfort. Our current knowledge indicates that the right atrium-coronary sinus lead configuration yields the lowest atrial defibrillation threshold. Investigation of internal atrial defibrillation has now moved to a second phase in which every aspect of the technique—exact lead size and location, extra electrodes, precise shock waveform and duration, antiarrhythmic drugs and ablation—is being examined in detail, in order to determine how much further the atrial defibrillation threshold can be lowered by optimization of these variables. A lowering of 50% from current levels would probably allow cardioversion to be performed without sedation in the majority of patients. Data available to date indicate a high degree of safety, if shocks are correctly synchronized to the R wave. Animal data suggest that the avoidance of shock delivery following short RR intervals or beats with prolonged repolarization would also be prudent.

The technique of atrial defibrillation has several potential applications, from acute use in the electrophysiology laboratory and intensive care unit, to the cardioversion of patients with AF that is resistant to other interventions. Most exciting is the use of the technique in implantable devices; several patients have already received the stand-alone atrial defibrillator, and future ICDs will probably have the capability to deliver shocks for atrial as well as ventricular fibrillation. The evolution of two families of implantable devices can be foreseen: (1) an atrial arrhythmia device that can use single or multisite pacing to prevent arrhythmias, antitachycardia pacing to terminate atrial flutter, and biatrial shocks to treat sustained episodes of AF; and (2) a ventricular ICD with dual chamber pacing and sensing that allows enhanced diagnostic capabilities for the detection and differentiation of atrial arrhythmias,[62] and that can terminate AF using conventional lead configurations or an extra electrode permitting the use of biatrial shocks (Fig. 7). The manner in which atrial defibrillation shocks are delivered will be crucial to their acceptability, and unless the atrial defibrillation threshold can be brought so low that it becomes imperceptible, some form of patient control or activation will be desirable. Ultimately, the future of implantable devices for the treatment of AF will depend firstly on economic considerations (a reasonable cost comparison would be with the strategy of AV nodal ablation and implantation

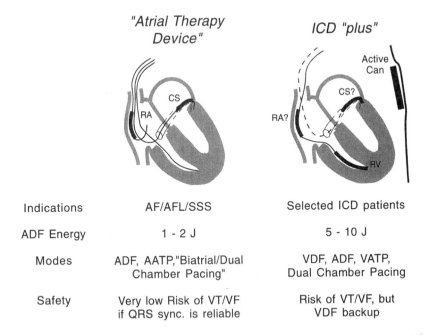

Figure 7. Possible future implantable defibrillators capable of treating atrial fibrillation. AATP = atrial antitachycardia pacing; ADF = atrial defibrillation; AF = atrial fibrillation; AFL = atrial flutter; SSS = sick sinus syndrome; VATP = ventricular antitachycardia pacing; VDF = ventricular defibrillation; VF = ventricular fibrillation; VT = ventricular tachycardia.

of a mode-switching pacemaker), secondly on the effects of each form of device therapy on the natural history of AF, and thirdly on the parallel developments of alternative strategies, such as catheter-based Maze procedures.

References

1. Lown B, Perlroth MG, Kaidbey S, et al. "Cardioversion" of atrial fibrillation: a report on the treatment of 65 episodes in 50 patients. N Engl J Med 1963;269:325–331.
2. Van Gelder IC, Crijns HJ, Van Gilst WH, et al. Prediction of uneventful cardioversion and maintenance of sinus rhythm from direct-current electrical cardioversion of chronic atrial fibrillation and flutter. Am J Cardiol 1991;68:41–46.
3. Kerber RE, Jensen SR, Grayzel J, et al. Elective cardioversion: influence of paddle-electrode location and size on success rates and energy requirements. N Engl J Med 1981;305:658–662.
4. Wharton JM, Wolf PD, Smith WM, et al. Cardiac potential and potential gradient fields generated by single, combined, and sequential shocks during ventricular defibrillation. Circulation 1992;85:1510–1523.
5. Chen PS, Wolf PD, Claydon FJ, et al. The potential gradient field created by epicardial defibrillation electrodes in dogs. Circulation 1986;74:626–636.
6. Dixon EG, Tang AS, Wolf PD, et al. Improved defibrillation thresholds with large contoured epicardial electrodes and biphasic waveforms. Circulation 1987;76:1176–1184.
7. Yamanouchi Y, Kumagai K, Tashiro N, et al. Transesophageal low-energy synchronous cardioversion of atrial flutter/fibrillation in the dog. Am Heart J 1992;123:417–420.
8. McNally EM, Meyer EC, Langendorf R. Elective countershock in unanesthetized patients with use of an esophageal electrode. Circulation 1966; 33:124–127.
9. McKeown PP, Croal S, Allen JD, et al. Transesophageal cardioversion. Am Heart J 1993;125:396–404.
10. Jain SC, Bhatnagar VM, Azami RU, Awasthey P. Elective countershock in atrial fibrillation with an intracardiac electrode: a preliminary report. J Assoc Physicians India 1970;18:821–824.
11. Hartzler GO, Kallock MJ. Low energy transvenous intracavitary cardioversion of tachycardias. In: Steinbach K, ed. Cardiac Pacing. Proceedings of the VIIth World Symposium on Cardiac Pacing. Darmstadt: Steinkopff; 1983:853–858.
12. Nathan AW, Bexton RS, Spurrell RAJ, Camm AJ. Internal transvenous low energy cardioversion for the treatment of cardiac arrhythmias. Br Heart J 1984;52:377–384.
13. Kumagai K, Yamanouchi Y, Hiroki T, Arakawa K. Effects of transcatheter cardioversion on chronic lone atrial fibrillation. PACE 1991;14:1571–1575.
14. Lévy S, Lacombe P, Cointe R, Bru P. High energy transcatheter cardioversion of chronic atrial fibrillation. J Am Coll Cardiol 1988;12:514–518.
15. Lévy S, Lauribe P, Dolla E, et al. A randomized comparison of external

and internal cardioversion of chronic atrial fibrillation (see comments). Circulation 1992;86:1415–1420.

16. Bardy GH, Coltorti F, Stewart RB, et al. Catheter-mediated electrical ablation: the relation between current and pulse width on voltage breakdown and shock-wave generation. Circ Res 1988;63:409–414.

17. Cooper RA, Alferness CA, Smith WM, Ideker RE. Internal cardioversion of atrial fibrillation in sheep. Circulation 1993;87:1673–1686.

18. Keane D, Boyd E, Anderson D, et al. Comparison of biphasic and monophasic waveforms in epicardial atrial defibrillation. J Am Coll Cardiol 1994; 24:171–176.

19. Murgatroyd FD, Slade AKB, Sopher SM, et al. Efficacy and tolerability of transvenous low energy cardioversion of paroxysmal atrial fibrillation in man. J Am Coll Cardiol 1995;25:1347–1353.

20. Alt E, Schmitt C, Ammer R, Coenen M, et al. Initial experience with intracardiac atrial defibrillation in patients with chronic atrial fibrillation. PACE 1994;17:1067–1078.

21. Sopher SM, Murgatroyd FD, Slade AKB, et al. Low energy internal cardioversion of atrial fibrillation resistant to transthoracic shocks. Heart 1996; 75:635–638.

22. Baker BM, Botteron GW, Smith JM. Low-energy internal cardioversion for atrial fibrillation resistant to external cardioversion. J Cardiovasc Electrophysiol 1995;6:44–47.

23. Min X, Mongeon L, Mehra R. Analysis of CS-RA, Can-RA, Can-RV and SVC-RV systems for atrial defibrillation by using finite element human thorax model and comparisons with the clinical studies. PACE 1996;19: 696. Abstract.

24. King BG. The effect of electric shock on heart action with special reference to varying susceptibility in different parts of the cardiac cycle. New York, NY: Columbia University; 1934. Thesis.

25. Wiggers CJ, Wegria R. Ventricular fibrillation due to single, localized induction and condenser shocks applied during the vulnerable phase of ventricular systole. Am J Physiol 1921;128:500–505.

26. Niwano S, Sokoloski MC, Ortiz J, et al. Evaluation of ventricular vulnerability and safety during atrial defibrillation via implanted transvenous catheters in the sterile pericarditis model. Circulation 1994;90:I-13. Abstract.

27. Ayers GM, Alferness CA, Ilina M, et al. Ventricular proarrhythmic effects of ventricular cycle length and shock strength in a sheep model of transvenous atrial defibrillation. Circulation 1994;89:413–422.

28. Keelan E, Krum E, Hare J, et al. Atrial defibrillation shocks synchronized to QRS complexes preceded by short-to-long cycles: minimal heart rate deceleration may protect against ventricular proarrhrhythmia. PACE 1996;19:647. Abstract.

29. Murgatroyd FD, Johnson EE, Cooper RA, et al. Safety of low energy transvenous atrial defibrillation: world experience. Circulation 1994;90: 14. Abstract.

30. Saksena S, Krol RB, Varanasi S, Mathew P. Internal atrial defibrillation in symptomatic atrial flutter/fibrillation. Circulation 1994;90:I-377. Abstract.

31. Dunbar DN, Tobler HG, Fetter J, et al. Intracavitary electrode catheter

cardioversion of atrial tachyarrhythmias in the dog. J Am Coll Cardiol 1986;7:1015-1027.

32. Kalman JM, Power JM, Chen JM, et al. Importance of electrode design, lead configuration and impedance for successful low energy transcatheter atrial defibrillation in dogs. J Am Coll Cardiol 1993;22:1199-1206.

33. Coltorti F, Bardy GH, Reichenbach D, et al. Effects of varying electrode configuration with catheter-mediated defibrillator pulses at the coronary sinus orifice in dogs. Circulation 1986;73:1321-1333.

34. Fisher JD, Brodman R, Kim SG, et al. Attempted nonsurgical electrical ablation of accessory pathways via the coronary sinus in the Wolff-Parkinson-White syndrome. J Am Coll Cardiol 1984;4:685-694.

35. Bardy GH, Allen MD, Mehra R, Johnson G. An effective and adaptable transvenous defibrillation system using the coronary sinus in humans. J Am Coll Cardiol 1990;16:887-895.

36. Bardy GH, Allen MD, Mehra R, et al. Transvenous defibrillation in humans via the coronary sinus. Circulation 1990;81:1252-1259.

37. Arnold AZ, Mick MJ, Mazurek RP, et al. Role of prophylactic anticoagulation for direct current cardioversion in patients with atrial fibrillation or atrial flutter. J Am Coll Cardiol 1992;19:851-855.

38. Bjerkelund CJ, Orning OM. The efficacy of anticoagulant therapy in preventing embolism related to DC electrical conversion of atrial fibrillation. Am J Cardiol 1969;23:208-216.

39. Laupacis A, Albers G, Dunn M, Feinberg WM. Antithrombotic therapy in atrial fibrillation. Chest 1992;102:426S-433S.

40. Manning WJ, Leeman DE, Gotch PJ, Come PC. Pulsed doppler evaluation of atrial mechanical function after electrical cardioversion of atrial fibrillation. J Am Coll Cardiol 1989;13:617-623.

41. Zipes DP, Jackman WM, Heger JJ, et al. Clinical transvenous cardioversion of recurrent life-threatening ventricular tachyarrhythmias: low energy synchronized cardioversion of ventricular tachycardia and termination of ventricular fibrillation in patients using a catheter electrode. Am Heart J 1982;103:789-794.

42. Saksena S, Mongeon L, Krol R, et al. Clinical efficacy and safety of atrial defibrillation using current nonthoracotomy endocardial lead configurations: a prospective randomized study. J Am Coll Cardiol 1994;23:125A. Abstract.

43. Steinhaus DM, Cardinal D, Mongeon L, et al. Atrial defibrillation: are low energy shocks acceptable to patients? PACE 1996;19:625. Abstract.

44. Cooper RA, Johnson EE, Yarger MD, et al. Comparison of multiple biphasic and monophasic waveforms for internal cardioversion of atrial fibrillation in humans. Circulation 1994;90:I-13. Abstract.

45. Cooper RA, Smith WM, Ideker RE. Atrial defibrillation with biphasic waveforms: a strength duration response for the second phase duration. PACE 1996;19:697. Abstract.

46. Cooper RA, Johnson EE, Wharton JM. The improved efficacy of asymmetric biphasic waveforms for internal cardioversion of atrial fibrillation in humans. PACE 1995;18:896. Abstract.

47. Mongeon L, Hill M, Mehra R. The effect of capacitance and tilt on atrial defibrillation in a sustained atrial fibrillation canine model. PACE 1996; 19:696. Abstract.

48. Barold H, Newby KH, Kearney MM, et al. Tilt-based transvenous atrial defibrillation in patients: improved efficacy with certain biphasic waveforms. Circulation 1995;I-473. Abstract.

49. Desai PK, Mongeon L, Conlon S, et al. Is energy for transvenous defibrillation of atrial fibrillation (AF) with active pectoral can feasible? Circulation 1994;90:I-376. Abstract.

50. Kalman JM, Jones EF, Doolan L, et al. Low energy endocardial cardioversion of atrial arrhythmias in humans. PACE 1995;18:1869–1875.

51. Geiger MJ, Mongeon L, Kearney MM, et al. Effects of an additional electrode on atrial defibrillation in patients. PACE 1996;19:624. Abstract.

52. Schmitt C, Ammer R, Plewan A, et al. Energy requirements for intracardiac low energy cardioversion of chronic atrial fibrillation: comparison of different lead positions. Circulation 1995;92:I-473. Abstract.

53. Lok N, Lau CP, Lee KLF, et al. Effect of different right atrial lead locations on the efficacy and tolerability of low energy transvenous atrial defibrillation with an implantable lead system. PACE 1996;19:633. Abstract.

54. Hillsley RE, Yarger MD, Greenfield RA, et al. Effect of catheter electrode length on internal atrial defibrillation thresholds in humans. Circulation 1995;92:I-473. Abstract.

55. Santini M, Pandozi C, Toscano S, et al. Changes in intracardiac atrial cardioversion threshold at rest and during exercise. PACE 1996;19:634. Abstract.

56. Baker BM, Botteron GW, Ambos D, et al. The effects of amiodarone, sotalol, and procainamide on internal atrial defibrillation threshold. Circulation 1996;92:I-473. Abstract.

57. Kalman JM, Olgin JE, Karch M, et al. Effect of right atrial linear lesions on atrial defibrillation threshold: implication for "hybrid therapy". PACE 1996;19:625. Abstract.

58. Ortiz J, Sokoloski MC, Ayers GM, et al. Atrial defibrillation using temporary epicardial defibrillation stainless steel wire electrodes: studies in the canine sterile pericarditis model. J Am Coll Cardiol 1995;26:1356–1364.

59. O'Nunain S, Roelke M, Trouton T, et al. Limitations and late complications of third-generation automatic cardioverter-defibrillators. Circulation 1995; 91:2204–2213.

60. Ayers GM, Griffin JC, Ilina MB, et al. An implantable atrial defibrillator: initial experience with a novel device. PACE 1994;17:769. Abstract.

61. Lau CP, Tse H, Lok N, et al. Initial clinical experience with an implantable human atrial defibrillator. PACE 1997;20–220–225.

62. Lavergne T, Daubert C, Chauvin M, et al. Preliminary experience with a dual chamber pacemaker defibrillator. PACE 1997;20:182–188.

63. Lévy S, Ricard P, Lau CP, et al. Multicenter low energy transvenous atrial defibrillation (XAD) trial. Circulation 1995;92:I-472. Abstract.

CHAPTER 31

How Can Atrial Defibrillation Be Made More Tolerable?

Gregory M. Ayers

Background

Defibrillation has long been used to treat atrial fibrillation (AF) with high-energy, high-voltage shocks delivered transthoracically.[1] These shocks can be quite uncomfortable, resulting in skin burns and musculoskeletal pain; therefore, general anesthesia has been required for the elective cardioversion of atrial arrhythmias. Research in the area of ventricular defibrillation has previously shown that termination of ventricular fibrillation and tachycardia can be accomplished at lower energies when the shocks are delivered to electrodes surrounding or inside the heart.[2-6] These promising results led to the development of present day implantable ventricular defibrillators that can deliver up to 35 joules (J) through electrodes in and around the heart. However, few patients with ventricular defibrillators used to treat ventricular fibrillation receive their shocks in the fully conscious state, due to the significant hemodynamic deterioration that usually results from this ventricular tachyarrhythmia; therefore the tolerability of such shocks, for the most part, remains unknown. However, in patients with ventricular tachycardia treated with an implantable defibrillator, some data exist pertaining to the tolerability of these shocks. Zipes et al. reported that shocks of an intensity of less than 0.5 J were generally well tolerated while shocks of greater than 0.5 J were less well tolerated.[7] They stated that, although the mechanism of the shock-related discomfort was not known, skeletal muscle contraction seen during delivery of the shock probably played a role in the patient-reported discomfort.

From *Nonpharmacological Management of Atrial Fibrillation*, edited by F.D. Murgatroyd and A.J. Camm. © 1997, Futura Publishing Co., Inc., Armonk, NY.

Internal Atrial Defibrillation

Internal atrial defibrillation may provide the medical community with a new method for the termination of atrial arrhythmias that is more tolerable than external defibrillation. Using this method to decrease the energy and voltage requirements for conversion of atrial arrhythmias with defibrillation shocks, patient tolerability and acceptance of therapy would be expected to improve since general anesthesia might no longer be needed and postconversion morbidity could be decreased.

A significant improvement in the efficacy of high-energy atrial defibrillation was seen using the technique described by Lévy et al.[8,9] This technique, using a single electrode on an electrophysiological mapping catheter floating in the right atrium, and a second electrode on the chest wall, resulted in high conversion rates of AF even in patients in whom external cardioversion had failed. However, due to the high shock intensities used for this technique, patient tolerance of this procedure would be expected to be poor.

Recent animal studies have shown that by positioning both electrodes within the heart or the vascular system, low-energy shocks of less than 1 J can be used to convert atrial arrhythmias.[10-20] Using this technique of internal atrial cardioversion, Keane et al. achieved good efficacy of conversion for a variety of atrial arrhythmias with low energy required for successful outcome.[21] They positioned catheter-based defibrillation electrodes in the distal coronary sinus and in the right atrium. Using a 4/4 msec biphasic waveform, they converted two patients with atrial flutter (mean energy 0.57 ± 0.44 J), five patients with short duration AF (3.3 ± 3.4 J), and eight patients with AF (6.7 ± 2.2 J). Using similar electrode locations, but with electrophysiological mapping style catheters instead, Johnson et al. converted patients with both short duration induced AF and spontaneous AF episodes at energies less than 3 J for biphasic waveforms, and less than 5 J for monophasic waveforms.[22-23] Murgatroyd et al. using a 3/3 biphasic waveform and distal coronary sinus to right atrium shock vector, attempted cardioversion in patients with paroxysmal AF.[24] They reported conversion in 19 of 19 patients with a mean threshold of 237 ± 55 V, 2.16 ± 1.02 J. Alt et al. compared the coronary sinus to right atrial shock vector to a left pulmonary artery to right atrium shock vector in patients with either cardioversion or drug resistant AF.[25,26] They found, in this difficult to manage population with AF, that 30 of 33 patients could be converted to sinus rhythm. They also found that the coronary sinus to right atrial shock vector had lower energy requirements (4.4 ± 2.5 J) as compared to using the left pulmonary artery (6.0 ± 2.6 J). Saksena et al. tested four shock vectors using electrodes in the right ventricle, left pulmonary artery, axilla, right atrium and coronary sinus.[27] Mean thresholds for the four shock vectors ranged from 20.1 ± 7.4 J for the right atrium to axilla vector, to 9.9 ± 7.7 J for shocks delivered from the right atrium to either the left pulmonary artery or coronary sinus. Only two thresholds were obtained using the right atrium to coronary sinus vector, and they were 2.0 and 7.5 J. These data, from the right atrium to the coronary sinus vector, were pooled with thresholds obtained from the right atrium to pulmonary artery vector, resulting in the higher mean threshold of 9.9 J. Lastly, Desai et al. found that in patients with chronic (N = 3) or short duration induced AF (N = 6), the coronary sinus to right atrium shock vector had the lowest energy requirement (1.8 J), and that patients with chronic AF had higher thresholds.[28] It appears that by using a shock vector that encompasses both atria and biphasic waveforms, atrial defibrillation can be accomplished with high efficacy and low energies in patients with both chronic or persistent, and paroxysmal AF. The lowest defibrillation thresholds are obtained with one electrode positioned in the distal coronary sinus and the second in the right atrium; although other shock vectors can be used, they tend to require higher intensity shocks.

Lower energy and voltage requirements, in combination with improved clinical efficacy associated with internal cardioversion of atrial arrhythmias, has spurred the development of techniques and equipment for the acute conversion of atrial arrhythmias with internal defibrillation shocks. These include removable wire electrodes for positioning around the heart in postoperative patients,[29,30] temporary catheters purposely built for acute positioning and cardioversion,[31] as well as implantable atrial defibrillators.[20,32] In an editorial, Camm and Lévy described the primary requirements for acceptance of an implantable atrial defibrillator—safety, efficacy, and patient tolerability of shock delivery.[33] The issue of patient tolerability is relevant for both conversion of acute episodes of AF with internal electrodes, and for an implanted device that treats recurrent episodes.

Saksena et al. reported that, in patients with AF, transvenous atrial cardioversion using shocks of greater than 3 J was found to be intolerable in 14 of 16 patients, and they concluded that tolerance for shocks greater than 2 J is limited.[27] Nathan et al. reported that in patients with atrial arrhythmias, 21 of 22 patients had some amount of discomfort for shocks delivered in the range of 0.1 J to 6.7 J.[34] In another study of transvenous atrial defibrillation, following a 20 V test shock, shocks of increasing intensity were delivered in 40 V increments.[24] Patients were initially unsedated and were asked to report pain on a scale of 1–5 following each shock. In this study, the largest shock delivered to a fully conscious patient was 116 ± 51 V; tolerable shock voltages varied in individual patients, from 60 V, 0.1 J in seven patients to 180 V, 1.1–1.2 J in six. Jung et al. reported that 73% of patients reported severe discomfort at shock energies of less than 1 J.[35] However, Toscano et al. reported conversion of 11 patients at or below 3 J with only mild discomfort.[36] These studies demonstrate that an exact threshold at which discomfort occurs is not well defined. Many factors may contribute to the mechanisms producing discomfort, including skeletal muscle contraction, direct nerve stimulation and a psychological component involving patient preparation for the shock.

Shock Intensity Units and Discomfort

To date, as well as in most of the reports cited in this chapter, the most commonly used unit of shock intensity to which discomfort was related was energy. Due to the work of Lapique, and others later, there is a well-defined relationship between pulse duration and pulse intensity (either energy or voltage) required for excitable tissue stimulation.[37] The relationship between pulse duration and threshold voltage and energy for stimulation is shown in Figure 1. As can be seen, at longer durations the voltage requirements for stimulation decrease, approaching rheobase, while the energy begins to climb after reaching a minimum. From this relationship, one could speculate that for nerve stimulation, which may result in either muscle contraction or sensory perception of pain, higher energies could be delivered at longer pulse durations and these pulses might not result in increased discomfort if the voltage threshold is not exceeded. Clinically, comparison of the discomfort of radiofrequency ablation versus direct current ablation provides a good example of this concept as it pertains to the delivery of energy to the heart. In radiofrequency ablation, an approximately 100-fold decrease in delivered voltage compared to that used for direct current ablation was possible, although approximately 10 times more energy is applied with radiofrequency ablation than direct current ablation. Despite the higher energy applied with radiofrequency ablation, this technique is known to be rather painless, whereas direct current ablation procedures are associated with significant pain and typically require heavy sedation or general anesthesia. These data suggest that, for energy applied to the heart through ablation catheters, voltage, rather than energy, may be the cause of the discomfort.

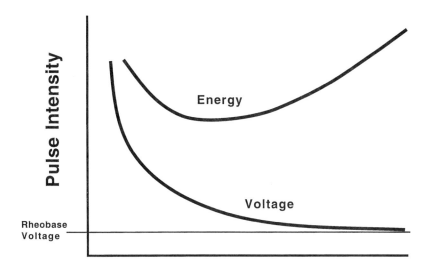

Pulse Duration

Figure 1. Graph of pulse voltage and energy versus pulse duration for excitable tissue stimulation. The graphs were generated from the Lapicque equations[37] and show that at longer durations the voltage required for stimulation approaches rheobase while the energy requirements of the pulse continues to increase.

Waveforms

It may be possible to decrease peak voltage by utilizing the relationship between pulse duration and capacitance for a truncated exponential waveform. If tilt can be maintained by increasing capacitance, peak voltage for an equal energy shock could be decreased (Fig. 2). Bourland et al. showed in sheep that for transvenous atrial defibrillation with square, biphasic waveforms, prolonging waveform duration resulted in decreased peak voltage for successful cardioversion.[17] Bourland further showed that delivered energy continues to climb, even as voltage requirements continue to decrease at the longer pulse durations; therefore, the voltage decrease may come at the expense of increased energy. If voltage causes discomfort associated with defibrillation shocks, a decrease in energy efficiency may be appropriate if patient tolerance of transvenous atrial defibrillation shocks is improved. Recent data suggest that for biphasic waveforms, the use of a limited range of durations (3/3 msec to 10/10 msec) and increased capacitance (to maintain equiva-

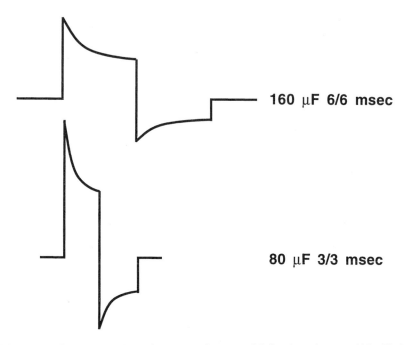

160 μF 6/6 msec

80 μF 3/3 msec

Figure 2. Representation of two equal energy biphasic pulses, a 160 μF, 6/6 msec pulse and a 80 μF 3/3 msec pulse. For equal energy delivered, the 160 μF, 6/6 msec waveform voltage is only 70% of the 80 μF 3/3 msec waveform voltage.

lent tilt) allows a decrease in peak voltage without significantly increasing the energy requirement.[38] In patients with chronic AF, the use of a longer duration, increased capacitance waveform with decreased peak voltage improves patient tolerability of atrial defibrillation shocks.[39]

Another possibility for reducing discomfort that may be associated with shocks is rounding of the leading edge of the defibrillation waveform (Fig. 3). In defibrillation therapy, the myocardium may not respond to the rapid onset of voltage in the initial peak of the first phase of the waveform; therefore this unusable energy could be "moved" from the peak to the latter portion of the waveform. Additionally, the "shift" in energy afforded by the rounding effect can permit prolongation of the waveform duration without increasing capacitance, an important consideration in implantable device use where capacitor size impacts device volume. Rounding was originally done with transthoracic defibrillators using inductors. For lower voltage implantable defibrillators or purposely built external atrial defibrillators, rounding can be per-

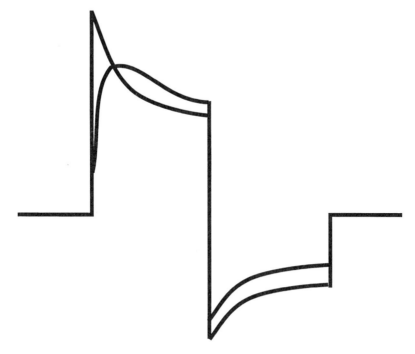

Figure 3. Representation of the waveforms before and after addition of rounding circuitry. The capacitor voltage was the same for both simulated discharges; however, with the rounding circuitry the peak voltage is diminished and the energy is "shifted" to the later phases of the waveform.

formed with analog components allowing for smaller size devices. Recent data from studies in sheep comparing capacitance, duration and the presence or absence of rounding indicate that rounded waveforms result in significantly lower peak voltage requirements with either similar[38] or decreased[40] atrial defibrillation energy requirements.

Electrode Positioning and Patient Posture

To date, atrial defibrillation studies have focused on evaluation of electrode positions, and therefore shock vectors that are either aimed at decreasing defibrillation threshold requirements or simplifying catheter placement.[11,15] Obviously, shock vectors such as those used for ventricular defibrillation (right ventricle to superior vena cava or right atrium) that have higher thresholds for atrial defibrillation would be expected to result in higher levels of discomfort.[27] However, as major nerves such as the phrenic, which in some part may be responsible for shock-related discomfort, course through or around the more successful atrial defibrillation electrode positions in the right atrium, pulmonary artery and coronary sinus, certain shock vectors made up of combinations of these locations may result in higher or lower patient tolerance. Lok et al. evaluated three right atrial electrode locations (lateral, inferomedial, and superior), with respect to both atrial cardioversion and shock discomfort thresholds.[41] In this study it was found that although the defibrillation requirements were lower for some of the electrode locations, there was no significant difference with respect to discomfort.

It may also be important to consider the effects of patient posture and stimuli from the surrounding environment on the tolerability of atrial defibrillation shocks, especially as they pertain to an implantable device that will be used in different settings. In the studies performed to date, patients studied in the catheterization laboratory were in the supine position. As position affects the relative locations of the electrical field with respect to the nerves and muscles, shocks delivered in the supine position may not replicate the perception of shocks delivered when the patient is in the upright or other position.

Pharmacological Agents

Pharmacological agents may play two important roles in decreasing discomfort associated with atrial defibrillation shocks. The first, and best established, is the use of antiarrhythmic agents to decrease either episode frequency or defibrillation threshold. Agents that decrease episode frequency would also decrease treatment frequency, and would therefore be especially important for patients treated with an implantable atrial defibrillator. By receiving fewer shocks, the patient's overall impression of the therapy with such a device would be expected to be more favorable. Agents that decrease atrial defibrillation thresholds have been studied to a limited extent in animal and clinical studies.[18,19,42,43] By decreasing defibrillation voltage and energy requirements, such agents would permit either the delivery of fewer shocks or at least shocks of lower intensity to terminate an episode of AF, thereby improving patient tolerance of therapy.

Secondly, pharmacological agents could be used to directly impact either anxiety or pain associated with atrial defibrillation shocks. Ideal for this purpose would be short-acting agents (sedative, hypnotic, or analgesic medications) delivered through transdermal, oral, or transnasal means, which would thus permit delivery in a variety of settings such as the physician's office, or potentially allow for patient self-medication. Although the onset and duration of action of these drugs would be critical to their successful use, their impact on defibrillation thresholds would also need to be determined. Patient self-medication would permit the delivery of these agents during patient preparation for implantable defibrillator therapeutic shock delivery, e.g., after a therapy warning or alert as described later in this chapter. In general, most studies to date have used intravenous sedative agents after patient report of discomfort, and their effect on discomfort has been sufficient to permit higher intensity shock delivery resulting in successful conversion of AF. Recent studies, as yet unreported in the literature, have shown that a transnasally delivered analgesic, prior to shock delivery, decreased shock- related discomfort such that nearly all patients tolerated shocks in excess of intensities previously reported to result in severe discomfort.[44]

Psychological Issues

The discomfort related to atrial defibrillation shocks may have both a centrally mediated anxiety component and a peripheral nervous system pain component. The predominance of these two components may be intensity related. Murgatroyd et al. reported that most patients perceived the delivery of very low-intensity shocks; however, most tolerated these shocks.[24] From these data, it is reasonable to assume that shocks of lower intensity probably produce a "startle" effect as well as potential anxiety associated with future shocks, and that higher intensity shocks are probably more causal of pain. Studies are underway that evaluate the different components of the discomfort with specific scales of anxiety (fear) and pain, as well as compare the effects of various pharmaceutical agents on these components. If the predominant component is more related to a startle effect or anxiety, these effects may abate with patient experience or may be treated with appropriate short-acting pharmaceuticals. Patient preparation could potentially decrease the startle response and may be accomplished with an implanted device through the use of a warning signal, such as a low-voltage shock. This warning shock could be of an adequate intensity to be felt by the patient, but of a low enough intensity not to be perceived as painful. In this way, the patient could prepare for the shock either through knowledge of the upcoming shock or through self-medication after a warning signal from the device.

Patient tolerance may also be related to the number of shocks required for cardioversion and individual shock intensities. Methods could be used that tailor therapy to individual patient preferences for number and intensity of shocks delivered. One approach is to use a limited number of higher intensity shocks to convert AF, with each shock having a high likelihood of success. With an implanted device, this approach would require patient willingness to receive fewer shocks with potentially greater discomfort associated with each shock. Another approach would be to deliver multiple shocks of increasing intensity, starting from a low intensity. Each shock individually would have a low probability of converting AF, but with multiple shocks of increasing intensity, successful conversion would eventually be achieved. Using this approach with an implanted device, some episodes would be converted with very low-intensity shocks and the patient might experience lower average shock intensities. The patient would have to be willing to accept multiple, but likely tolerable, shocks, both from an individual and cumulative sense. Some data exist that evaluate shock intensity and number of shocks delivered for successful atrial defibrillation. In the previously discussed study by Murgatroyd et al., the maximum shock intensity without sedation was about 120 V.[24] Based on the protocol followed in the study, patients would have received approximately 3 to 4 shocks before requesting sedation. Recent data suggest patients tolerate about the same number of shocks when starting from a voltage near the defibrillation threshold, despite the higher intensity of these shocks as compared to those used in the Murgatroyd study.[41] These data suggest patients may better tolerate delivery of fewer higher-intensity shocks rather than a greater number of lower-intensity shocks.

Lastly, the psychological effects of stimuli from the outside world during shock delivery may play a role in patient perception of the shock. To date, most shock delivery and patient questioning pertaining to discomfort has taken place in the catheterization laboratory, where all attention is focused on the shock delivery. This setting can be devoid of significant outside stimuli. As patients with an implantable device may receive the treatment in a different setting, such as in the home or physician's office, the somewhat distracting effects of such stimuli may indeed alter the patient's perception of the shocks. These issues merit clinical evaluation as the effects may be either positive or negative with respect to patient shock tolerance.

Conclusion

Many patients presently tolerate transvenous cardioversion of AF. Additional studies are required to evaluate whether the decreases in peak voltage requirements that are possible with current technology can decrease discomfort in patients who do not tolerate transvenous cardioversion. Palliative efforts, both pharmacological and psychological, will continue to play a role in improving patient tolerance of transvenous cardioversion. As has been observed through experience with other arrhythmias, continued technological advances will only serve to increase our understanding of AF, help address tolerability of atrial defibrillation shock, and thereby improve patient care.

References

1. Lown B, Perroth MG, Kaidbey S, et al. "Cardioversion" of atrial fibrillation. New Engl J Med 1963;269:325–331.
2. Mirowski M, Mower M, Staewen W, et al. Standby automatic defibrillator: an approach to prevention of sudden coronary death. Arch Intern Med 1970;126:158–161.
3. Schuder JC, Steoeckle H, Gold JH, et al. Experimental ventricular defibrillation with an automatic and completely implanted system. Trans Am Soc Amil In Organs 1970;16:207.
4. Mirowski M, Mower M, Staewen W, Denniston RH, et al. Ventricular defibrillation through a single intravascular catheter electrode system. Clin Res 1971;19:328.
5. Mirowski M, Mower M, Staewen WS, et al. The development of the transvenous automatic defibrillator. Arch Intern Med 1972;239:773–779.
6. Mirowski M, Mower M, Gott VL, et al. Feasibility and effectiveness of low-energy catheter defibrillation in man. Circulation 1973;47:79–85.
7. Zipes DP, Jackman WM, Heger JJ, et al. Clinical transvenous cardioversion of recurrent life-threatening ventricular tachyarrhythmias: low energy synchronized cardioversion of ventricular tachycardia and termination of ventricular fibrillation in patients using a catheter electrode. Am Heart J 1982;103:789–794.
8. Lévy S, Lacombe R, Cointe R, et al. High energy transcatheter cardioversion of chronic atrial fibrillation. J Am Coll Cardiol 1988;12:514–518.
9. Lévy S, Lauribe P, Dolle E, et al. A randomized comparison of external and internal cardioversion of chronic atrial fibrillation. Circulation 1992; 86:1415–1420.
10. Powell A, Garan H, McGovern B, et al. Low energy conversion of atrial fibrillation in the sheep. J Am Coll Cardiol 1992;20:707–711.
11. Ayers G, Ilina M, Wagner D, Kreyenhagen P, et al. Cardiac vein electrode locations for transvenous atrial defibrillation. J Am Coll Cardiol 1993;21: 306A.
12. Cooper RA, Alferness CA, Smith WM, et al. Internal cardioversion of atrial fibrillation in sheep. Circulation 1993;87:1673–1686.
13. Kalman JM, Power JM, Jin-Ming C, et al. Importance of electrode design, lead configuration and impedance for successful low energy transcatheter atrial defibrillation dogs. Am Coll Cardiol 1993;22:1199–1206.
14. Ayers GM, Alferness CA, Ilina M, et al. Ventricular proarrhythmic effects

of ventricular cycle length and shock strength in a sheep model of transvenous atrial defibrillation. Circulation 1994;89:413–422.
15. Ayers GM, Ilina MI, Wagner DO, et al. Right atrial electrode location for transvenous atrial defibrillation. J Am Coll Cardiol 1994;23:484A.
16. Benditt DG, Dunbar D, Fetter J, et al. Low energy transvenous cardioversion defibrillation of atrial tachyarrhythmias in the canine: an assessment of electrode configurations and monophasic pulse sequencing. Am Heart J 1994;127:994–1002.
17. Bourland JD, Ayers GM, Tacker WA, et al. Transvenous atrial fibrillation curves in sheep. PACE 1994;17:68.
18. Kumagai K, Niwano S, Sokoloski MC, et al. Effect of quinidine, d-sotalol and digoxin on atrial defibrillation thresholds during intraatrial transcatheter cardioversion in the sterile pericarditis model. PACE 1995;18:851.
19. Niwano S, Sokoloski MC, Ortiz J. Effects of digoxin and sotalol on atrial defibrillation thresholds via implanted transvenous catheter electrodes. J Am Coll Cardiol 1995:109A. Abstract.
20. Ayers GM, Griffin JC, Ilina MB, et al. An implantable atrial defibrillator: initial animal experience with a novel device. PACE 1994;17:769.
21. Keane D, Sulke N, Cooke R, et al. Endocardial cardioversion of atrial flutter and fibrillation. PACE 1993;16:928.
22. Johnson E, Yarger M, Wharton J. Monophasic and biphasic waveforms for low energy cardioversion of atrial fibrillation in humans. Circulation 1993; 88:3184.
23. Johnson E, Smith W, Yarger MD, et al. Clinical predictors of low-energy defibrillation thresholds in patients undergoing internal cardioversion of atrial fibrillation. PACE 1994;17:742.
24. Murgatroyd FD, Slade AKB, Slade SM, et al. Efficacy and tolerability of transvenous low energy cardioversion of paroxysmal atrial fibrillation in humans. J Am Coll Cardiol 1995;25:1347–1353.
25. Alt E, Schmitt C, Ammer R, et al. Initial experience with intracardiac atrial defibrillation in patients with chronic atrial fibrillation. PACE 1994;17: 1067–1078.
26. Alt E, Ammer R, Plewan A, et al. Energy requirements for intracardiac low-energy cardioversion of chronic atrial fibrillation: comparison of different lead positions. Circulation 1994;92:I-473.
27. Saksena S, Prakash A, Mangeon L, et al. Clinical efficacy and safety of atrial defibrillation using biphasic shocks and current nonthoracotomy endocardial lead configurations. Am J Cardiol 1995;76:913–921.
28. Desai PK, Mongeon L, Conlon S, et al. Is energy for transvenous defibrillation of atrial fibrillation with active pectoral can feasible? Circulation 1995; 90:1–376.
29. Ortiz J, Sokoloski MC, Niwano S, et al. Successful atrial defibrillation using temporary pericardial electrodes. J Am Coll Cardiol 1994;23:125A.
30. Mehma H, Haisch G, Lange R, et al. Temporary atrial patch electrode (TAPE): first report of a new method to treat supraventricular tachycardias after heart surgery. PACE 1995;18:901.
31. Alt E. Personal communication. 1996.
32. Sra J, Wharton M, Biblo L, et al. Feasibility of METRIX™ atrial defibrillation system in humans with atrial fibrillation. JACC 1996;27:375A.

33. Lévy S, Camm AJ. An implantable atrial defibrillator: an impossible dream? Circulation 1993;87:1769–1771.
34. Nathan AW, Bexton RS, Spurrell RA, Camm AJ. Internal transvenous low energy cardioversion for the treatment of cardiac arrhythmias. Br Heart J 1984;52:377–384.
35. Jung W, Pfeiffer D, Wolpert C, et al. Which patients do benefit from an implantable atrial defibrillator? JACC 1996;27:(2)301A.
36. Toscano S, Pandozi C, Castro A, et al. Low-energy endocavitary cardioversion for paroxysmal and chronic atrial arrhythmias. Eur Heart J 1995;16: 245.
37. Lapicque, L. Definition experimental de l'excitation. Comptes Rendus Acad Sci 1909;67(2):280–285.
38. Gonzales X, Ayers GM, Wagner DO, et al. Waveforms to reduce peak voltages for internal atrial defibrillation. PACE 1996;19:696. Abstract.
39. Ammer R, Alt E, Ayers GM, Schmitt C, et al. Pain threshold for low energy intracardiac cardioversion of atrial fibrillation with little or no sedation. PACE 1996;19:230–236.
40. Harbinson M, Allen JD, Iman Z, et al. Rounded biphasic waveform reduces energy requirements for transvenous catheter cardioversion of atrial fibrillation and flutter. PACE 1997;20:226–229.
41. Lok NS, Lau CP, Lee KLF, et al. Effect of different right atrial lead locations on the efficacy and tolerability of low energy transvenous atrial defibrillation with an implantable lead system. PACE 1996;19:633. Abstract.
42. Lok NS, Lau CP, Leung WH. Effect of sotalol on transvenous atrial defibrillation for acute and chronic atrial fibrillation. JACC 1995;25:109A.
43. Baker BM, Botteron GW, Ambos HD, et al. The effects of amiodarone, sotalol, and procainamide on internal atrial defibrillation threshold. Circulation 1995;92:I-473.
44. Timmermans C, Wellens HJJ. Personal communication. 1996.

CHAPTER 32

How Can Atrial Defibrillation Be Made Safe?

John Adams, Harley White, Jerry C. Griffin

Transthoracic atrial defibrillation is a routine procedure that has, with little change, been performed safely in human cardioversion since Lown et al.[1] demonstrated the principles of external R-wave synchronized direct current (DC) cardioversion in 1962. Recently, interest has grown in transvenous atrial defibrillation[2] and the possibility of an implantable atrial defibrillator.[3] An early attempt at transvenous atrial defibrillation in humans reported one case of a synchronized atrial defibrillation shock resulting in ventricular fibrillation (VF).[4] Other attempts at transvenous low-energy cardioversion of atrial fibrillation (AF)[5] and ventricular tachycardia (VT)[6] have resulted in proarrhythmic events, as has routine experience with modern implantable cardioverter defibrillators (ICDs) that treat VT.[7] With this background, the question "How can atrial defibrillation with an implanted atrial defibrillator be made safe?" is a very important one, especially in the context of the implanted atrial defibrillator as a single chamber device.

We will attempt to describe what we have learned both in the past and more recently about the known parameters of transvenous atrial defibrillation that can lead to an accelerated arrhythmia. We will then describe the design features that have been incorporated into one atrial defibrillator to address these issues, and finally, summarize the specific measurements to date that assess the performance of those features.

Previous Experience

Published reports of the inadequacy of synchronized cardioversion of the atrium to prevent proarrhythmia have been rare. Perhaps exter-

From *Nonpharmacological Management of Atrial Fibrillation*, edited by F.D. Murgatroyd and A.J. Camm. © 1997, Futura Publishing Co., Inc., Armonk, NY.

nal cardioversion of the atrium, simultaneously, fully defibrillates the ventricle, thereby eliminating the probability of a ventricular proarrhythmic effect. In any case, the only report known to the authors is the one quoted above[4] in which the cardioversion attempt used transvenous electrodes. Unlike external cardioversion, sufficient energy may not be provided with transvenous electrodes to defibrillate the ventricles even though the atrial tissue is fully depolarized. In 1992, our group, while performing routine transvenous atrial defibrillation in a sheep model from the right atrium (RA) to the coronary sinus (CS), experienced a case of VF in the animal (Fig. 1).

Careful analysis of the recordings revealed that the shock was precisely timed to an R wave as recorded on the right ventricular electrogram. Like the 1984 report of Nathan et al.,[4] our shock was synchronized to an R wave, and yet, VF resulted. This rare event was repeated a few weeks later. A detailed study was initiated to understand the mechanism of this surprising outcome since, at that time, synchronized cardioversion of the atrium was "known" to be safe from years of experience. In an implanted atrial defibrillator, which will be cardioverting

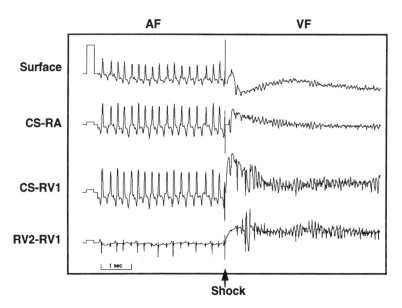

Figure 1. In a sheep model of AF, a shock synchronized to RV2–RV1 electrogram accelerates to VF. CS = coronary sinus; RA = right atrium; RV = right ventricle. (Same abbreviations in Figs. 2–6.)

a patient many times in a lifetime, even a rare event like this would be too often.

Our investigation, published in 1994,[8] determined that not all R waves were equal for timing a transvenous synchronized cardioversion shock. In the sheep model, we found proarrhythmia following approximately 1.1% of the shocks synchronized to R waves following the previous R wave by 300 ms or less. Equally important, all shocks delivered on longer cycles were not proarrhythmic. A quotation from the article best summarizes our conclusion:

> "It is logical to assume that if enough time has elapsed since the last beat for all ventricular cells to fully repolarize, none of the ventricle myocardium should be vulnerable."

Though our study did not provide the mechanistic proof, it seemed clear that the problem resulted from the fact that short coupled beats encroached on the relative refractory period of the preceding beat. Analysis of recordings from the initial sheep experiences of acceleration and the report of Nathan et al.[4] showed that the proarrhythmic synchronized shocks were indeed on short RR intervals.

Other reports in different models followed this one both in the baseline state as well as in the presence of different antiarrhythmic drugs. These studies all generally confirmed the same basic results. Kumagai et al.[9] reported that, in addition to short cycle lengths being vulnerable, an S1S2S3 protocol, where S2 is long relative to S3, was even worse in terms of vulnerability to proarrhythmia. AF, of course, results in many ventricular intervals with long-short combinations. Li et al. reported that, in dogs, a wide QRS complex, such as a PVC or bundle branch block, is followed by a longer period of vulnerability to atrial defibrillation shocks than is a normally conducted beat.[10] Natale et al. reported that patients with AF and a history of VT did not accelerate when AF alone was shocked synchronously, but did accelerate when the AF was shocked synchronously to a VT rhythm.[11] In an earlier report Saksena et al.[12] reported that cardioversion of AF in a VT patient resulted in a brief, slow unsustained wide complex rhythm after a shock of over 10 J.

The effects of digoxin and quinidine on the vulnerability of the ventricle to atrial shocks have been reported as well.[13,14] Digoxin was shown to have virtually no effect, while quinidine reduced the vulnerability to proarrhythmia under the conditions of low-energy, short cycle length shocks.

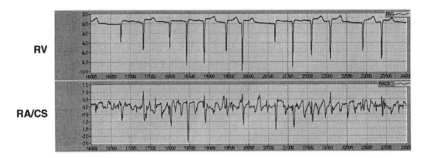

Figure 2. Bipolar RV electrogram interval and amplitude are variable in AF. Note some intervals are less than 500 ms.

Device Assessment of Proper Shock Timing

For avoidance of potential proarrhythmia, cardiac rhythm management devices of all levels of output, including pacemakers, coordinate energy delivery with ventricular depolarization. The studies above demonstrate that additional protection from proarrhythmic risk of transvenously delivered electrical shocks to the atrium can be achieved by avoiding certain situations; namely, very short cycle lengths and those in a long-short sequence. Fortunately, as shown in Figure 2, AF provides a large selection of RR interval cycle lengths from which an implanted atrial defibrillator may choose. The electronics of an atrial defibrillator can easily monitor the time since the last R wave and only permit shock delivery to occur if this elapsed time exceeds a programmed minimum, typically 500–600 ms. As can be seen in Figure 2, some of the intervals do not meet this criterion and would therefore be rejected as not being "optimal for shock" by the METRIX™ 3000 (InControl, Redmond, WA) implantable atrial defibrillator. Delays to cardioversion are minimal[15] and of no consequence in the treatment of this arrhythmia.

In order to accurately synchronize with the R wave and accurately time intervals between R waves, the device should be extremely specific in the identification of R waves, though not necessarily sensitive, and extremely sensitive to events occurring in the ventricles, though not necessarily specific. Although this may appear to be somewhat contradictory, it is the basis for the highly robust synchronization system of the METRIX™ 3000. The device is able to achieve this by being both highly sensitive to events occurring in the ventricles as well as very accurate in examining a group of events clustered in time and determining if they constitute a ventricular depolarization. Measuring the time between R waves has been possible since the first demand pacemaker. However, in an atrial defibrillator as described here, it is very important that every R wave is detected prior to shock delivery in order to assure that adequate time has passed since the last R wave. In Figure 2, it can be seen that considerable amplitude variation may also be present in the bipolar right ventricular (RV) electrogram while AF is occurring. Some of the low-amplitude signals are followed by short cycle lengths. Yokoyama[16] reported a similar variation in RV amplitude in patients with chronic bipolar RV pacing electrodes. If the low-amplitude signals are undersensed by the atrial defibrillator, proper interval measurement and minimum interval criteria application would be compromised even though all the R waves that are detected are genuine. In order to assure that all shocks are delivered on only long intervals, all R-wave events must be detected prior to the shock delivery. This will prevent the device from undercounting events (high sensitivity) at the expense of occasionally detecting events that may not be part of an R wave (high specificity). On the other hand, if synchronized shock delivery is to be performed, the device must select an event upon which to deliver a shock that is highly probable of actually being an R wave (specific) even if the process rejects a considerable number of candidates in the process. Thus if the shock is to be synchronized to an R wave and an adequate safe interval is required, all R waves must be detected.

In order to fully achieve these objectives, the METRIX™ 3000 implantable atrial defibrillator contains a second R-wave amplifier, detector circuit, and logic software as shown in Figure 3. The additional amplifier monitors the ventricular electrogram between the RV tip and

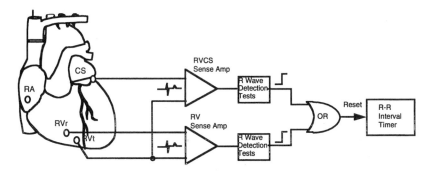

Figure 3. Either channel of the dual R-wave sense amplifiers can reset R-R interval timer.

Table 1
EGM Amplitude Variability in AF With
Temporary Leads

RV max/min = 2.8 mean
RVCS max/min = 1.8 mean

the CS electrode to provide a second view of the ventricles. The second amplifier is connected to the second R-wave detector, which is then coupled to the interval timer with a logical "OR" connection. If either R-wave detector detects an event, the interval timer is reset to zero time. The interval timer must reach 600 ms (the actual number is programmable), for example, without being reset by either R-wave detector in order to permit shock delivery. As implemented in the METRIX™ 3000, shock delivery is in synchronization to the next following R wave.

The RV/CS electrogram has amplitude variation during AF also, but not as prevalently as the RV electrogram. Table 1 shows the mean of the amplitude variation (maximum R-wave amplitude/minimum amplitude) for these two vectors in several patients with temporary leads. The provision of these two R-wave monitoring systems and their interrelation as described above provides additional security that all R waves will be detected and that the interval timer will be measuring true intervals.

Figure 4 illustrates the RV and RV/CS electrograms with the implanted device detection markers for each channel as telemetered from a METRIX™ 3000 implantable atrial defibrillator to the programmer. On the left-center of the electrograms, we can see an incidence where an R wave is not detected in the RV channel, while the same R wave is detected in the RV/CS channel. Thus, even with the considerable electrogram amplitude variation that can occur during AF, the interval timer is able to function properly since the "dual reset" function of the timer is more sensitive than a single reset with either channel alone.

To deliver the shock synchronized to an R wave, one would intuitively conclude that a highly sensitive detector would be best for detection of every R wave. However, counterintuitively, a more specific R-wave detector is preferred to avoid an oversensing condition that might cause a T wave to be detected at this time. To provide more specific R-wave detection for the actual shock delivery, the two R-wave detection circuits are interrelated in a logical "AND" connection as shown in Figure 5. Both R-wave detectors must determine that an R wave has occurred before a shock may be delivered.

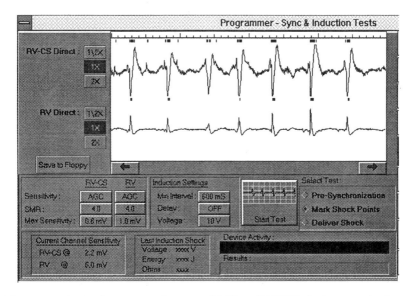

Figure 4. A simultaneous, telemetered RV and RV/CS electrogram is shown with R-wave detection marks around the traces. Note the third RV complex was not detected while the RV/CS channel detected the R wave.

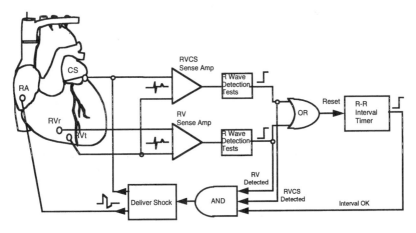

Figure 5. A dual R-wave sense amplifier connected for synchronization requiring both channels to deliver a synchronized shock.

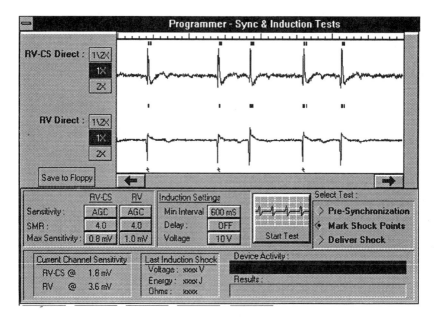

Figure 6. Shockable R waves are shown with "lightning bolt". Note only long cycle lengths are marked shockable.

In the METRIX® 3000, before an atrial cardioversion shock is delivered, a minimum time must elapse since the sensitive detection of a last R wave, and the shock is then synchronized to the next, more specifically detected, R wave. This unique combination provides both very specific and sensitive R-wave detection for the purpose of determining when the optimum atrial shock synchronization conditions are satisfied.

Figure 6 shows telemetered electrograms of the RV and RV/CS channels with the R-wave detection marks shown above each electrogram. In addition, at the bottom of the traces are synchronization or shock markers showing which R waves satisfy the synchronization conditions as shockable. These markers are the small lightning bolts. Short electrogram intervals are rejected. Long electrogram intervals with R-wave detection in both channels are indicated as acceptable.

In Vitro Test Results

The synchronization algorithm system has been tested with digitally recorded electrograms from the same vectors as those intended for the permanent locations. Electrograms from 32 patients containing 17,271 R waves were evaluated by the METRIX™ 3000 System for "marking" acceptable R waves. Forty-nine percent of these R waves occurred while the patients were in AF. 4,839 R waves (28%) were marked as "shockable", meeting all the criteria. One-hundred percent of all shock markers (marked R waves) were synchronous to an R wave and completed an RR interval greater than 500 ms duration.

Clinical Testing

The implanted system was tested externally under an Investigational Device Exemption (IDE) approved study in the USA on 15 patients with AF. In this study, 2,391 R waves were tested with the synchronizer algorithm described above. The patients were in AF for 64% of these R waves. In this case, 1,135 R-wave markers (47%) were generated indicating each corresponding R wave as being shockable, again with 100% of the markers being within the R wave and completing an interval greater than 500 ms in duration. This same group of patients were shocked by the METRIX™ System 64 times with no proarrhythmia.[17] Early reports on the first five patients permanently implanted with the device show over 11,000 R waves have been analyzed with 37% meeting the synchronizer criteria and all being marked accurately.

Conclusion

A dual R-wave synchronizer and a long RR interval criterion have been shown to be accurate. Shocks delivered in the first external clinical trial using this system were without any proarrhythmia. At this time, this device remains in clinical trials.

References

1. Lown B, Amarasingham R, Neuman J. New method for terminating cardiac arrhythmias. JAMA 1962;182:548–555.
2. Cooper RA, Alferness CA, Smith WM, et al. Internal cardioversion of atrial fibrillation in sheep. Circulation 1993;87:1673–1686.
3. Levy S, Camm AJ. An implantable atrial defibrillator: an impossible dream? Circulation 1993;87:1769–1771.
4. Nathan AW, Bexton RS, Spurrell RA, Camm AJ. Internal transvenous low energy cardioversion for the treatment of cardiac arrhythmias. Br Heart J 1984;52:377–384.

5. Osswald S, Trouton TG, Roelke M, et al. Efficacy and limitations of single lead low energy conversion of atrial fibrillation in cardiomyopathy model. PACE 1994;17:817.
6. Zipes DP, Jackman WM, Heger JJ, et al. Clinical transvenous cardioversion of recurrent life-threatening ventricular tachyarrhythmias: low energy synchronized cardioversion of ventricular tachycardia and termination of ventricular fibrillation in patients using a catheter electrode. Am Heart J 1982;103:789–794.
7. Bardy G. A prospective randomized repeat-crossover comparison of antitachycardia pacing with low-energy cardioversion. Circulation 1993;87: 1889–1896.
8. Ayers GM, Alferness CA, Ilina M, et al. Ventricular proarrhythmic effects of ventricular cycle length and shock strength in a sheep model of transvenous atrial defibrillation. Circulation 1994;89:413–422.
9. Kumagai K, Niwano S, Ayers GM, et al. Effects of the preceding R-R interval on the safety of atrial defibrillation via transvenous catheter electrodes in the sterile pericarditis model. J Am Coll Cardiol 1995;(special issue): 15A. Abstract.
10. Li H, Hare J, Mughai K, et al. Safety of atrial defibrillation: the importance of pre-shock R-R intervals and the risk of premature ventricular contractions. J Am Coll Cardiol 1996;27:301A. Abstract.
11. Natale A, Kearney MM, Brandon J, et al. Safety of transvenous atrial defibrillation in patients with monomorphic ventricular tachycardia and heart disease. J Am Coll Cardiol 1996;27:302A. Abstract.
12. Saksena S, Prakash A, Mangeon L, et al. Clinical efficacy and safety of atrial defibrillation using biphasic shocks and current nonthoractomy endocardial lead configurations. Am J Coll Cardiol 1995;76:913–920.
13. Niwano S, Sokoloski MC, Ortiz J. Effects of digoxin and sotalol on atrial defibrillation thresholds via implanted transvenous catheter electrodes. J Am Coll Cardiol 1995:109A. Abstract.
14. Kumagai K, Niwano S, Sokoloski MC, et al. Effect of quinidine on ventricular vulnerability during intraatrial transcatheter cardioversion in the canine sterile percarditis model. PACE 1995;18:941. Abstract.
15. Hnatkove K, Murgatroyd F, Alferness C, et al. Distribution of episodes with short ventricular cycles during paroxysmal atrial fibrillation. PACE 1995;18:1125. Abstract.
16. Yokoyama M, Nitta S. A shorter R-R inverval causes a larger endocardial R-wave amplitude. PACE 1995;18:2180–2182.
17. Sra J, Wharton M, Biblo L, for the METRIX™ System External Defibrillation Study Invesitgators. Feasibility of the METRIX™ Atrial Defibrillation System in humans with atrial fibrillation. J Am Coll Cardiol 1996;27:375A. Abstract.

CHAPTER 33

Who Needs an Atrial Defibrillator?

Samuel Lévy, Philippe Ricard

Atrial fibrillation (AF) is an extremely common arrhythmia seen in clinical practice as shown by a number of epidemiological studies.[1,2] Pharmacological therapy is usually the treatment of first choice, and a number of patients respond favorably, at least for a given period of time.[3] However, a significant number of patients have recurrent attacks of AF despite pharmacological therapy, or are controlled but the drug is discontinued as the patient develops intolerable side effects. Symptoms related to the arrhythmia may be due to the rapid ventricular response and/or irregular rhythm. Other symptoms or complications include: a deleterious effect on cardiac function, reduced cardiac output, and peripheral emboli. The embolic risk averages 3% to 5% per year and depends on the age of the patient, presence and type of underlying heart disease, and ventricular function.[4,4a]

The success of the automatic implantable cardioverter defibrillator (ICD) for the treatment of ventricular life-threatening tachyarrhythmias has led to the idea that a device capable of detecting and automatically terminating AF may be useful. The validity of such a concept was addressed in a recent editorial.[5] The feasibility and safety of such a device must be discussed together with the possible need for an implantable atrial defibrillator and its role among the therapeutic strategies for AF.

The indications of an atrial defibrillator must be assessed in light of the currently available device (METRIX™ 3000, InControl, Inc., Redmond, WA, USA) and our current understanding and knowledge of AF and defibrillation. Therefore, the indications outlined in this chapter will be revised and extended in the future. The longer term may see the development of a small device capable of double chamber sensing and pacing and double chamber defibrillation.

From *Nonpharmacological Management of Atrial Fibrillation*, edited by F.D. Murgatroyd and A.J. Camm. © 1997, Futura Publishing Co., Inc., Armonk, NY.

Background on Low-Energy Defibrillation

As detailed in an earlier chapter, low-energy defibrillation is possible in more than 75% of patients with AF with energy lower than 5 joules (J). Most studies[6-8] have dealt with induced AF. The multicenter Low Energy Transvenous Atrial Defibrillation trial (XAD)[14] included various types of AF: induced, paroxysmal, intermediate, and chronic. In our own series of patients with spontaneous AF,[9] successful low-energy cardioversion was obtained in 22 of 28 patients (78%) with chronic AF with a mean energy level of 3.3 ± 1.3 J. In paroxysmal AF, 11 of 14 patients (78%) were successfully cardioverted with a mean energy level of 1.8 ± 0.7 J and the difference between the groups was statistically significant. Considering the right atrium-coronary sinus electrode configuration, 27 of 30 patients (84%) had restoration of sinus rhythm with a mean voltage of 256 ± 51 V and a mean energy of 2.4 ± 0.9 J. The right atrium-left pulmonary configuration restored sinus rhythm in 6 of 10 patients and required a conversion voltage of 325 ± 74 V and a mean energy of 4.2 ± 2.0 J. As the right atrium-coronary sinus configuration is the one used in the current device, most patients with paroxysmal AF, and a number of patients with chronic AF, may be defibrillated with less than 300 V, the current maximum of the device. A safety margin should be considered and successful defibrillation with 240 V or less is required. Therefore, the candidate for an atrial defibrillator should be reproducibly cardioverted with a conversion voltage of 240 V or less. At present, very little is known on the reproducibility of low-energy defibrillation either during the same session or at different sessions. Although there are some data suggesting that repeat low-energy cardioversion after a period of sinus rhythm is associated with a lower defibrillation threshold compared with cardioversion from chronic AF, the reproducibility in the same session of the defibrillation voltage needs to be evaluated. In the protocol adopted in the clinical trial of METRIX™ 3000, more than three successful defibrillation attempts with 240 V or less are required. In fact, failure of the device at its maximal output is less crucial than for ventricular implantable defibrillators as AF is not an immediately lethal arrhythmia.

A major concern with an implantable atrial defibrillator is its safety, i.e., the potential risk of inducing ventricular tachycardia or fibrillation when delivering a shock to convert AF. Obviously, the shock delivered to the right atrium should be synchronized to the ventricular electrogram recorded through an electrode positioned in the right ventricle. Such an electrode catheter may also be useful for pacing the ventricles in case of shock-related bradycardia (asystole or AV block).

The concern for safety was addressed in a previous chapter. To our knowledge, there has been no case of sustained ventricular proarrhythmia observed with low-energy atrial defibrillation using properly synchronized shocks. However, safety remains an important aspect to be assessed during the clinical trial. It justifies an initial phase of 1 year for a physician-activated device before allowing the use of the atrial defibrillator programmed on the automatic mode.

The issue of pain-related shocks has also been discussed previously in this book. It needs to be assessed for every patient on an individual basis and may vary from country to country as pain may have a cultural component. The patient may tolerate shock-related discomfort more easily if AF is poorly tolerated and perceived by the patient as altering his/her quality of life.

Which Arrhythmias May Be Treated with an Atrial Defibrillator?

At present, AF is the only atrial arrhythmias to be correctly recognized and treated. The detection algorithms of the device and the programmed shortest RR interval preceding shocks will not allow the delivery of shocks for atrial flutter.

The clinical presentation of AF is quite heterogeneous, and a classification system has recently been proposed (Table 1).[10] It seems appropriate to define different types of AF although such definitions may be

---

Table 1
Proposed Clinical Classification of Atrial
Fibrillation

CLASS I. First attack of AF.
    A. Spontaneous termination.
    B. Pharmacological or electrical cardioversion.
CLASS II. Recurrent attacks of AF (untreated).
    A. Asymptomatic.
    B. Less than 1 attack/3 months.
    C. More than 1 attack/3 months.
CLASS III. Recurrent attacks of AF (treated).
    A. Asymptomatic.
    B. Less than 1 attack/3 months.
    C. More than 1 attack/3 months.

AF = Atrial fibrillation.

arbitrary. Atrial fibrillation is usually subdivided into the paroxysmal form and the established or chronic form. The paroxysmal form may be self-terminating in less than 48 hours, or persistent, lasting more than 48 hours. By definition, the paroxysmal form will have a duration of less than 7 days. If AF lasts 7 days or more it will be defined as established. The term "chronic" is used more in the literature than the term "established", and is defined as having a duration ranging from more than 7 days to more than 1 month. The term intermediate AF is sometimes used for AF lasting more than 7 days and less than 1 month. Electrical cardioversion of AF may be indicated in patients with paroxysmal persistent AF or in patients with established AF. Only a subset of patients with either type of AF may benefit from an atrial defibrillator. Patients with paroxysmal AF may be categorized according to a classification system for AF presented in Table 1.

Which Patients May Be Treated with an Atrial Defibrillator?

Obviously, symptomatic patients in class III, i.e., patients who experience symptomatic episodes of AF despite the use of antiarrhythmic agents (sodium channel blockers and potassium channel blockers), are potential candidates. The number and duration of episodes should be taken into account in the indications. Patients with frequent episodes (several episodes per day) must be excluded, as an implantable atrial defibrillator may result in too frequent discharges, patient discomfort, and rapid battery depletion. Similarly, patients with episodes of short duration and spontaneous termination may not be good candidates. The severity of patient symptom(s) and arrhythmia tolerance must be taken into account. Selected patients with infrequent attacks (fewer than 1 episode per 3-month period) may benefit from an implantable atrial defibrillator, particularly those patients with long-lasting episodes of AF that require pharmacological or electrical reversion. It is not known whether there is an indication for an implantable atrial defibrillator in patients with asymptomatic AF and a history of embolic complications. Candidates for an implantable atrial defibrillator should undergo a complete work-up including transesophageal echocardiogram to rule out intracavitary thrombus as well as atheromatous plaques on the ascending aorta which may be responsible for platelet aggregation and clots. These patients have been excluded in the initial protocol of evaluation of an implantable atrial defibrillator. However, it may appear from clinical trials, as believed by many investigators, that restoring and maintaining sinus rhythm represents the best prevention of AF-associated embolic complications, particularly stroke. The use of anticoagulant therapy is indicated in patients with a history of embolic events. Whether this should be the case in every patient who undergoes an automatic atrial defibrillator implantation is not known. It is usually believed that termination of AF of less than 2 days duration is not associated with embolic event. In the initial phase of the physician-activated devices, we believe that oral anticoagulant therapy is generally indicated. Intravenous heparin is indicated if the decision is made after implantation not to use long-term anticoagulation.

A selected group of patients with established AF may benefit from an implantable atrial defibrillator e.g., patients who underwent successful external cardioversion and who experienced recurrence after a period of time ranging from 1 to 6 months. Obviously, this time period is an arbitrary example, and should be assessed for each patient on an individual basis.

The underlying heart disease may play a role in the indication of an implantable atrial defibrillator. Patients with significant valvular heart disease may not be good candidates for an implantable atrial defibrillator. The appropriate and early treatment of the valvular lesion may prevent recurrences of AF. Similarly, patients with idiopathic dilated cardiomyopathy and depressed ventricular function (ejection fraction <0.20) should be excluded from the study. In contrast, patients with hypertrophic cardiomyopathy and rapid paroxysmal AF resulting in hemodynamic compromise may benefit from rapid conversion to sinus rhythm. The presence of hypertension with or without left ventricular hypertrophy may not represent a contraindication to an implantable atrial defibrillator. Although the incidence of AF is higher in patients with hypertension, the cause and effect relationship is not clear. Atrial fibrillation is a known precipitating factor of pulmonary edema in patients with hypertension, but AF in this context is usually transient and often terminates with the treatment of heart failure. Similarly, patients with hyperthyroidism often convert spontaneously after treatment of thyrotoxicosis. Following elective cardioversion and treatment of the underlying disorder, the rate of recurrence is low. Although correlation does exist between the rate of successful cardioversion and the size of the left atrium, the latter should not be a limiting factor as the correlation is poor. However, an atrial size above 60 mm should, in our point of view, be a contraindication to an implantable atrial defibrillator.

At this stage of evaluation of the efficacy as well as the safety of the device, it is advisable to avoid implantation of an implantable atrial defibrillator in patients with AF and coronary artery disease associated with myocardial ischemia. It is not known if termination of AF in a patient with coronary insufficiency may be proarrhythmic.

Patients with so-called "lone AF" or idiopathic AF should provide the bulk of the patient group for evaluation of the device, at least at the initial phase. However, presence of an underlying heart disease should not be a contraindication in the longer term.

As the available device does not prevent AF, the use of antiarrhythmic agents to prevent recurrences may not be an exclusion criterion for the evaluation study. Some antiarrhythmic agents may decrease the frequency of episodes and shock delivery and may allow some patients with frequent episodes (Class IIC or IIIC) to become candidates.

Alternative nonpharmacological therapies are discussed in other chapters of this book. When control of ventricular rate and symptoms cannot be achieved with pharmacological treatment, (atrioventricular) AV nodal ablation with pacemaker implantation may be an alternative. Recently, AV nodal modification has been proposed and may obviate the need for pacemaker implantation in a large number of patients.[11] Preliminary results are encouraging; however long-term results are still needed. Catheter ablation of AF is still experimental. Surgery for AF prevention includes the "Corridor" and the "Maze" operations.[12,13] Although the results reported are impressive, this major surgery carries a significant operative mortality and long-term results on mortality and morbidity in a large series are not yet available.

Conclusion

Potential indications for an implantable atrial defibrillator do exist. Patients with recurrent attacks of AF (Class IIIB or IIIC) resistant to antiarrhythmic therapy are potential candidates, as are patients with infrequent attacks, or poorly tolerated or long-lasting attacks requiring medical intervention. Most of the technical problems related to AF detection and atrial defibrillation have been solved.

A clinical trial aimed at assessing the efficacy and safety of the currently available device (METRIX 3000) is ongoing and includes a physician-activated device phase. As the technology is refined and experience is gained, more concrete indications are likely to evolve.

References

1. Kannel WB, Abbott RD, Savage DD, et al. Epidemiologic features of chronic atrial fibrillation: the Framingham study. N Engl J Med 1982;306:1018–1022.

2. Bialy D, Lehmann MH, Schumacher DM, et al. Hospitalization for arrhythmias in the United States: importance of atrial fibrillation. J Am Coll Cardiol 1992;19:41A.
3. Pritchett ELC. Management of atrial fibrillation. N Engl J Med 1992;326: 1264–1271.
4. Cabin HS, Clubb KS, Hall C, et al. Risk for systemic embolization of atrial fibrillation without mitral stenosis. Am J Cardiol 1990;61:714–717.
4a. Godtfredsen J. Embolic complications in paroxysmal atrial fibrillation. Stroke 1986;17:622–626.
5. Lévy S, Camm AJ. An implantable atrial défibrillator: an impossible dream? Circulation 1993;87:1769–1772.
6. Murgatroyd F, Slade AKB, Sopher M, et al. Efficacy and tolerability of transvenous low energy cardioversion of paroxysmal atrial fibrillation in humans. J Am Coll Cardiol 1995;25:1347–1353.
7. Keane D, Sulke N, Cooke R, et al. Endocardial cardioversion of atrial flutter and fibrillation. PACE 1993;16:928.
8. Johnson E, Smith W, Yarger M, et al. Clinical predictors of low energy defibrillation thresholds in patients undergoing internal cardioversion of atrial fibrillation. PACE 1994;17:742. Abstract.
9. Lévy S, Ricard Ph. Low energy cardioversion of spontaneous atrial fibrillation: immediate and long-term results. Circulation 1997. In press.
10. Lévy S, Novella P, Ricard Ph, et al. Paroxysmal atrial fibrillation: a need for classification. J Cardiovasc Electrophysiol 1995;6:69–74.
11. Williamson BD, Ching Man K, Daoud E, et al. Radiofrequency catheter modification of atrioventricular conduction to control the ventricular rate during atrial fibrillation. N Engl J Med 1994;331:910–917.
12. Leitch JW, Klein G, Yee R, et al. Sinus node-atrioventricular node isolation: long term results with the "corridor" operation for atrial fibrillation. J Am Coll Cardiol 1991;17:970–975.
13. Cox JL, Schuessler RB, D'Agostino HJ, et al. The surgical treatment of atrial fibrillation III. Development of a definitive surgical procedure. J Thorac Cardiovascular Surg 1991;101:509–583.
14. Lévy S, Ricard P, Lau CP, Lok N, et al. Multicenter low energy transvenous atrial defibrillation (XAD) trial: results in different subsets of atrial fibrillation. J Am Coll Cardiol 1997. In press.

CHAPTER 34

Antiarrhythmic Trial Design in Atrial Fibrillation

Jeffrey L. Anderson

Introduction

This treatise on trial design derives from 20 years of clinical trial experience by the author, and, for the past 4 years, service on the regulatory ledger as member and currently Chair, Cardiovascular and Renal Advisory Committee, United States Food and Drug Administration (FDA). Past clinical trials have primarily involved pharmacological agents for cardiac conditions, including atrial fibrillation (AF). Device and procedure therapy of AF are relatively new and experience is limited, but the future will be replete with nonpharmacological therapies. Innovative and efficient means of establishing efficacy and safety will be required. However, much can be learned from general principles and past experience.

FDA approval of a new therapy requires substantial evidence of effectiveness, or indication that a new drug (or other therapy) will have the effect it is claimed to have. This "substantial evidence" must include evidence from "adequate and well controlled" trials. A premise of this treatise is that trial design forms an important basis on which clinical and statistical inference is formed about therapies, including antiarrhythmic therapy of AF. Thus, careful and prospective attention to the details of study design is imperative. Table 1 summarizes study designs that have been frequently used in medical trials, including trials of antiarrhythmic therapies.[1] These include observational, nonrandomized controlled, and randomized controlled study designs.

Observational Studies

Observational studies describe outcomes of patient series given a new therapy. There is no formal control group. Comparisons with the

From *Nonpharmacological Management of Atrial Fibrillation*, edited by F.D. Murgatroyd and A.J. Camm. © 1997, Futura Publishing Co., Inc., Armonk, NY.

Table 1
Study Designs Frequently Used in
Antiarrhythmic Trials

- Observational design
- Historical control design
- Nonrandomized concurrent control design
- Matched, concurrent control design
- Randomized, parallel group design
- Cross-over design
- Positive control design

readers' past experiences and with textbook overviews of the disease-course are implied. Examples of observational studies of therapies to prevent recurrence of AF include a staged-care approach using propafenone and sotalol[2] and low-dose amiodarone.[3] At the end of ≥ 1 year, 40–60% of patients remained in sinus rhythm. This study design, however, does not demonstrate whether outcome was better (and to what degree) than untreated or alternatively treated patients with the same characteristics.

The Good-Responder Syndrome

An example of how an observational study using a risk-stratifying procedure to "guide" therapy can be misleading has been provided by Hallstrom et al.[4] Holter monitoring to assess arrhythmia suppression is considered as an example, as with postinfarction ventricular arrhythmias in the Cardiac Arrhythmia Suppression Trial (CAST).[5] (The same considerations might also apply to suppression of sustained tachyarrhythmias at electrophysiological study[6] or to AF suppression on transtelephonic monitoring.) The example starts with 100 patients with an expected annual rate of arrhythmia recurrence or mortality of 40% (Fig. 1). Antiarrhythmic therapy is given and therapy is "guided" with Holter monitoring; 50 patients "suppress" in-hospital and 50 are "nonsuppressed". Of suppressed patients, five have events and 45 do not, whereas of 50 nonsuppressed patients, 35 have events and only 15 are without events after 1 year. The event rate in suppressed patients is only 10%, compared with 70% among nonsuppressed patients. Although at first it appears that an excellent therapeutic strategy has been devised, the overall event rate in the 100 patients is still 40%

Hypothetical Example:
Electrophysiologic-Guided or Holter-Guided Therapy

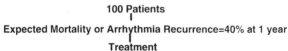

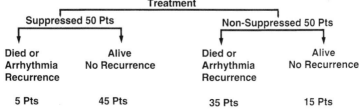

Figure 1. Hypothetical example of the "healthy responder" phenomenon. (Adapted from Hallstrom et al.[4])

(10% + 70% / 2). The approach has had no impact in the group as a whole. Moreover, in the absence of randomization to treatment versus placebo in the whole group, the impact of therapy cannot be assessed in either the suppressed or the unsuppressed stratum. The difference in the suppressed versus nonsuppressed groups may be due entirely to the risk-stratifying test (Holter suppression) and not to therapy. In the CAST study, patients who did best were those who showed the "good-responder phenomenon" of suppression on Holter but subsequently were given placebo.[5] Indeed, continuing active therapy *increased* subsequent event rates. Thus, the "guided" but observational study design does not allow an inference as to whether therapy improved, had no effect, or even worsened the prognosis. The absence of a control group is a major limitation this design.

Historical Control Studies

The easiest solution to the need for a control group is a previous (historical) series of patients given "standard" treatment. By definition, these controls are nonconcurrent and nonrandomized. The design is the easiest of the controlled designs to perform. Physicians become involved in studies because of the potential benefits of a new therapy and, in turn, motivate their patients regarding the new approach. Because no concurrent controls are recruited, the sample size is half as large. The consent process is easier because it does not require acceptance of randomization. The design, however, is severely limited by the potential for bias. Over time, populations change, even within the same institution, and the management approaches evolve. Only a few comparisons of baseline factors can be made although other, often uncontrolled, factors may play a role. Coronary heart disease mortality has been decreasing over the past two decades,[7] for uncertain reasons. Thus, a comparison of a currently treated patient group with a previous one would likely show a better outcome, even if a newly added therapy was ineffective. Pocock[8] evaluated 19 instances where two consecutive series were reported for the same intervention from the same center. Differences in mortality ranged from −46% to +24%, with 4 (21%) being "significant" (P<.05). This highlights the severe limitations of historical control trials. A useful role of this study design is to provide an easy, inexpensive initial impression of a new therapy, including nonpharmacological approaches to AF. After observational evaluation, unpromising therapies can be discarded or modified and promising ones tested further in randomized studies. Historical control studies thus may supplement, but rarely replace, randomized ones.

Nonconcurrent, nonrandomized historical series may be derived from the literature. Preferably, the historical series is from the same institution. Geographic variation in the patient population is then avoided, baseline characteristics are available, and the standard approach to treatment is generally more comparable (or at least better defined) than when the control series is derived from the literature or a different institution. A well-characterized, prospectively collected, computerized data bank forms perhaps the ideal resource for historical control groups.

Nonrandomized Concurrent Control Studies

In this study design, selection of treatment also is not done by randomization. However, controls are subjects who are treated at the same time as the intervention group, from a concurrent literature series, from a neighboring hospital, or by a different physician group at the same hospital. The design is easier to perform than a randomized design, again because all patients receive the new therapy and the randomization process is avoided. Again, however, the lack of assurance of comparability is a problem. Comparability of a few (known)

Table 2
ICD Versus Drug Therapy for VT/VF Using a Nonrandomized
(Concurrent or Recent Historical) Design

	% Mortality at 1 Year	
	*ICD (N = 270)**	*Amiodarone (N = 462)†*
Sudden Cardiac Death	4	21
Other Deaths	22	41
Total Mortality	26	62

* From Winkle et al.[9]; † From Herre et al.[10].
ICD = implantable cardioverter defibrillator; VT/VF = ventricular tachycardia/ventricular fibrillation.

baseline variables can be assessed and adjustment for differences approached statistically. However, other or unknown variables may not be assessed and adjustment for differences between groups is imperfect. An example of a nonrandomized concurrent (or recent historical) treatment comparison between drug and device (implantable cardioverter defibrillator [ICD]) therapy for ventricular tachycardia or fibrillation (VT/VF) is shown in Table 2. The ICD series[9] demonstrates a substantially reduced sudden death rate at 5 years (4% vs. 21%), as well as a marked reduction in total mortality (26% vs. 62%) compared with amiodarone.[10] However, other deaths are also substantially lower in the ICD series (22% versus 41%). Because an ICD should not impact nonsudden death mortality, a likely explanation for the difference in outcomes is the selection of a sicker patient group for medical than device therapy.

Matched, Concurrent Control Studies

The matched, concurrent control study design is a variation of a concurrent control design in which one or more controls are selected for each patient receiving new therapy, from a data base of patients receiving standard therapy. Controls are selected for comparability in a few key baseline variables (e.g., age, gender, type of structural heart disease, left ventricular function, presenting arrhythmia). Matching can also be used for historical control patients when a large and well-defined data base of patients treated in a standard fashion is available. This matching process improves comparability of groups, but bias is not entirely eliminated. Unknown or unmeasured (and unmatched) characteristics also may be of importance. Furthermore, the design is not "intention to treat"; for example, patients considered for interventional therapy that was aborted for various reasons would not be evaluated in the interventional group.

VT/VF Trials

The study of Choue et al.[11] provides an example of concurrent patient groups that were selected for similarity in left ventricular ejection fraction, gender, and diagnosis. Unlike the studies of Winkle and Herre[9,10] (Table 2), the outcomes of medical and ICD therapy were similar. Newman et al.[12] compared total mortality in patients with a history of VT/VF treated with an ICD with matched concurrent controls (Fig. 2). Initially, ICD therapy tended to be superior, but after 2 to 3 years, events rates were comparable. The hypothesis that the ICD may provide early benefit compared with medical therapy in VT/VF patients is now being tested in two randomized studies (Antiarrhythmics Versus Implantable Defibrillators (AVID),[27] Canadian Implantable Defibrillator Study (CIDS)[29]), modeling the statistical analysis after these observed event rates.[13]

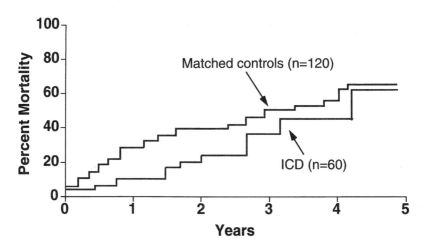

Figure 2. Total mortality over time in patients treated with an implantable cardioverter defibrillator (ICD) and in matched, concurrent, medically treated controls. (Reproduced with permission from Newman et al.[12])

Digitalis

Digitalis has formed standard therapy for AF for most of this century. Digitalis-associated cardiac mortality has been assessed in several historical or concurrent control series. Moss et al.[14] evaluated digitalis-associated cardiac mortality among 812 postinfarction patients. Differences in mortality between digitalis-treated and untreated patients was modeled using important predictive variables in a logistical regression equation. After other risk predictors were adjusted for, digitalis was still associated with a 31% excess in mortality (90% confidence interval, 18%–42%). Very recently, the DIG trial has evaluated the mortality effect of digitalis in a double-blind, placebo control study in almost 8,000 patients with congestive heart failure. The impact on mortality after 3 years was neutral (risk ratio 1.00, 95% confidence interval 0.93–1.02, $P = 0.92$).[15] Although the postinfarction heart failure patients may differ somewhat from those in DIG, a likely explanation for much of the mortality excess found with the use of digitalis in older, nonrandomized studies is unadjusted baseline bias. That is, digitalis-treated patients were sicker, but their excess baseline risk was only partially adjusted for.

Calcium Channel Blockers

A recent controversy has risen over the use of calcium channel blockers for treatment of hypertension.[16] The FDA Advisory Committee was asked to review information with respect to the potential of these agents to increase the risk of myocardial infarction (MI) and mortality, compared with other therapies such as beta-blockade for hypertension. Three key epidemiological studies (concurrent control studies) were reviewed. The study of Psaty et al.[16] found a risk ratio for MI of 1.6 (95% confidence interval, 1.1–2.3), compared with beta-blockade, with no difference among calcium channel blockers (nifidipine = verapamil = diltiazem). However, in an unpublished study from another group, the risk ratio for MI was <1. In a third study,[17] mortality with calcium channel blockers in elderly, hypertensive patients tended to be slightly better (verapamil, 0.8), relatively neutral (diltiazem, 1.3), or worse (nifedipine, 1.7, confidence interval 1.1–2.7), depending on which agent was used. Other data have suggested that short-acting nifedipine may increase mortality when given for acute MI,[18] the presumed mechanism being induction of excessive hypotension and sympathetic activation. The Advisory Committee recommended avoidance of short-acting nifedipine for treatment of hypertension (an indication for which it was never approved) and acute MI (also an unapproved indication). For longer-acting calcium channel blockers (which do not reflexively activate the sympathetic nervous system), additional safety studies (e.g., ALLHAT) will be needed to justify a change in labeling. This experience suggests that "in general, case-control studies . . . simply cannot test definitively whether there are small to moderate risks or benefits of a class of drugs".[19] (Small to moderate risks or benefits are those with odds ratios of <2–3 compared with control.)

Randomized Parallel Design Studies

The randomized parallel study design is the "gold standard" for evaluation of medical therapies. Its major advantages over nonrandomized designs are: (1) It removes potential biases in allocation; (2) It tends to produce comparable groups; and (3) The validity of statistical testing is guaranteed.[1] This is true even when the randomized groups are not precisely identical, because the probability of these differences is taken into account.[1] In addition, blinding of treatment allocation (with a placebo, for example) adds to design strength, and is especially preferable when endpoints are subject to assessment bias.[1,20] The problem of blinding is problematic with devices and procedures, and may not always be possible. However, "sham" procedures may be used in some situations, and devices, although implanted, may be programmed ("blindly") to an off-mode (see cross-over design below).

Postmyocardial Infarction Arrhythmias

A classical example of the utility of the blinded, randomized parallel design in antiarrhythmic therapy is provided by the CAST study.[5] After demonstration of arrhythmia suppressibility, patients were randomized to active or placebo treatment. A significant advantage was shown with placebo therapy, a result that has revolutionized the approach to antiarrhythmic therapy. An observational study likely would have entirely missed this result because the annual mortality rate with therapy of 8% was exactly that predicted from historical control trials. Further, those that suppressed and were treated did better than those who were not suppressed,[21] seemingly supporting "guided therapy" (but see Fig. 1). The key result in CAST was not how poorly actively treated patients fared, but how well those who showed suppressibility did on placebo, a result only achievable using a blinded, randomized control design.

Digoxin for AF

Digoxin was compared with placebo for conversion of acutely occurring AF by Falk et al.[22] Thirty-six patients with AF for <7 days were randomized to digoxin or placebo; nine (50%) of the digoxin patients converted to normal rhythm at a mean of 5.1 hours. This ostensibly positive result was put into perspective by the placebo limb, however: eight patients (44%) also converted to normal rhythm at a mean of 3.3 hours. Overall, digoxin had no effect on conversion of AF. A more recent experience has confirmed this result, although it did show moderate effects of digoxin on ventricular rate.[23]

Approval Basis for Ibutilide

Recently, the FDA Advisory Committee reviewed a submission for ibutilide, a new class III antiarrhythmic agent, proposed as acute IV therapy for conversion of AF or flutter. Ibutilide has a unique mechanism of action (sodium-channel opener) that causes increases in monophasic action potential and effective refractory periods of atrium and ventricle with increases in electrocardiographic QT and QTc intervals. The studies submitted, involving only a few hundred patients, were randomized and placebo-controlled. In the AF group (AF duration, 3 hours-45 days), ibutilide doses of 1.5–2 mg IV led to conversion within 3 hours in 31% of AF (28/90) compared with only 2% (1/43) of placebo patients ($P<0.001$). Results with atrial flutter were more impressive: 56% (50/90) converted, compared with 2% (1/43) of placebo patients ($P<0.0001$). Thus, carefully controlled trials in a relatively small patient group allowed efficacy to be demonstrated unequivocally, even though the level of efficacy was only moderate (and consistent with that seen with both digoxin and placebo in another study[22]—note that only the placebo group response rates changed). Accordingly, ibutilide was approved and marketed in the USA from April, 1996.

Bias in Controlled Trials

Even in controlled trials, the risk of bias exists that must be carefully guarded against. Shultz et al.[20] evaluated 250 controlled trials for methods of concealing treatment allocation and blinding of treatment assignment, then associated the methods for randomization and blinding with the outcomes by multiple logistic regression. Trials with inadequate concealment of treatment allocation (i.e., with faulty randomization procedures) demonstrated a substantially exaggerated treatment effect, averaging 41% ($P<.001$) compared with trials with adequate concealment. An example of faulty concealment is when the investigator is aware of the next treatment assignment (e.g., a list may be posted in which the order of assignment of consecutive patients is given). Faulty concealment allows bias to enter in and patients may be selected who are deemed to best "fit" the next treatment allocation. Similarly, trials that were not double blind also exaggerated the treatment effect (by 17%, $P = 0.01$). Knowing the treatment assignment might introduce a bias in the assessment of "soft" endpoints or encourage the cross-over of patients from one therapy to the other (preferred) therapy. Thus, careful concealment of treatment allocation until after consent has been obtained and the randomization procedure undertaken is critical to study integrity. Further, blinding of treatment throughout the course of the study adds to study integrity (especially for endpoints other than total mortality).

A standards group for trial reporting has suggested four areas of concern in reporting (and designing) randomized control trials: participant assignment, masking of therapy, participant follow-up, and approaches to statistical analysis.[24] Several aspects of randomization are important to the integrity of studies and require thoughtful consideration and planning in advance (Table 3, A). Of equal importance are methods of masking intervention (Table 3, B), to prevent the provider, participant, outcomes assessor, and analyst from being aware of treatment allocation. Only when these issues are appropriately dealt with can the scientific strengths and benefits of the randomized, controlled clinical trial be realized.

Cross-Over Study Design

The cross-over design is a specialized case of the randomized control trial.[1] In this case, each subject serves as his/her own control. As a result, within-subject variability is essentially eliminated. Sample size can be reduced because each subject participates both in active and placebo (control) phases of therapy. Study design is simplified, and recruitment of patients is easier. Each patient is evaluated on active

Table 3
Issues of Treatment Assignment and Masking*

A. Issues Related to Participant Assignment
  • Unit of assignment (individual, cluster, site)\
  • Method to generate assignment (table, computer)
  • Method to conceal assignment schedule
  • Method to separate generator and executor of assignment
  • Process of executing assignment (should be describable, auditable)
  • Ability to identify, compare baseline characteristics

B. Issues of Masking Intervention
  • Method of masking
  • Frequency of provider awareness of treatment allocation
  • Frequency of participant awareness of treatment allocation
  • Frequency of awareness of outcome assessor of allocation
  • Awareness of allocation by analyst when data entered into database

* Modified from Ref. 24, from the Standards of Reporting Trials Group.

therapy. Despite these many advantages, the cross-over design is limited by the possibility of carry-over effects (i.e., treatment in phase 1 may carry over to and confound treatment during phase 2). This may be of particular relevance to procedure or device-based therapy. For example, if patients undergo an ablation for an arrhythmia (including AF) in phase 1, the possibility of assessing the outcome of medical therapy in that patient during a second observation period is eliminated. Similarly, if a device is placed for cardioversion of AF (atrial ICD) during phase 1, the possibility of testing therapy without the device is complicated (although not impossible; for example, an implanted device could be activated during the second phase of the study in a way that blinds the patient as well as the primary investigator). Even when cross-over is successful, problems with statistical analysis may be present: the statistical test for period-intervention interaction is weak,[1] leaving open the possibility of at least modest confounding by carry-over effects.

The Efficacy of Flecainide for Paroxsymal AF

The primary efficacy study for FDA approval of flecainide for paroxsymal AF used a randomized, blinded, cross-over design (Fig. 3).[25] After an initial open-label, dose-finding phase, patients were randomly as-

PAF STUDY DESIGN

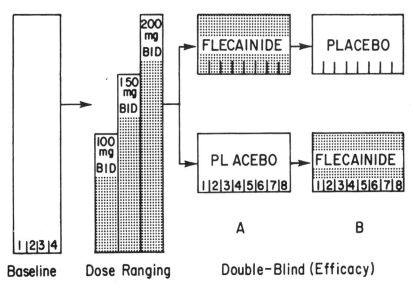

Figure 3. Study design for the evaluation of flecainide for suppression of symptomatic paroxymal atrial fibrillation (PAF). (Reproduced with permission from Anderson et al.[25])

signed to receive 8 weeks of either placebo or flecainide after which they were reassigned to the alternative treatment. However, results were presented to the FDA in the less controversial parallel design format, using time-to-failure analysis (Fig. 4), avoiding concerns about carry-over effects. (The cross-over analysis, comparing within-patient responses, also favored flecainide). The randomized, blinded treatment approach also allowed assessment of subjective symptoms of AF. Thus, perhaps for the first time, an objective analysis of the impact of therapy on aspects of quality of life (AF-associated symptoms) could be quantitatively evaluated.[25,26] Within the past 2 years, propafenone has also been favorably reviewed by the FDA Advisory Committee for treatment of paroxsymal atrial tachyarrhythmias based on a similar blinded treatment design using transtelephonic monitoring to confirm symptomatic recurrences.

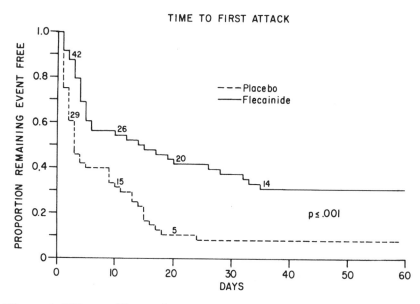

Figure 4. Efficacy of flecainide versus placebo for suppression of symptomatic paroxysmal atrial fibrillation using Kaplan-Meier (time-to-failure) method. (Reproduced with permission from Anderson et al.[25])

Model Trial Designs and Statistical Analyses for AF Studies

This recent FDA experience suggests that one successful trial design for pharmacological trials in AF involves beginning with patients in sinus rhythm (achieved either spontaneously or with cardioversion), and then assigning blinded therapy (active or placebo) in a random fashion. Treatment groups are followed over time for endpoint assessment (i.e, AF recurrence or death). Recurrences of symptomatic AF may be documented efficiently by outpatient event monitors. Results are then analyzed by actuarial methods.[25]

For trials using time-to-failure (Kaplan-Meier) methods (currently, a preferred approach except for studies with limited and uniform observation periods), statistical analysis may use either the log rank test or a generalized Wilcoxon test.[13] The log rank statistic is the most commonly used test when time-to-failure is the measure of response. It is the most powerful test for the proportional hazards model when the hazard ratio remains >1 (or, alternatively, <1) throughout the trial period. It also is a good statistic when one curve continually remains above another. On the other hand, a generalized Wilcoxon test (for example, the Peto-Prentice version) deals better with the situation when the hazard ratio shifts from above to below 1 (or vice-versa) during the trial. It is superior for detecting early differences between trials and less powerful (assigns less weight) for later differences. Examples of results favoring each analytical approach are shown in Figure 5. Modeling for the Antiarrhythmic Versus Internal Defibrillator (AVID) study was based on the hypothesis that differences between device and drug will occur primarily in the first 2 years after therapy.[13,27] Accordingly, a generalized Wilcoxon test will be used.

Randomized, Positive Control Studies

Instead of a placebo, a "positive" control may be used in trial design. This is a standard active therapy against which the new therapy is compared. The parallel control study is thus a variation of the randomized parallel study design. It is attractive from an ethical standpoint, because all patients receive an active, presumably effective, therapy. It is logistically attractive in that it is easy to recruit patients when both therapies can be enthusiastically endorsed by the physician. Also, an acceptable goal of a positive control study is to show that the new therapy is at least comparable (if not better) than the more standard therapy, a less demanding task than demonstrating superiority. In the recent ibutilide submission to FDA, positive control study data for sotalol, compared with ibutilide, and, separately, procainamide with ibutilide, were presented. These data formed supportive although not primary trial data for approval. A positive control study design is particularly appealing for nonpharmacological therapies of AF because it allows treatment with the new device or intervention to be compared with the most favorable medical therapy available.

Despite growing use and enthusiasm for positive control trials, a number of design issues and practical problems exist, as identified by Temple.[28] First, there is a lack of agreement on a test for statistical significance. The question becomes, what is the chance of incorrectly failing to reject the null hypothesis when the drugs are really different, i.e., what is the beta-error? In contrast, there is much better agreement on tests for statistical significance when a difference is expected (i.e., an alpha of <.05). Secondly, there is less incentive to perform an excellent study in positive control trials. A reasonable goal is only that

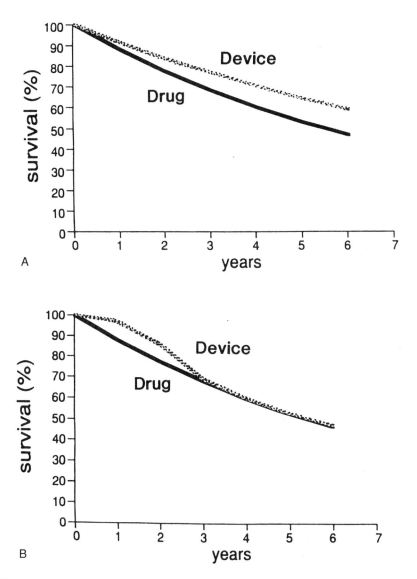

Figure 5. A: Proportional (exponential) and **B**: nonproportional (nonexponential) hazards models for arrhythmic event occurrence in randomized trials. (From the AVID Investigators.[27])

Table 4
Trials Comparing a New Antidepressant, Imipramine, and Placebo*

Study	(N)	Baseline	New Rx	Imipramine	Placebo
1	102	24	13	13	15
2	105	26	13	13	14
3	35	28	19	20	19
4	22	30	7	10	24†
5	23	38	22	22	22
6	105	26	11	11	11

* Data abstracted from Temple[28]; † Difference among placebo, new Rx, and imipramine significant; Rx = treatment.

"everyone does well", rather than to show that one treatment is better. Sloppiness in study execution, poor compliance, high cross-over rates and incomplete ascertainment of endpoints all lend themselves to equivalence in a study, whereas to show a difference, careful control of all these variables is needed. Finally, demonstrating that two therapies are equivalent does not show that either is effective. Control therapy may not be performing in an effective manner in the study population tested. Temple[28] has demonstrated this to be the case for a series of trials of antidepressants (Table 4). Note that compared with baseline, both new therapy and imipramine were substantially and equally effective, reducing the depression score by about half. Fortunately, the inclusion of a parallel placebo group prevented the inappropriate conclusion of substantial benefit: only one of six trials showed an overall benefit of active therapies; in five, placebo patients showed similar improvements from baseline.

The challenge of a positive control design is summarized by Temple as follows:

"if one cannot be very certain the positive control in a study would have beaten a placebo group, had one been present, then the fundamental assumption of a positive-control study cannot be made. Any condition in which large spontaneous placebo-responses occur, or where there is great variability in response, or in which treatment responses are difficult to distinguish from placebo should be considered a poor candidate for positive control study."[28]

Thus, positive-control studies present significant challenges, even though they lend themselves to the current era of incremental advancement in medical therapies, including therapy of AF.

The AFFIRM Study

In 1996, The National Institutes of Health initiated a randomized trial in AF comparing two treatment strategies (positive control design). The goals of strategy 1 are heart rate control and anticoagulation, whereas the goal of strategy 2 is to maintain normal rhythm with antiarrhythmic drugs. The primary endpoint is all-cause mortality, with a recruitment goal of 5,000 patients. AFFIRM (Atrial Fibrillation Follow-up: Interventions in Rhythm Management) has completed its pilot phase and began its full-scale, mortality phase in 1996, with almost 1,000 patients recruited by March 1997. AFFIRM will be faced with all of the problems of a positive-control (and unblinded) study, but will incorporate a large patient population with a mortality endpoint.

Caveats for Development of Devices and Procedures for AF

Previous AF trial experience, summarized here, derives primarily from pharmacological studies, whereas future development will concern itself increasingly with procedures (e.g., a frequency catheter ablation) and devices (e.g., atrial defibrillators, multisite pacing, etc.). Guidelines for these studies are currently under development by the FDA, and only preliminary conclusions and caveats can be provided. Obviously, these therapies present new challenges for study design with respect to randomization, blinding, size, and expense.

Technology issues have more recently been subdivided into: (1) evaluation of existing therapies; (2) evaluation of evolutionary therapies (i.e., improved pacemakers or defibrillators), and; (3) evaluation of novel therapies (i.e., first assessment of an atrial defibrillator, first assessment of AF ablation therapy, etc.). As therapies become increasingly novel, greater clinical trial experience is required. For example, an atrial defibrillator developer may wish to pursue a claim of superiority over medical management. Preclinical studies would include bench and animal work. Clinical studies would require a relatively large comparison of device-based versus medical management using a concurrent, randomized design with follow-up of at least 6–12 months in at least 150 patients. The choice of a primary endpoint is challenging.

Preferably, improved survival would be demonstrated, but, realistically, trials of perhaps thousands of patients (e.g., 5,000 patients in AFFIRM) would be required, and would be difficult for new device companies to fund. Thus, a composite of morbidity (arrhythmia recurrence, quality of life) and mortality may be necessary.

Concluding Thought

Despite the many and very real issues in clinical trial design, it is clear that the development of cardiovascular therapies has undergone gradual but steady improvement in the past 20 years. The result is greater certainty about the true efficacy of new treatments with an improved ability to discern real from chance observations. Issues of safety continue to be a challenge as experience with at least 1,000–2,000 patients is necessary to adequately define relatively uncommon but important adverse effects of therapy. Certainly, the future will present new challenges as nonpharmacological therapies of AF undergo evaluation. However, with an appreciation of study design issues and limitations, what has and has not been learned during development becomes clear, to the benefit of patients as well as a better understanding of a most challenging disease, atrial fibrillation.

References

1. Friedman LM, Furberg CD, DeMets DL. Basic study design. In: Wright J, ed. Fundamentals of Clinical Trials. Boston, MA: PSG Inc; 1982:28–39.
2. Antman EM, Beamer AD, Cantillon C, et al. Therapy of refractory symptomatic atrial fibrillation and atrial flutter: a staged care approach with new antiarrhythmic drugs. J Am Coll Cardiol 1990;15:698–707.
3. Gosselink ATM, Crijns HJGM, Van Gelder IC, et al. Low-dose amiodarone for maintenance of sinus rhythm after cardioversion of atrial fibrillation or flutter JAMA 1992;267:3289–3293.
4. Hallstrom AP, Greene HL, Huther ML. The healthy responder phenomenon in non-randomized clinical trials. Stat Med 1991;10:1621–1631.
5. Epstein AE, Hallstrom AP, Rogers WJ, et al, for the CAST Investigators. Mortality following ventricular arrhythmia suppression by encainide, flecainide, and moricizine after myocardial infarction: the original design concept of the Cardiac Arrhythmia Suppression Trial (CAST). JAMA 1993; 270:2451–2455.
6. Mason JW, for the ESVEM Investigators. A comparison of electrophysiologic testing with Holter monitoring to predict antiarrhythmic-drug efficacy for ventricular tachyarrhythmias. N Engl J Med 1993;329:445–451.
7. McGovern PG, Pankow JS, Shahar E, et al for the Minnesota Heart Survey

Investigators. Recent trends in acute coronary heart disease. N Engl J Med 1996;334:884–890.

8. Pocock SJ. Letter to the editor. Br Med J 1977;1:1661.

9. Winkle RA, Mead RH, Ruder MA, et al. Long-term outcome with the automatic implantable cardioverter-defibrillator. JACC 1989;13:1353–1361.

10. Herre JM, Sauve MJ, Malone P, et al. Long-term results of amiodarone therapy in patients with recurrent sustained ventricular tachycardia or ventricular fibrillation. JACC 1989;13:442–449.

11. Choue CW, Kim SG, Fisher JD, et al. Comparison of defibrillator therapy and other therapeutic modalities for sustained ventricular tachycardia or ventricular fibrillation associated with coronary artery disease. Am J Cardiol 1994;73:1075–1079.

12. Newman D, Sauve MJ, Herre J, et al. Survival after implantation of the cardioverter defibrillator. Am J Cardiol 1992;69:899–903.

13. Brooks MM, Hallstrom A, Peckova M. A simulation study used to design the sequential monitoring plan for a clinical trial. Stat Med 1995;14: 2227–2237.

14. Moss AJ, Davis HT, Conard DL, et al. Digitalis associated cardiac mortality after myocardial infarction. Circulation 1981;64:1150.

15. Anonymous. Rationale, design, implementation and baseline characteristics of patients in the DIG trial: a large long-term trial to evaluate the effect of digitalis on mortality in heart failure. Control Clin Trials 1996; 17(1):77–97.

16. Psaty BM, Heckbert SR, Koepsell TD, et al. The risk of myocardial infarction associated with antihypertensive drug therapies. JAMA 1995; 274: 620–625.

17. Pahor M, Guralnik JM, Corti MC, et al. Long-term survival and use of antihypertensive medications in older persons. J Am Geriatr Soc 1995;43: 1191–1197.

18. Furberg DC, Psaty BM, Meyer JV. Nifedipine: dose-related increase in mortality in patients with coronary heart disease. Circulation 1995;92: 1326–1331.

19. Buring JE, Glynn RJ, Hennekens CH. Calcium channel blockers and myocardial infarction. JAMA 1995;274:654–655.

20. Schulz KF, Chalmers I, Hayes RJ, Altman DG. Empirical evidence of bias. JAMA 1995;273:408.

21. Hallstrom A, Pratt CM, Greene HL, et al. for the CAST Investigators. Relations between heart failure, ejection fraction, arrhythmia suppression and mortality: analysis of the Cardiac Arrhythmia Suppression Trial. J Am Coll Cardiol 1995;25:1250–1257.

22. Falk RH, Knowlton AA, Bernard SA, et al. Digoxin for converting recent-onset atrial fibrillation to sinus rhythm: a randomized, double-blinded trial. Ann Intern Med 1987;106:503–506.

23. Hornestam B, Carlsson T, Falk L, et al. for the DAAF study group. Effects of intravenously administered digoxin in acute atrial fibrillation compared to placebo. Circulation 1995;92:I-774.

24. The Standards of Reporting Trials Group. A proposal for structured reporting of randomized controlled trials. JAMA 1994;272:1926–1931.

25. Anderson JL, Gilbert EM, Alpert BL, et al. Prevention of symptomatic recurrences of paroxysmal atrial fibrillation in patients initially tolerating

antiarrhythmic therapy: a multicenter, double-blind, crossover study of flecainide and placebo. Circulation 1989;80:1557–1570.

26. Bhandari AK, Anderson JL, Gilbert EM, et al. Correlation of symptoms with occurrence of paroxysmal supraventricular tachycardia or atrial fibrillation: a transtelephonic monitoring study. Am Heart J 1992;124:381–386.

27. The AVID Investigators. Antiarrhythmics versus implantable defibrillators (AVID): rationale, design, and methods. Am J Cardiol 1995; 75: 470–476.

28. Temple R. Difficulties in evaluating positive control trials. Biopharmaceutical section, Proceedings of the American Statistical Association. 1983: 1–7.

29. The CIDS Investigators. Canadian Implantable Defibrillator Study (CIDS): study design and organization. Am J Cardiol 1993;72(16):103F-108F.

Index

529